MANUAL FOR STAGING OF CANCER

This manual was prepared and published through the support of American Cancer Society Grant CCG #99V and Grant Number CA110612 awarded by the National Cancer Institute, National Institutes of Health.

Edited by

OLIVER H. BEAHRS, M.D.
Mayo Clinic and Mayo Foundation
Professor of Surgery, Emeritus
Mayo Medical School
Rochester, Minnesota

DONALD EARL HENSON, M.D.
U.S. Public Health Service
Division of Cancer Prevention and Control
National Cancer Institute
Bethesda, Maryland

ROBERT V. P. HUTTER, M.D.
Chairman, Department of Pathology
St. Barnabas Medical Center
Livingston, New Jersey

MAX H. MYERS, Ph.D.
Statistical Consultant
Gaithersburg, Maryland

MANUAL FOR STAGING OF CANCER

THIRD EDITION

AMERICAN JOINT COMMITTEE ON CANCER

*Executive Office
55 East Erie Street
Chicago, Illinois 60611*

SPONSORING ORGANIZATIONS

*American Cancer Society
National Cancer Institute
College of American Pathologists
American College of Physicians
American College of Radiology
American College of Surgeons*

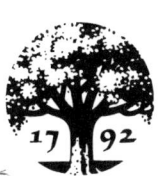

J. B. LIPPINCOTT COMPANY

PHILADELPHIA
London, Mexico City, New York, St. Louis, São Paulo, Sydney

Acquisitions Editor: J. Stuart Freeman
Sponsoring Editor: Sanford J. Robinson
Manuscript Editor: Jody A. DeMatteo
Design Coordinator: Michelle Gerdes
Production Manager: Carol A. Florence
Production Coordinator: Charlene Catlett Squibb
Compositor: McFarland Graphics & Design, Inc.
Printer/Binder: The Murray Printing Company

The authors and publisher have exerted every effort to ensure that drug selection and dosage set forth in this text are in accord with current recommendations and practice at the time of publication. However, in view of ongoing research, changes in government regulations, and the constant flow of information relating to drug therapy and drug reactions, the reader is urged to check the package insert for each drug for any change in indications and dosage and for added warnings and precautions. This is particularly important when the recommended agent is a new or infrequently employed drug.

THIRD EDITION

Copyright © 1988, by J. B. Lippincott Company. All rights reserved. No part of this book may be used or reproduced in any manner whatsoever without written permission except for brief quotations embodied in critical articles and reviews. Printed in the United States of America. For information write J. B. Lippincott Company, East Washington Square, Philadelphia, Pennsylvania 19105.

3   5   6   4   2

First printing 1977
Revised and reprinted 1978
Reprinted 1980
Second edition 1983
Third edition 1988

Library of Congress
Cataloging-in-Publication Data

Manual for staging of cancer.

"Prepared and published through the support of American Cancer Society grant CCG # 99V and grant number CA110612 awarded by the National Cancer Institute, National Institutes of Health."
  Includes bibliographies.
  1. Tumors—Classification.   2. Cancer—Diagnosis. I. Beahrs, Oliver Howard, 1914-
II. American Joint Committee on Cancer.
III. American Cancer Society.   IV. Title: Staging of cancer.   [DNLM: 1. Neoplasm Staging.
2. Neoplasms—classification. QZ 241 M293]
RC258.M36   1988   616.99'4'0012   87-22538
ISBN 0-397-50916-2

THIRD EDITION

Dedicated to the memory of
W. A. D. Anderson, M.D.
Marvin Polland, M.D.
Paul Sherlock, M.D.

and

All others who contributed greatly to the deliberations of the American Joint Committee and to the recommendations on Staging of Cancer.

SECOND EDITION

Dedicated to the memory of
Murray M. Copeland, M.D.

The first chairman of
The American Joint Committee on
Cancer Staging and End-Results Reporting

A native of McDonough, Georgia, Murray Copeland received his medical degree from Johns Hopkins University School of Medicine in 1927, followed by training in surgery and oncology at the Mayo Clinic, Memorial Hospital in New York City, and Union Memorial Hospital in Baltimore.

Among Dr. Copeland's numerous distinctions were his leadership positions as national president of the American Cancer Society in 1965 and secretary general of the 1970 UICC Cancer Congress.

He was known and loved by physicians around the world for his willingness and ability to support organizations designed to facilitate the spread of knowledge about cancer.

Murray Copeland was internationally acclaimed for his superior knowledge of and efforts against large bowel cancer and bone cancer.

Preface

The editors of this, the third edition of the *Manual for Staging of Cancer* of the American Joint Committee on Cancer, wish to recognize the contributions of 400 participants who have volunteered their time over 25 years in the evolution of the recommendations for staging cancer. Retrospective studies were carried out for cancer at some anatomic sites and many hours were spent reviewing available literature and information from personal experience of participants as well as reviewing staging recommendations previously brought forward by others. These deliberations led to the recommendations published in the first comprehensive *Manual* in 1977.

Subsequently, the Committee has continued to review its definitions and fine tune the recommendations and stage grouping at all anatomic sites with the hope that staging of cancer will be most helpful in arriving at decisions regarding appropriate treatment of malignant tumors and in determining prognosis and end results.

Unfortunately, recommendations regarding staging of cancer by individual researchers, specialties, committees, and other groups have not been uniform. This has been true in some instances between the published reports of the TNM Committee of the International Union Against Cancer (UICC) and the American Joint Committee on Cancer (AJCC). Under the leadership of Dr. Harvey Baker as Chairman of the AJCC, discussions were first undertaken with the TNM Committee to reach uniform recommendations of the two groups so that one system of staging might be used worldwide. These efforts have been actively pursued under the subsequent chairmanship of Dr. Robert Hutter with the cooperation of Dr. Leslie Sobin, Chairman of the TNM Committee, and with the aid of Professor Paul Hermanek and his associates.

Through multiple meetings on both sides of the

Atlantic Ocean, agreements have been reached on all definitions of T, N, and M and on stage groupings for cancers at all anatomic sites. The recommendations of the AJCC in this revised *Manual* and the publications of the UICC, published in 1987, are identical. Thus, an international system of staging cancer is available. Using this system will make possible appropriate decisions regarding treatment and, more importantly, evaluation of end results and comparability of data.

Credit is due all members of the American Joint Committee and its Task Forces on cancer for individual anatomic sites. Special credit is given to those in leadership positions and to staff support persons, in particular, Rosemarie Clive, Margaret David, Kathleen Collins, and LeAnn Krueger. Personnel of J. B. Lippincott Company have been most cooperative and helpful, including J. Stuart Freeman, Jody DeMatteo, and others. The interest and help of the publisher is greatly appreciated.

Oliver H. Beahrs, M.D.
Donald Earl Henson, M.D.
Robert V. P. Hutter, M.D.
Max H. Myers, Ph.D.

Introduction

This manual brings together all currently available information on staging of cancer at various anatomic sites as developed by the American Joint Committee on Cancer (AJCC) in cooperation with the TNM Committee of the International Union Against Cancer (UICC). All of the schemes included here are uniform between the two organizations. The manual permits consistency in describing the extent of the neoplastic diseases in different anatomic parts, systems, or organs.

Proper classification and staging of cancer will allow the physician to determine treatment more appropriately, to evaluate results of management more reliably, and to compare worldwide statistics reported from various institutions on a local, regional, and national basis more confidently.

Staging of cancer is not a fixed science. As new information becomes available about etiology and various methods of diagnosis and treatment, the classification and staging of cancer will change. Periodically, this manual will be revised to reflect the changing knowledge, but revisions will occur only at reasonable periods. At the present time the anatomic extent of the cancer is the primary basis for staging; the extent of differentiation of the tumor and the age of the patient are also factors in some tumors. In the future, biologic markers and other factors may play a part.

It is hoped that the staging recommendations included in this manual may be used as published—or at least modified only minimally—so that consistency in data gathering will be possible. The recommendations in the manual are to be used in the cancer programs approved by the Commission on Cancer of the American College of Surgeons. Also, future reports by the Surveillance, Epidemiology, and End-Results program (SEER) of the National Cancer Institute (NCI) will be based on the classifications recommended by the AJCC.

The AJCC was first organized on January 9, 1959, as the American Joint Committee for Cancer Staging and End-Results Reporting (AJC), for the purpose of developing a system of clinical staging for cancer acceptable to the American medical profession. The sponsoring organizations are the American College of Surgeons, the American College of Radiology, the College of American Pathologists, the American College of Physicians, the American Cancer Society, and the National Cancer Institute. Each of the sponsoring organizations designates three representatives to the Committee. The American College of Surgeons serves as administrative sponsor. Subcommittees, called "task forces," have been established to consider malignant neoplasms of selected anatomic sites in order to develop classifications. Each task force is composed of committee members and other professional appointees whose special interests and skills are appropriate to the site under consideration.

During its 28 years of activity, various special consultants have worked with the Committee, as well as liaison representatives from the American Academy of Pediatrics, the American College of Obstetricians and Gynecologists, the American Urological Association, the Association of American Cancer Institutes, and the SEER program of the NCI. More than 400 individuals have contributed to the work of the various task forces. Dr. Murray Copeland was Chairman from the inception until 1969, Dr. W. A. D. Anderson from 1969 to 1974, Dr. Oliver H. Beahrs from 1974 to 1979, Dr. David T. Carr from 1979 to 1982, and Dr. Harvey W. Baker from 1982 to 1985. The current Chairman is Dr. Robert V. P. Hutter.

Pioneer work on the clinical classification of cancer was done by the League of Nations Health Organization (1929), the International Commission on Stage Grouping and Presentation of Results (ICPR) of the International Congress of Radiology (1953), and the International Union Against Cancer (Union Internationale Contre le Cancer, UICC). The latter organization became most active in the field through its Committee on Clinical Stage Classification and Applied Statistics (1954), later known as the TNM Committee.

The AJC decided to use the TNM system, when applicable, to describe the anatomic extent of the cancer at the time of diagnosis (before the application of definitive treatment), and from this to develop classification into stages, which would serve as a guide for treatment and prognosis and for comparing the end results of treatment. Subsequently, the system has been extended to other periods during the natural history and treatment of a cancer. Task forces to accomplish this extension were established to focus on particular sites of cancer. Retrospective studies have resulted in recommendations for stage classifications for cancer at various sites or systems, which have been published and distributed in separate fascicles and articles.

The AJC sponsored a National Cancer Conference on Classification and Staging in Atlanta on March 27-28, 1976. This conference delineated the accomplishments to that time and brought into focus future needs and activities.

In January 1970, a revised statement of the "Objectives, Rules and Regulations of the American Joint Committee" was adopted. Among other things, it broadened the scope of the Committee by including in its objectives the formulation and publication of systems of classification of cancer not limited to but including staging and end-results reporting.

It was recognized that for cancer of certain sites the information made available by observation at the time of a surgical procedure, as well as information from the pathologic examination of the surgically removed cancer, could form the basis for useful classifications. From this evolved a "surgical evaluative staging" and a "postsurgical treatment-pathologic staging." Surgical evaluative staging has subsequently been dropped. Information obtained during surgical exploration may be used for clinical staging.

Further consideration of the chronology of staging has led to two main time periods. First is the Diagnostic Stage, which uses all data available to the first definitive treatment. Second is the Pathologic Stage, which can be established if a completely resected specimen of the lesion is available.

It also became evident that in certain organs (e.g., thyroid), the biologic potential of different histologic types of cancer is such that different types cannot be mixed together in a meaningful classification. Therefore, cases should be analyzed separately by histologic type. In some kinds of cancer, such as

Introduction

soft-tissue sarcomas, histologic grading is of such significance that it becomes a necessary component of the classification system. For certain cancers, widely used and accepted classifications, such as the Ann Arbor classification of Hodgkin's disease and the FIGO classification for carcinoma of the cervix, are considered in the recommendations. Whenever possible, established and accepted classifications are considered.

The various data in previously published individual-site fascicles, with revisions and the addition of other material, were brought together to form a *Manual for Staging of Cancer*, the first edition of which was published in 1977. A second printing, slightly revised, appeared in 1978. The 1983 edition of the *Manual* updated the earlier publications and included additional sites. Also, the recommendations were brought more closely in conformity with those of the TNM Committee.

The need for a staging form for use in the staging system of each site has been recognized for some years. Such forms ensure the recording of the data necessary for stage classification. Recent emphasis has been given to the development of a checklist for each cancer site for which there is a stage classification and to the availability of such checklists as a part of each staging recommendation.

The expanding role of the Committee in a variety of cancer classifications, including its significance and value and the promotion of indicated usage in cancer diagnosis and therapy, suggested that the original name of the Committee no longer portrayed the broader scope of its interests and activities. The name was therefore changed in 1980 to the American Joint Committee on Cancer (AJCC). The publication of this new edition of the *Manual* reflects the widening interests and activities of the Committee.

The TNM Committee of the UICC and the AJCC have been working along similar lines and with similar objectives. In the past, points of view and methods have occasionally differed. Cooperation between the two groups during 1982–1987 has resulted in uniform and identical definitions and stage grouping of cancers for all anatomic sites so that a universal system is now available.

Members of the AJCC, its task forces and its committees, as well as the sponsoring organizations, owe a debt of gratitude to the many physicians and others who have voluntarily contributed to this effort in the hope that patients with cancer would survive and that the quality of life of the cancer patient could be as near normal as possible. The contributions of the TNM Committee of the UICC and other international organizations are gratefully acknowledged.

Introduction to the Second Edition

Sixty thousand copies of the first two printings of the *Manual for Staging of Cancer 1977* and *1978* have been distributed. Based on the demand for the manual and for the subsequently published separate pamphlets on Reporting of Cancer Survival and End Results and Staging for Cancer of Head and Neck Sites, Melanoma, Lung, Gynecologic Sites, and Soft-Tissue Sarcoma, there is an indication that the staging of cancer at the time of diagnosis and management is more universally applied now than previously. The Commission on Cancer of the American College of Surgeons, with 900 approved cancer programs, has recently requested that the recommendations of the American Joint Committee on Cancer (AJCC) be used in their programs and cancer registries. This will lead to further uniformity in recording the extent of cancers at the time of diagnosis and treatment and will make statistical data on follow-up and end results more meaningful.

This second edition of the *Manual* contains some revised recommendations based on new and added information. In a few instances, arbitrary changes have been made to make the recommendations of the AJCC consistent with those of the TNM Committee of the International Union Against Cancer (UICC). Consistency at all anatomic sites has not as yet been achieved.

The data-collecting forms have been modified to reflect more usefully the information required to stage cancer. These forms can become part of the patient's record but are not considered to be a replacement for history, treatment, or follow-up data forms. In some instances they list the information essential for staging as well as data that may be useful for future staging systems or research studies.

The AJCC wishes to thank all of those physicians, nurses, registrars, and others who have made suggestions regarding the contents of this manual, but in particular all of the more than 400 persons who, over 20 years, have contributed so greatly to the evaluation of the material and recommendations made in this revision. Likewise, great credit and thanks go to Mr. Robert Rowan and J.B. Lippincott Company for their cooperation and help in undertaking this *Manual for Staging of Cancer* for the American Joint Committee on Cancer.

Foreword

More than 20,000 copies of the second edition of the *Manual for Staging of Cancer* have been distributed. The Commission on Cancer of the American College of Surgeons has recommended to its over 1100 approved cancer programs that the AJCC system of staging cancer be used in their programs and registries. Likewise, the Commission uses the *Manual* in its Cancer Management Course. Other societies and groups are requiring the use of the recommendations in their meetings and published reports.

Most importantly, in this, the third edition of the *Manual*, all definitions and stage groupings of cancer at all anatomic sites are identical with those of the TNM Committee of the UICC. Thus, a worldwide system of staging is available. If used, it will lead to improved management of the cancer patient and make end-results reporting meaningful.

Contents

PART I	GENERAL INFORMATION ON CANCER STAGING AND END-RESULTS REPORTING	1
1	Purposes and Principles of Staging	3
	Philosophy of Classification and Staging by the TNM System	3
	Nomenclature in Morphology of Cancer	4
	General Rules for Staging of Cancer	6
	General Rules of the TNM System	6
	Cancer Staging Form	9
	Screening for the Early Detection of Cancer	10
2	Reporting of Cancer Survival and End Results	11
PART II	STAGING OF CANCER AT SPECIFIC ANATOMIC SITES	25
	Head and Neck Sites	27
3	Lip and Oral Cavity	27
4	Pharynx (including base of tongue, soft palate, and uvula)	33

5	Larynx	39
6	Maxillary Sinus	45
7	Salivary Glands (including parotid, submaxillary, and sublingual)	51
8	Thyroid Gland	57

Digestive System Sites — 63

9	Esophagus	63
10	Stomach	69
11	Colon and Rectum	75
12	Anal Canal	81
13	Liver (including intrahepatic bile ducts)	87
14	Gallbladder	93
15	Extrahepatic Bile Ducts	99
16	Ampulla of Vater	105
17	Exocrine Pancreas	109
18	*Lung*	115

Musculoskeletal Sites — 123

19	Bone	123
20	Soft Tissues	127
21	Carcinoma of the Skin (excluding eyelid, vulva, and penis)	133
22	Melanoma of the Skin (excluding eyelid)	139
23	*Breast*	145

Gynecologic Sites — 151

24	Cervix Uteri	151
25	Corpus Uteri	157
26	Ovary	163
27	Vagina	169
28	Vulva	173

Genitourinary Sites — 177

29	Prostate	177
30	Testis	183

31	Penis	189
32	Urinary Bladder	193
33	Kidney	199
34	Renal Pelvis and Ureter	205
35	Urethra	209
	Ophthalmic Tumors	213
36	Carcinoma of the Eyelid	213
37	Melanoma of the Eyelid	217
38	Carcinoma of the Conjunctiva	223
39	Melanoma of the Conjunctiva	227
40	Melanoma of the Uvea	231
41	Retinoblastoma	237
42	Sarcoma of the Orbit	241
43	Carcinoma of the Lacrimal Gland	245
44	*Brain*	249

Contents

Hodgkin's and Non-Hodgkin's Lymphoma — 255

45	Hodgkin's Disease	255
46	Non-Hodgkin's Lymphoma	259

Pediatric Cancers — 265

47	Nephroblastoma (Wilms' Tumor)	265
48	Neuroblastoma	271
49	Soft-Tissue Sarcoma—Pediatric	277

PART III	PERSONNEL OF THE AMERICAN JOINT COMMITTEE ON CANCER	283
APPENDIX	Sites, Subsites, and ICD-O Code Numbers	287

PART I

GENERAL INFORMATION ON CANCER STAGING AND END-RESULTS REPORTING

1

Purposes and Principles of Staging

Philosophy of Classification and Staging by the TNM System

A classification scheme for cancer must encompass all attributes of the tumor that define its life history. The American Joint Committee on Cancer (AJCC) classification is based on the premise that cancers of similar histology or site of origin share similar patterns of growth and extension.

The size of the untreated primary cancer or tumor (T) increases progressively, and at some point in time regional lymph node involvement (N) and, finally, distant metastases (M) occur. A simple classification scheme, which can be incorporated into a form for staging and universally applied, is the goal of the TNM system as proposed by the AJCC. This classification is identical with that of the Union Internationale Contre le Cancer (UICC) and is a distillate of several existing systems.

For most cancer sites the staging recommendations in this manual are concerned only with anatomic extent of disease, but in several instances grade (soft-tissue sarcoma) and age (thyroid cancer) are factors that must be considered. In the future, biologic markers and other parameters may have to be added to those of anatomic extent in classifying cancer, but they are not necessarily components of stage.

As the primary tumor increases in size throughout its time span, at some point (probably early) local invasion occurs, followed by spread to the regional lymph nodes draining the area of the tumor. The period when this spread is manifest or discernible by available methods of clinical examination is thus another significant marker in the progression of the cancer (N). It is usually later, and often in the middle or older period of the life span of the cancer, that distant spread or metastasis (M) becomes evident from clinical examination. Thus, metastasis (M) is the third and usually the latest time marker.

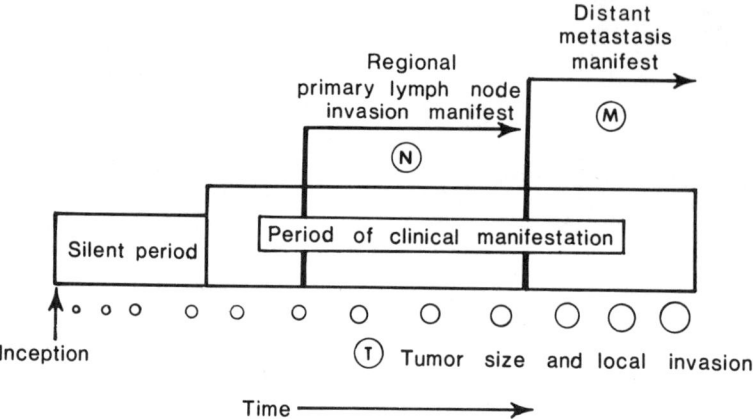

These three significant events in the life history of a cancer—tumor growth (T), spread to primary lymph nodes (N), and metastasis (M)—are used as they appear (or do not appear) on clinical examination, before definitive therapy begins, to indicate the extension of the cancer. This shorthand method of indicating the extension of disease at a particular designated time is the stage of the cancer in its evolution. It may be used, however, sometimes with other features added, in a scheme of stage classification. When retrospective or prospective studies of cases show that certain groupings of TNM or other features can be identified that have valid significance for staging, a stage classification may be devised.

Events such as local spread, including spread to primary regional lymph nodes, and distant metastasis sometimes occur before they are discernible by clinical examination. Thus, examination at the time of a surgical procedure and histologic examination of the surgically removed tissues may identify the significant markers of the life history of the cancer (T, N, and M) as being different from what could be discerned clinically before therapy. Although this may be the basis of a stage classification (pathological, based on examination of a surgically resected specimen), it should be identified separately from clinical classification. Nevertheless, it may be a more accurate depiction of the period in the life history of the cancer and may be valuable for prognostic purposes.

Therapeutic procedures, even if not curative, may alter the course and life history of cancer. Although cancers that recur after therapy may be staged with the same markers as are used in pretreatment clinical staging, the significance of cancer markers may not be the same. Hence the stage classification of recurrent cancer must be considered separately for therapeutic guidance, prognosis, and end-results reporting.

The significance of the marker points in their life history differs for tumors of different sites and of different histologic types. Therefore, the marker points, even if T, N, and M, must be defined for each type of tumor in order to be valid and to have maximum significance. In certain types of tumors, such as Hodgkin's disease and lymphomas, a different system for designating the extent of the disease and for classifying its stage is necessary to accomplish the goal of usefulness. In these cases other symbols or descriptive markers are used rather than T, N, and M.

Classification and stage-grouping is thus a method of designating the extent of a cancer and is related to the natural course of the particular type of cancer. It is intended to provide a way by which this information can be readily communicated to others, to assist in decisions regarding treatment, and to be a factor in determining prognosis. Ultimately, it provides a mechanism for comparing groups of cases, particularly in regard to the results of different therapeutic procedures.

In addition to anatomic extent, the histologic analysis and grade of the tumor may be important determinants in classification. The type of tumor and the grade are also most important variables affecting choices of treatment. For sarcomas the tumor grade may prove to be the most important index.

Nomenclature in Morphology of Cancer

Cancer therapy decisions are made after an assessment of the patient and tumor, using many methods that often include sophisticated technical procedures. For most types of cancer, the extent to which the disease has spread is probably the most important factor determining prognosis and must be given prime consideration in evaluating and comparing different therapeutic regimens.

Staging classifications are based on description of the extent of disease, and their design requires a thorough knowledge of the natural history of each type of cancer. Such knowledge has been and continues to be derived primarily from morphologic studies, which also provide us with the definitions and classifications of tumor types.

An accurate histologic diagnosis, therefore, is an essential element in a meaningful evaluation of the tumor patient. In certain types of cancer, biochemical or immunologic measurements of normal or abnormal cellular function have become important elements in typing tumors precisely. Increasingly, definitions and classifications should include function as a component of the pathologist's anatomic diagnosis. One may also anticipate that special techniques in histochemistry, cytogenetics, and tissue culture will be used more routinely for typing and characterizing tumor behavior.

The most complete and best known compendium of tumor definitions and illustrations in English is the *Atlas of Tumor Pathology*, published in many volumes by the Armed Forces Institute of Pathology in Washington, D.C. These are under constant revision and are used as a basic reference by pathologists throughout the world.

RELATED CLASSIFICATIONS

Since 1958 the World Health Organization (WHO) has been involved in a program aimed at providing internationally acceptable criteria for the histologic diagnosis of tumors. This has resulted in the International Histological Classification of Tumours, which contains, in an illustrated 25-volume series, definitions of tumor types and a proposed nomenclature.

The WHO *International Classification of Diseases for Oncology* (ICD-O) was developed as a coding system for neoplasms by topography and morphology and for indicating behavior (*e.g.*, malignant, benign, *in situ*). This coded nomenclature is identical in the morphology field for neoplasms with the Systematized Nomenclature of Medicine (SNOMED) published by the College of American Pathologists in 1976.

In the interest of promoting national and international collaboration in cancer research and specifically to facilitate cooperation in clinical investigations, it is recommended to use the International Histological Classification of Tumours for classification and definition of tumor types and the ICD-O code for storage and retrieval of data.

BIBLIOGRAPHY

1. Atlas of Tumor Pathology: Washington, DC, Armed Forces Institute of Pathology
2. World Health Organization: ICD-O—International Classification of Diseases for Oncology, 1st ed. Geneva, WHO, 1976
3. World Health Organization: International Histological Classification of Tumours, Vol 1–25. Geneva, WHO, 1967 to 1981

General Rules for Staging of Cancer

The practice of dividing cancer cases into groups according to "stages" arose from the fact that survival rates were higher for cases in which the disease was localized than for those in which the disease had extended beyond the organ or site of origin. These groups were often referred to as "early cases" and "late cases," implying some regular progression with time. Actually, the stage of disease at the time of diagnosis may be a reflection not only of the rate of growth and extension of the neoplasm but also of the type of tumor and of the tumor–host relationship.

The staging of cancer is hallowed by tradition, and, for the purpose of analysis of groups of patients, it is often necessary to use such a method. It is preferable to reach agreement on the recording of accurate information on the extent of the disease for each site because the precise clinical description and histopathological classification (when possible) of malignant neoplasms may serve a number of related objectives, namely

1. To aid the clinician in the planning of treatment
2. To give some indication of prognosis
3. To assist in evaluation of the results of treatment
4. To facilitate the exchange of information between treatment centers
5. To contribute to the continuing investigation of human cancers

The principal purpose to be served by international agreement on the classification of cancer cases by extent of disease, however, is to provide a method of conveying clinical experience to others without ambiguity.

There are many bases or axes of classification: for example, the anatomic site and the clinical and pathologic extent of disease; the reported duration of symptoms or signs; the sex and age of the patient; and the histologic type and grade. All of these represent variables that are known to have an influence on the outcome of the disease. Classification by anatomic extent of disease as determined clinically and histopathologically (when possible) is the classification to which the attention of the AJCC and the UICC is primarily directed.

The clinician's immediate task is to make a decision as to the most effective course of treatment and to make a judgment as to prognosis. This decision and this judgment require, among other things, an objective assessment of the anatomic extent of the disease. In accomplishing this, the trend is away from staging and toward meaningful description, with or without some form of summarization.

To meet the stated objectives, we need a system of classification

1. Whose basic principles are applicable to all sites regardless of treatment; and
2. Which may be supplemented later by information that becomes available from histopathology and/or surgery.

The TNM system meets these requirements.

General Rules of the TNM System

The TNM system for describing the anatomic extent of disease is based on the assessment of three components:

T   The extent of the primary tumor
N   The absence or presence and extent of regional lymph node metastasis
M   The absence or presence of distant metastasis

The addition of numbers to these three components indicates the extent of the malignant disease, thus showing progressive increase in tumor size or involvement:

T0, T1, T2, T3, T4   N0, N1, N2, N3   M0, M1

In effect, the system is a shorthand notation for describing the clinical extent of a particular malignant tumor.

The general rules applicable to all sites are as follows:

1. All cases should be confirmed histologically. Any cases not confirmed must be reported separately.
2. Four classifications are described for each site, namely:
   Clinical Classification, designated cTNM or TNM. Clinical classification is based on evidence acquired before treatment. Such evidence arises from physical examination, imaging, endoscopy, biopsy, surgical exploration, and other relevant findings. In other words, all information available prior to first definitive treatment is used.
   Pathologic Classification, designated pTNM. Pathologic classification is based on the evidence acquired before treatment, supplemented or modified by the additional evidence acquired from pathologic examination

Purposes and Principles of Staging

of a resected specimen. The pathologic assessment of the primary tumor (pT) entails a resection of the primary tumor or biopsy adequate to evaluate the highest pT category. The pathologic assessment of the regional lymph nodes (pN) entails removal of nodes adequate to validate the absence of regional lymph node metastasis (pN0) and sufficient to evaluate the highest pN category. The pathologic assessment of distant metastasis (pM) implies microscopic examination of distant lesions.

Retreatment Classification. Retreatment classification is used after a disease-free interval and when further definitive treatment is planned. All information available at the time of retreatment should be used in determining the stage of the recurrent tumor (rTNM). Biopsy confirmation of the cancer is required.

Autopsy Classification. If classification of a cancer is done after the death of a patient and a post-mortem examination has been done, all pathologic information should be used. The chronologic stage should be indicated as aTNM.

3. After assigning T, N, and M and/or pT, pN, and pM categories, these may be grouped into stages. The TNM classification and stage grouping, once established, must remain unchanged in the medical records. The clinical stage is essential to select and evaluate therapy, and the pathologic stage provides the most precise data to estimate prognosis and calculate end results.
4. If there is doubt concerning the correct T, N, or M category to which a particular case should be allotted, then the lower (less advanced) category should be chosen. This will also be reflected in the stage-grouping.
5. In the case of multiple, simultaneous tumors in one organ, the tumor with the highest T category should be identified and the multiplicity be indicated in parenthesis: for example, T2(m). In simultaneous bilateral cancers of paired organs, each tumor should be classified independently. In tumors of the thyroid and liver, multiplicity is a criterion of T classification but is not reflected in the stage-grouping.

THE ANATOMIC REGIONS AND SITES

The sites in this classification are listed by code number of the *International Classification of Diseases for Oncology* (ICD-O, World Health Organization, 1976).

Each chapter devoted to a specific form of cancer will be constructed according to the following outline:

Introduction
Anatomy
  Primary site
  Regional lymph nodes
  Metastatic sites
Rules for Classification
  Clinical (TNM or cTNM)
  Pathologic (pTNM)
Definition of TNM
  T Primary tumor size/extent
  N Regional lymph node involvement
  M Distant metastasis absent/present
Stage Grouping
Differences Between the 2nd and 3rd Editions
Histopathologic Type
Histopathologic Grade

TNM CLINICAL CLASSIFICATION

The following general definitions are used throughout:

Primary Tumor (T)

TX Primary tumor cannot be assessed
T0 No evidence of primary tumor
Tis Carcinoma *in situ*
T1, T2, T3, T4 Increasing size and/or local extent of the primary tumor

Regional Lymph Nodes (N)

NX Regional lymph nodes cannot be assessed
N0 No regional lymph node metastasis
N1, N2, N3 Increasing involvement of regional lymph nodes

Note: Direct extension of the primary tumor into lymph nodes is classified as lymph node metastasis.

Note: Metastasis in any lymph node other than regional is classified as a distant metastasis.

Distant Metastasis (M)

MX Presence of distant metastasis cannot be assessed
M0 No distant metastasis
M1 Distant metastasis

The category M1 may be further specified according to the following notation:

Pulmonary PUL
Osseous OSS

Hepatic HEP
Brain BRA
Lymph Nodes LYM
Bone Marrow MAR
Pleura PLE
Peritoneum PER
Skin SKI
Other OTH

Subdivisions of TNM. Subdivisions of some main categories are available for those who need greater specificity (*e.g.,* T1a, 1b or N2a, 2b).

HISTOPATHOLOGIC TYPE

The histopathologic type is a *qualitative* assessment whereby a tumor is categorized (typed) according to the normal tissue type or cell type it most closely resembles (*e.g.,* lobular carcinoma, osteosarcoma, squamous cell carcinoma).

HISTOPATHOLOGIC GRADE (G)

The histopathologic grade is a *quantitative* assessment of the extent to which a tumor resembles the normal tissue of its histopathologic type, expressed in numerical grades of differentiation (*e.g.,* squamous cell carcinoma, Grade 2, moderately differentiated).

GX Grade cannot be assessed
G1 Well differentiated
G2 Moderately well differentiated
G3 Poorly differentiated
G4 Undifferentiated

ADDITIONAL DESCRIPTORS

The use of the following descriptors is optional and does not affect stage classification in any way.

cTNM (or TNM) Should be used when the classification is clinical
pTNM Should be used when the classification is pathologic
rTNM Indicates retreatment classification for recurrence of tumor after a disease-free interval
aTNM Designates that classification is first determined at autopsy

m Symbol. The suffix m, in parenthesis, should be used to indicate the presence of multiple tumors.

y Symbol. In those cases in which classification is performed during or following initial multimodality therapy, the TNM or pTNM categories are identified by a y prefix.

r Symbol. Recurrent tumors, when staged after a disease-free interval, are identified by the prefix r.

Lymphatic Invasion (L)

LX Lymphatic invasion cannot be assessed
L0 No evidence of lymphatic invasion
L1 Evidence of invasion of superficial lymphatics
L2 Evidence of invasion of deep lymphatics

Venous Invasion (V)

VX Venous invasion cannot be assessed
V0 Veins do not contain tumor
V1 Efferent veins contain tumor
V2 Distant veins contain tumor

The UICC suggests the optional use of a C factor that reflects the validity of the classification, but this is not a component of the AJCC.

Residual Tumor (R) Classification (optional)

The absence or presence of residual tumor after treatment is described by the symbol R:

RX Presence of residual tumor at the primary site cannot be assessed
R0 No residual tumor
R1 Microscopic residual tumor
R2 Macroscopic residual tumor

STAGE GROUPING

Classification by the TNM system achieves reasonably precise description and recording of the apparent anatomic extent of disease. A tumor with four degrees of T, three degrees of N, and two degrees of M will have 24 TNM categories. For purposes of tabulation and analysis, except in very large series, it is necessary to condense these categories into a convenient number of TNM stage-groupings. Carcinoma *in situ* is categorized Stage 0, cases with distant metastasis are categorized Stage IV. The grouping adopted is such as to ensure, as far as possible, that each group is more or less homogeneous in respect to survival, and that the survival rates of these groups for each cancer site are distinctive.

HOST PERFORMANCE SCALE

The host performance status or the condition of the patient does not enter into determination of

Purposes and Principles of Staging

stage of the tumor but may be a factor in deciding type and time of treatment. Three suggested scales are illustrated. The simplified AJCC scale is preferred. The Karnofsky scale and the Eastern Cooperative Oncology Group (ECOG) scale are frequently used to record the physical state of patients and are listed for information and comparison.

Host (AJCC)

- H The physical state (performance scale) of the patient, considering all cofactors determined at the time of stage classification and subsequent follow-up examinations
- H0 Normal activity
- H1 Symptomatic and ambulatory; cares for self
- H2 Ambulatory more than 50% of time; occasionally needs assistance
- H3 Ambulatory 50% or less of time; nursing care needed
- H4 Bedridden; may need hospitalization

Karnofsky Scale: Criteria of Performance Status (PS)

Able to carry on normal activity; requires no special care	100	Normal; no complaints; no evidence of disease
	90	Able to carry on normal activity; minor signs or symptoms of disease
	80	Able to carry on normal activity with effort; some signs or symptoms of disease
Unable to work; able to live at home and care for most personal needs; requires a varying amount of assistance	70	Cares for self; unable to carry on normal activity or to do active work
	60	Requires occasional assistance but is able to care for most of own needs
	50	Requires considerable assistance and frequent medical care
Unable to care for self; requires equivalent of institutional or hospital care; disease may be progressing rapidly	40	Disabled; requires special care and assistance
	30	Severely disabled; hospitalization indicated although death not imminent
	20	Very sick; hospitalization necessary; active supportive treatment necessary
	10	Moribund, fatal processes progressing rapidly
	0	Dead

Eastern Cooperative Oncology Group Scale (ECOG)

GRADE
- 0 Fully active, able to carry on all predisease activities without restriction (Karnofsky 90–100)
- 1 Restricted in physically strenuous activity but ambulatory and able to carry out work of a light or sedentary nature, for example, light housework or office work (Karnofsky 70–80)
- 2 Ambulatory and capable of all self-care but unable to carry out any work activities. Up and about more than 50% of waking hours (Karnofsky 50–60)
- 3 Capable of only limited self-care, confined to bed or chair 50% or more of waking hours (Karnofsky 30–40)
- 4 Completely disabled, cannot carry on any self-care, totally confined to bed or chair (Karnofsky 10–20)

Cancer Staging Form

Each site staging form is to be used for recording the classification of the tumor and the stage of the cancer. The anatomic site of the cancer should be indicated, as well as the histologic cell type and grade. The appropriate period of the chronology of classification must be recorded. If a cancer is staged during several time periods in the chronology, separate forms must be used for each time period.

The T, N, and M classification can be checked opposite the appropriate definitions of the extent of the primary tumor, the regional nodes, and distant metastasis. The lesion(s) can be marked on the diagram and, finally, the stage can be checked according to the grouping of TNM. In some instances information regarding other characteristics of the tumor (not leading to stage) might be requested. These data may be pertinent in deciding management of the cancer. On the reverse side of the staging form is information and definitions that are important in proper classification of a cancer.

The cancer staging form is not a replacement for

history, treatment, or follow-up records but should become part of the patient file. The cancer staging form may be duplicated for individual or local institutional use.

Screening for the Early Detection of Cancer

The entire concept of cancer staging is built upon the foundation of progression of disease from clinically undetectable cancer to very limited disease, to involvement by direct extension of immediately adjacent organs or tissues, to metastatic spread of disease into regional lymph nodes or into distant sites or lymph nodes. The literature on cancer patient survival is filled with reports reflecting the survival advantage of patients whose cancer was diagnosed before direct extension or metastatic spread had taken place. Thus, one approach to improving overall survival for patients who develop cancer is to diagnose it while it can be managed more effectively with currently available therapeutic modalities. This idea has led to the search for methods of detecting cancers that heretofore could not be identified by routine clinical examination. The Pap smear for detection of cervical abnormality or cancer, mammography for detection of breast cancer, sputum cytology for detection of lung cancer, and the fetal occult blood test for early diagnosis of colon cancer are examples of methods currently being used.

There is substantial evidence that the Pap smear has been instrumental in reducing mortality due to carcinoma of the cervix. Mammography, in addition to clinical examination, has been shown by means of a randomized trial to be effective in reducing mortality due to breast cancer in women ages 50 to 60 years. The other two methods are currently being evaluated by controlled trials. Results from these studies are demonstrating that earlier detection is possible for cancers of the lung and colon, two of the most frequently occurring cancers.

The American Joint Committee on Cancer supports efforts to develop and evaluate early detection methods for these and other cancers as rapidly as possible, so that screening can be offered to a wide segment of the population. Thus, persons who are unaware of the existence of small cancers could have them identified and treated before the cancers have had the chance to grow and disseminate.

Reporting of Cancer Survival and End Results

To evaluate the efficacy of treatment and to provide a sound base for therapeutic planning for cancer patients, it is necessary to describe in comparable form the survival and the results of treatment of different patient groups. The objective of this report is to define several widely used methods of reporting end results. Throughout this chapter, the term *survival time* is used, although the guidelines apply equally to reporting length of response time, time to recurrence of disease, time to development of tumor following exposure to a risk factor, or any other function of time until the event of interest.

Certain basic information must be included in every report on cancer survival and end results. Such information should include

1. A description of the cancer patients whose survival experience is to be summarized, including basic demographic characteristics such as age, race, and sex, as well as a description of the disease in terms of basis of diagnosis, histology, anatomic site, extent of disease (or stage), treatment, and calendar year of observation
2. The size of the study group and the number of patients lost to follow-up or the percent of patients successfully followed up
3. A definition of the starting time or "zero" time for the measurement of survival
4. An explanation of the method used in calculating survival rates

DESCRIPTION OF CASE MATERIAL

Before any meaningful interpretation of survival data can be made, the case material from which the data are derived must be described. A fact not adequately appreciated is that the description of the case material is as important as the description of the actual mechanics of handling the data and method of calculating survival rates.

In organizing the material for presentation, consideration should be given to the following:

1. Reports should account for every case diagnosed as having the particular cancer under consideration. If some cases are excluded, the characteristics and number of these cases should be stated. The report should give the dates during which the patients were studied and should state whether the results are based on the experience of an entire institution, on the experience of a single clinic or hospital service, or on the experience of a single physician or group of physicians. The general nature of the institution and the general characteristics of the patients should be indicated, because factors such as race and socioeconomic status may influence end results.
2. All diagnoses should be confirmed histologically or cytologically. Those not confirmed at any time during the course of the disease or at autopsy should be reported and tabulated separately. When indicated, the findings for histologically distinct types of cancers should be reported separately. So that the effects of morphology on survival may be appreciated, reports should be stratified by histologic type when it is indicated.
3. The clinical or pathologic extent of disease or stage at the time of diagnosis is of particular importance in evaluating treatment and in making valid comparisons of end results reported from different sources. When it is applicable, patients should be stratified by stage of disease. The TNM system provides a convenient and widely used language for categorizing the primary lesion and the extent of involvement.

   The TNM assignments are grouped into appropriate summary combinations to create a small number of stages, usually four, so that the force of mortality increases from one stage to the next.

   Specific criteria modify this system according to the primary site. The *clinical* classification for cancer at certain accessible sites, such as the uterine cervix, includes all diagnostic and evaluative information (including surgical exploration) obtained up to the date that tumor-directed treatment begins or the decision for no treatment is made. Information obtained by surgical resection and histopathologic studies is used in describing extent of disease at sites inaccessible to *clinical* evaluation, such as carcinoma of the ovary, kidney, and stomach. Extent of disease for these cancers is usually reported in terms of the *pathologic* classification.
4. Data on groups of patients previously treated should be presented separately from the data on patients not previously treated. Retreated patients should be classified according to stage at retreatment.
5. The number of groups into which a patient series is subdivided will depend on the total number of patients, the purpose of the study, and the nature of the case material. For example, in reporting on cancer of the prostate, the patients might be grouped into three age groups, such as under 60, 60 to 69, and 70 and over. An entirely different age grouping would be used in reporting on patients with leukemia. For most sites it is desirable to subdivide with respect to histologic type, sex, stage, and treatment, although this is not always possible with small numbers of patients.

DEFINITION OF STARTING TIME

The starting time for determining survival of patients depends on the purpose of the study. For example, the starting time for studying the natural history of a particular cancer might be defined in reference to the appearance of the first symptom. Various reference dates are commonly used as starting times for evaluating the effects of therapy. These include (1) date of diagnosis; (2) date of first visit to physician or clinic; (3) date of hospital admission; and (4) date of treatment initiation. If the time to recurrence of a tumor after apparent complete remission is being studied, the starting time is the date of apparent complete remission. The specific reference date used should be clearly specified in every report.

The date of initiation of therapy should be used as the starting time for evaluating therapy. For untreated patients, the most comparable date is the time at which it was decided that no tumor-directed treatment would be given. For both treated and untreated patients, the above times from which survival rates are calculated will usually coincide with the date of the initial staging of cancer.

VITAL STATUS

At any given time the vital status of each patient is defined as alive, dead, or unknown (*i.e.*, lost to follow-up). The end point of each patient's participation in the study is either (1) a specified "terminal event" such as death, (2) survival to the completion of the study, or (3) loss to follow-up. In each case, survival time is the time from the starting point to the terminal event, to the end of the study, or to the date of last observation. This survival time may be further described in terms of patient status at the end point such as

Alive; tumor-free; no recurrence
Alive; tumor-free; after recurrence
Alive with persistent, recurrent, or metastatic disease
Alive with primary tumor
Dead; tumor-free
Dead; with cancer (primary, recurrent, or metastatic disease)
Dead; postoperative
Unknown; lost to follow-up

Completeness of the follow-up is crucial in any study of survival time because even a small number of patients lost to follow-up may bias the data. The maximum possible effects of bias from patients lost to follow-up may be ascertained by calculating a maximum survival rate, assuming that all lost patients lived to the end of the study. A minimum survival rate may be calculated by assuming that all patients lost to follow-up died at the time they were lost.

SURVIVAL INTERVALS

The total survival time is broken up into intervals in units of weeks, months, or years. This provides a description of the population under study with respect to the dynamics of survival over a specified time. The time interval used should be selected with regard to the natural history of the disease under consideration. In diseases with a long natural history, the duration of study could be 5 to 20 years and survival intervals of 6 to 12 months will provide a meaningful description of the survival dynamics. If the population being studied has a very poor prognosis (*e.g.,* patients with carcinoma of the esophagus or pancreas), the total duration of study may be 2 to 3 years and the survival intervals described in terms of 1 to 3 months. In interpreting survival rates one must also take into account the number of individuals entering a survival interval. Survival rates probably should not be computed for intervals in which fewer than 10 patients enter the interval alive.

CALCULATION OF SURVIVAL RATES

A properly calculated survival rate is the best single statistical index available for measuring the efficacy of one cancer therapy compared with another, administered to a comparable group of patients who also have similar disease characteristics. The basic concept is simple: Of a given number of patients, what percentage will be alive at the end of a specified interval, such as 5 years? For example, let us begin with 1,000 patients in a defined diagnostic category such as stage I carcinoma of the uterine cervix. If we observe each member of this group until death and enumerate those alive 5 years, 10 years, and 15 years after initiation of therapy, then the ratios of these numbers to the original 1,000 patients give the respective 5-year, 10-year, and 15-year survival rates. In practice, however, we do not begin literally with a given group and follow them all continuously until death before calculating survival rates. In a body of actual data, the group considered would generally contain persons who were treated at different times, so that different persons would have been observed for different lengths of time. On the closing date of the study, some would be known to be dead, others known to be alive, and some would have been lost to follow-up, and it would not be known whether they are alive or dead.

To illustrate the approach to dealing with this type of situation, let us consider in detail a small series of patients. Table 2-1 lists 40 patients with Stage II colon cancer treated in one hospital during the 8-year period from January 1975 to December 1982. The survival experience of these patients is to be assessed on the basis of information available through March 1986. For each patient, the table provides the following basic information:

1. Sex
2. Race
3. Age at initiation of treatment
4. Primary site
5. Histologic type
6. Treatment
7. Date treatment started (month and year)
8. Date of last contact (month and year)
9. Vital status at date of last contact (alive or dead)
10. Presence of colon cancer at date of last contact (yes or no)

Patients are listed consecutively by date of first treatment.

Calculation by the Direct Method. The simplest procedure for summarizing patient survival is to calculate the percentage of patients alive at the end of a specified interval, such as 5 years, using for this purpose only patients at risk of dying for at least 5 years. This approach is known as the *direct method.*

When we closed the study in March 1986, the

Table 2-1. Stage II Colon Cancer Patients Diagnosed: 1975–1982

OBS	RACE	SEX	AGE	SITE	HISTOL	TREAT	RX DATE	FUP DATE	CANCER STATUS	VITAL STATUS	SURV
1	WHITE	F	67	153.6	8140	S	02-75	01-77	YES	D	01Y-11M
2	WHITE	M	79	153.7	8140	S	06-75	09-75	NO	D	00Y-03M
3	WHITE	M	63	153.2	8140	S	10-75	03-81	YES	D	05Y-05M
4	WHITE	F	65	153.3	8010	S	05-76	10-85	NO	A	09Y-05M
5	WHITE	M	66	153.3	8140	S	06-76	02-77	YES	D	00Y-08M
6	WHITE	M	77	153.4	8140	S	07-76	10-78	YES	D	02Y-03M
7	WHITE	M	55	153.2	8140	S	08-76	10-85	NO	A	09Y-02M
8	WHITE	F	78	153.1	8140	S C	09-76	10-84	UNK	A	08Y-01M
9	WHITE	M	83	153.3	8140	S	09-76	05-81	NO	D	04Y-08M
10	WHITE	F	71	153.3	8140	S	12-76	03-82	YES	D	05Y-03M
11	WHITE	M	92	153.3	8140	S	01-77	06-84	NO	A	07Y-05M
12	WHITE	F	80	153.6	8140	S	05-77	05-84	NO	A	07Y-00M
13	WHITE	F	85	153.3	8140	S	01-78	12-81	YES	D	03Y-11M
14	WHITE	F	67	153.4	8140	S	02-78	07-80	NO	D	02Y-05M
15	WHITE	F	72	153.4	8140	S	02-78	06-79	NO	D	01Y-04M
16	WHITE	F	96	153.0	8140	S	03-78	03-81	NO	D	03Y-00M
17	WHITE	F	56	153.2	8140	S	05-78	12-85	NO	A	07Y-07M
18	WHITE	M	65	153.4	8140	S C	10-78	04-85	NO	A	06Y-06M
19	WHITE	F	62	153.3	8140	SR	01-79	06-85	NO	A	06Y-05M
20	WHITE	M	82	153.3	8480	S	02-79	01-82	NO	D	02Y-11M
21	WHITE	M	78	153.3	8140	S	02-79	08-84	YES	D	05Y-06M
22	WHITE	M	71	153.3	8140	S	05-79	06-85	NO	A	06Y-01M
23	WHITE	F	64	153.3	8140	S	06-79	09-85	NO	A	06Y-03M
24	WHITE	F	72	153.6	8140	S	07-79	08-82	NO	A	03Y-01M
25	WHITE	M	66	153.3	8140	SR	01-80	06-84	YES	D	04Y-05M
26	WHITE	M	68	153.1	8140	S	05-80	07-85	NO	A	05Y-02M
27	WHITE	M	86	153.6	8140	S	05-80	12-84	NO	A	04Y-07M
28	WHITE	F	71	153.6	8140	S	10-80	02-85	YES	D	04Y-04M
29	WHITE	M	67	153.4	8140	S	12-80	10-84	YES	D	03Y-10M
30	WHITE	F	66	153.1	8140	S	12-80	04-85	NO	A	04Y-04M
31	WHITE	F	45	153.3	8140	S	03-81	01-84	NO	A	02Y-10M
32	WHITE	F	61	153.4	8480	S	05-81	05-85	NO	A	04Y-00M
33	WHITE	M	70	153.4	8140	S	05-81	06-82	NO	D	01Y-01M
34	WHITE	F	79	153.1	8140	S	07-81	10-85	YES	A	04Y-03M
35	WHITE	F	66	153.4	8140	NONE	08-81	09-81	YES	D	00Y-01M
36	WHITE	F	66	153.1	8140	S C	10-81	05-83	YES	D	01Y-07M
37	WHITE	F	81	153.6	8140	S	11-81	10-84	UNK	A	02Y-11M
38	WHITE	M	66	153.1	8480	S	03-82	01-83	YES	D	00Y-10M
39	WHITE	F	65	153.0	8140	S	10-82	02-86	NO	A	03Y-04M
40	WHITE	M	68	153.2	8140	S	12-82	07-85	NO	A	02Y-07M

latest available follow-up information was from February 1986. Therefore, patients must have been treated in February 1981 or earlier in order to be at risk of dying for 5 years. Patients 1–30 all were diagnosed at least 5 years prior; however, patients 24, 27, and 30 have not had 5 full years of follow-up (in a strict statistical sense, these were lost to follow-up because their vital status was alive and their date of last contact was prior to the close of the study, March 1986). This means that 13 of the 40 patients (patients 24, 27, and 30–40) must be excluded from the calculation by the direct method.

Examining the entries in the "vital status" column in Table 2-1 for the 27 patients at risk for at least 5 years, we find that 11 patients were alive at last contact and 16 had died before February 1986. However, patient 3, although known to have died in March 1981, had been alive on his fifth anniversary. Patients 10 and 21 also lived at least 5 years. Therefore, we have 14 of the 27 patients alive 5 years after their respective dates of first treatment and, thus, the 5-year survival rate is 52%.

Calculation by the Actuarial Method. The direct method may be difficult for many hospital tumor registrars to use because of the limited number of patients with a particular type of disease who have been under follow-up for a full 5 years. In addition, the direct method does not provide for utilization of the survival information available on the most recently treated patients. For example, we know that patient 39 lived for 2 years and 9 months after treatment was started. Such information is valuable, but could not be used under the rules for the direct method because this patient was treated after February 1981.

The *actuarial*, or *life-table*, method provides a means for using all follow-up information accumu-

Reporting of Cancer Survival and End Results

John Doe	63	W	M	October, 1975
(Name)	(Age)	(Race)	(Sex)	(Date Treatment Started)
March, 1981		Dead		Yes
(Date of Last Contact)		(Vital Status)		(Colon Cancer Present?)
Descending Colon		Adenocarcinoma	Stage II	Surgery
(Site)		(Type)	(Stage)	(Treatment)
Survival Time	Age at Entry		Year of Entry	Expected Survival Probability
5 yrs. 5 mos.	63		1975	0.834

Fig. 2-1. Data card: Patient 3, Table 2-1

lated up to the closing date of the study. The actuarial method has the further advantage of providing information on the survival pattern, that is, the manner in which the patient group was depleted during the total period of observation. For example, do most patients die during the first year or is there a uniform death rate over 5 years?

The procedures described here are designed for the individual investigator who wants to analyze carefully the survival experience of a series of patients either manually or by using a computer.

Patient Information. Both the manual and computer approaches to survival analysis require recording on a data card, magnetic tape, or a disk, basic information on the patient, his disease, and outcome.

For purposes of clarifying the methodology and principles underlying the actuarial approach, we shall illustrate the steps in the manual approach to calculating survival rates. This might be done by employing a data card such as the one shown in Figure 2-1 with data fields providing for the following information:

1. Name or case number
2. Age: completed years of age at time of initiation of treatment
3. Race and sex
4. Dates of first treatment and of last contact: month and year
5. Survival time (years–months)
6. Vital status and presence of disease: reliable information on presence or absence of cancer at time of death is highly desirable
7. Diagnosis: site of the tumor, histologic type, and stage of disease
8. Treatment: brief summary

Observed Survival Rate. The life-table method of calculating a survival rate, using all the follow-up information available on the 40 patients under study, is illustrated in Table 2-2. There are seven steps necessary in preparing such a table:

1. The number of intervals and the length of each interval for survival time are chosen. One-year intervals were chosen for this example. The first interval is defined as up to but not including 1 year (survival years = 0), the second interval is surviving 1 year up to but not including 2 years (survival years = 1), and so on.
2. The patient data are tallied for vital status and survival time (columns 3 and 4). The sum of the totals for columns 3 and 4 must equal the total number of patients alive at the beginning of the study.

Table 2-2. Calculation of Observed Survival Rate by the Actuarial (Life-Table) Method

INTERVAL OF LAST OBSERVATION (YEARS) (1)	NO. ALIVE AT BEGINNING OF YEAR (2) l	NO. DYING DURING YEAR (3) d	NO. LAST SEEN ALIVE DURING YEAR (4) w	EFFECTIVE NO. EXPOSED TO RISK OF DYING (5) l'	PROPORTION DYING DURING YEAR (6) q	PROPORTION SURVIVING THE YEAR (7) p	PROP. SURV. FROM 1ST RX TO END OF INTERVAL (8) CP
0 — <1	40	4	0	40.0	0.100	0.900	0.900
1 — <2	36	4	0	36.0	0.111	0.889	0.800
2 — <3	32	3	3	30.5	0.098	0.902	0.722
3 — <4	26	3	2	25.0	0.120	0.880	0.635
4 — <5	21	3	4	19.0	0.158	0.842	0.535
5 or more	14	3	11				
Total		20	20				

3. The number of patients alive at the beginning of each year is entered in column 2 and is obtained by successive subtraction of patients dying or last seen alive during the previous year. Thus, of 40 patients alive at start of treatment, that is, at the beginning of the first year of observation, 4 died during the first year and 36 were alive at the beginning of the second year.
4. The "effective number exposed to risk of dying" (column 5) is based on the assumption that patients last seen alive during any year of follow-up were, on the average, observed for one-half of that year. Thus, for the third interval the "effective number" is $32 - (1/2 \times 3) = 30.5$ and for the fourth interval it is $26 - (1/2 \times 2) = 25.0$. This is equivalent to person–years at risk.
5. The proportion dying during any year (column 6) is found by dividing the entry in column 3 by the entry in column 5. Thus, for the first interval, the proportion dying is $4 \div 40 = 0.100$ and for the second interval it is $4 \div 36 = 0.111$.
6. The proportion surviving the year (column 7), that is, the observed *annual* survival rate, is obtained by subtracting the proportion dying (column 6) from 1,000.
7. The proportion surviving from first treatment to the end of each year (column 8), that is, the observed *cumulative* survival rate, is the product of the annual survival rates for the given year and all preceding years. For example, for the fifth interval the proportion 0.535 is the product of all entries in column 7 from the first through the fifth years.

The 5-year survival rate calculated by the life-table method is 0.535 or 54%. In this instance, the calculation obtained by using the information available on all 40 patients agrees well with the rate (52%) based on the 27 patients eligible for inclusion in the calculation by the direct method. Such close agreement by the two methods usually will not occur when patients are excluded from the calculation of a survival rate by the direct method. In such instances, the life-table method is more reliable because it is based on more information.

The cumulative rates in column 8 may be used to plot a survival curve and therefore provide a pictorial description of the survival pattern as shown in Figure 2-2. In Figure 2-3, the survival pattern for patients with colon cancer (based on a large series) is compared with the patterns for cancer of the lung and melanoma of the skin for a 10-year period of observation.

The same set of survival rates was plotted in Figure 2-4 using a logarithmic scale, which provides a

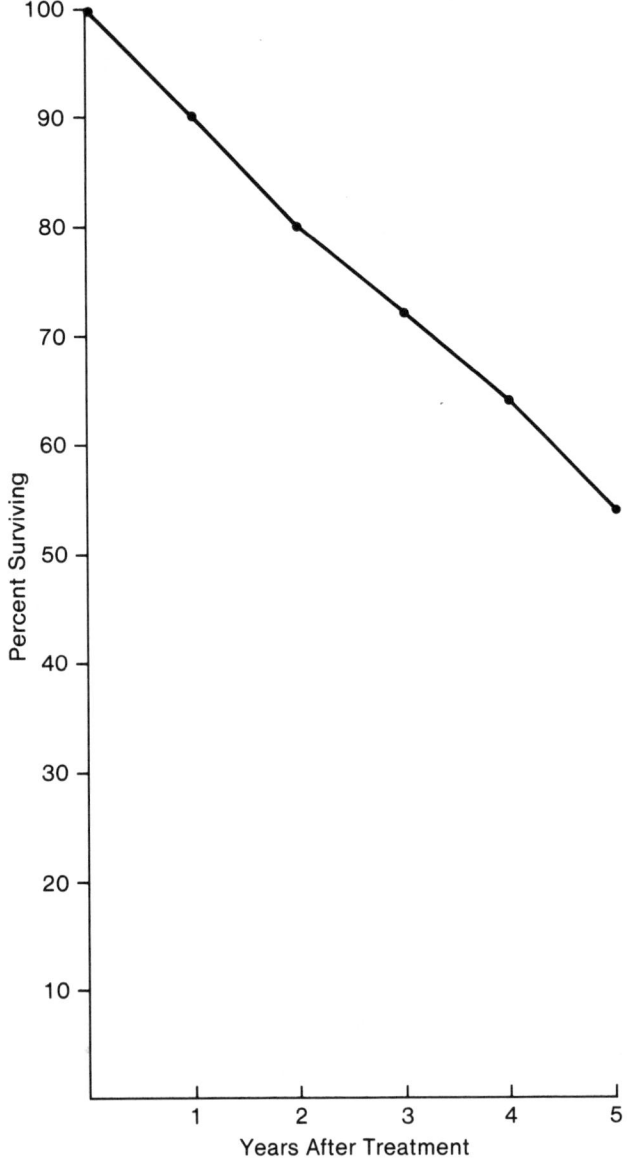

Fig. 2-2. Survival curve for 40 Stage II colon cancer patients

pictorial representation of changes in the rate at which patients died—a steep slope indicates a high rate, a shallow slope indicates a low rate. For each disease group, the death rate slowed appreciably after the third year and the slope of each curve became shallower. However, it is clear from Figure 2-4 that patients with lung cancer were dying at a greater rate from the third through the tenth years than patients with cancer of the colon or with melanoma. In contrast, examination of Figure 2-3 might lead one to the erroneous conclusion that beyond the third year, lung cancer patients died at a lower rate. This is because Figure 2-3 portrays

Reporting of Cancer Survival and End Results

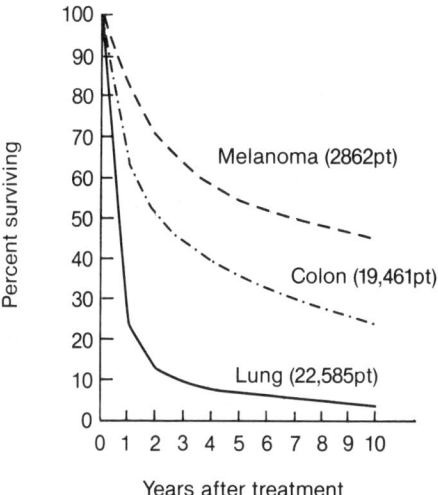

Fig. 2-3. Survival curves for patients with melanoma, colon cancer, and lung cancer: arithmetic scale. (Data from End-Results Group: End Results in Cancer, Report No. 4, DHEW Publication NIH 73-272. Bethesda, MD, National Cancer Institute, 1972)

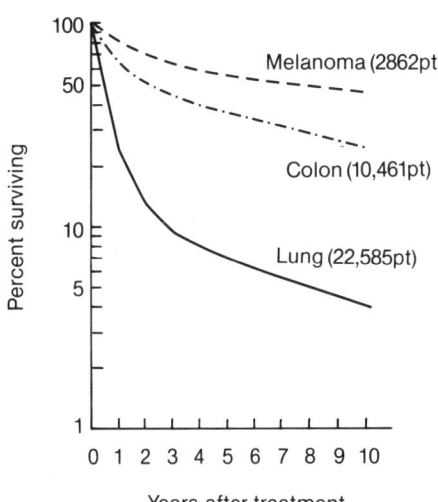

Fig. 2-4. Survival curves for patients with melanoma, colon cancer, and lung cancer: logarithmic scale. (Data from End-Results Group: End Results in Cancer, Report No. 4, DHEW Publication NIH 73-272. Bethesda, MD, National Cancer Institute, 1972)

absolute changes, while Figure 2-4 provides a true picture of *relative* changes.

Adjusted Survival Rate. The *observed* survival rate described above accounts for all deaths, regardless of cause. Although this is a true reflection of total mortality in the patient group, we are frequently interested in describing mortality attributable to the disease under study. The *adjusted* survival rate is the proportion of the initial patient group that escaped death due to cancer if all other causes of death were not operating. Examination of Table 2-1 reveals that in seven instances colon cancer was not present at time of death (patients 2, 9, 14, 15, 16, 20, and 33). All of these deaths occurred within the first 5 years of follow-up and thus influenced the 5-year *observed* survival rate calculated in Table 2-2.

Whenever reliable information on cause of death is available, an adjustment can be made for deaths due to causes other than the disease under study. The procedure is shown in Table 2-3. Observed deaths are recorded as "with disease" (column 3a) or "without disease" (column 3b). Patients who died without disease are treated in the same manner as patients "last seen alive during year" (column 4), that is, both groups are withdrawn from the risk of dying from colon cancer. Thus, "the effective number exposed to risk of dying" (from colon cancer) in the third year of observation is $32 - (1/2\,[2 + 3]) = 29.5$.

The 5-year *adjusted* survival rate is 69% compared to an *observed* rate of 54%. The adjusted rate indicates that 69% of patients with colon cancer escaped the risk of death from colon cancer for 5 years after treatment.

Table 2-3. Calculation of Adjusted Survival Rate

INTERVAL OF LAST OBSERVATION (1)	NO. ALIVE AT BEGINNING OF YEAR (2)	NO. DYING DURING YEAR WITH DISEASE (3a)	NO. DYING DURING YEAR WITHOUT DISEASE (3b)	NO. LAST SEEN ALIVE DURING YEAR (4)	EFFECTIVE NO. EXPOSED TO RISK OF DYING (5)	PROPORTION DYING DURING YEAR (6)	PROPORTION SURVIVING TO END OF YEAR (7)	CUMULATIVE PROPORTION SURVIVING (8)
Years								
1	40	3	1	0	39.5	.076	.924	.924
2	36	2	2	0	35	.057	.943	.871
3	32	1	2	3	29.5	.034	.966	.842
4	26	2	1	2	24.5	.082	.918	.773
5	21	2	1	4	18.5	.108	.892	.689
≥6	14	3	—	11				
Total		13	7	20				

Use of the adjusted rate is particularly important in comparing patient groups that may differ with respect to factors such as sex, age, race, and socioeconomic status. Of the 40 patients listed in Table 2-1, 18 are males and 22 are females. The observed survival curves are plotted in the upper part of Figure 2-5. There is an apparent difference in survival between male and female patients. However, 4 of the 9 males who died during the first 5 years of observation had no evidence of colon cancer at time of death. Colon cancer was present at time of death in 5 of the 8 females who died. The effect of the adjustment for cause of death is shown in the lower portion of Figure 2-5. The survival curve for males is now very close to that for females. The 5-year adjusted survival rate is 66% for males and 71% for females. The corresponding observed rates are 48% and 59%, a much larger difference.

Relative Survival Rates. Information on cause of death is sometimes unavailable or unreliable. Under such circumstances, it is not possible to compute an adjusted survival rate. However, it is possible to account for differences among patient groups in "normal mortality expectation," that is, differences in the risk of dying from causes other than the disease under study. This can be done by means of the relative survival rate, which is the ratio of the observed survival rate to the expected rate for a group of people in the general population similar to the patient group with respect to race, sex, age, and calendar period of observation.

Table 2-4 provides 5-year expected survival probabilities for white males and females in the United States, based on mortality experience in calendar years 1950, 1955, 1960, 1965, 1970, 1975, and 1980. The appropriate probability, depending on the sex and age of the patient and the calendar year of entry to observation, is taken from this table and entered in the lower portion of the patient data card (Figure 2-1). Thus, for example, for patient 3 (Table 2-1), who is a 63-year-old man with a 1975 date of entry, the 5-year expected survival probability is 0.834. For patient 17, a 56-year-old woman who entered observation in 1978, the expected survival probability is 0.966. Thus, for the hypothetical group of patients in Table 2-1, the average expected 5-year survival probability is the sum of the individual expected probabilities (31.241) divided by the number of patients (40), and equals 0.781. The ratio of the observed (0.535) to the expected (0.781) survival rate is 0.685 or 69%. This is the relative rate and in this instance is identical with the adjusted rate.

Although in this illustration 5-year results were used to depict the relative survival rate calculation, it is conventional to calculate relative survival rates for each interval and cumulatively for successive follow-up intervals. For detailed analysis, one must consult more extensive expected rate tables and more explicit methodology (see bibliography entry 8). In publishing relative survival rates, it is important to report the method used for calculation and the source of expected rates.

In Figure 2-6, comparison is made between the survival curves based on the observed, adjusted, and relative rates on a logarithmic scale. It can be seen that the values along the adjusted and relative

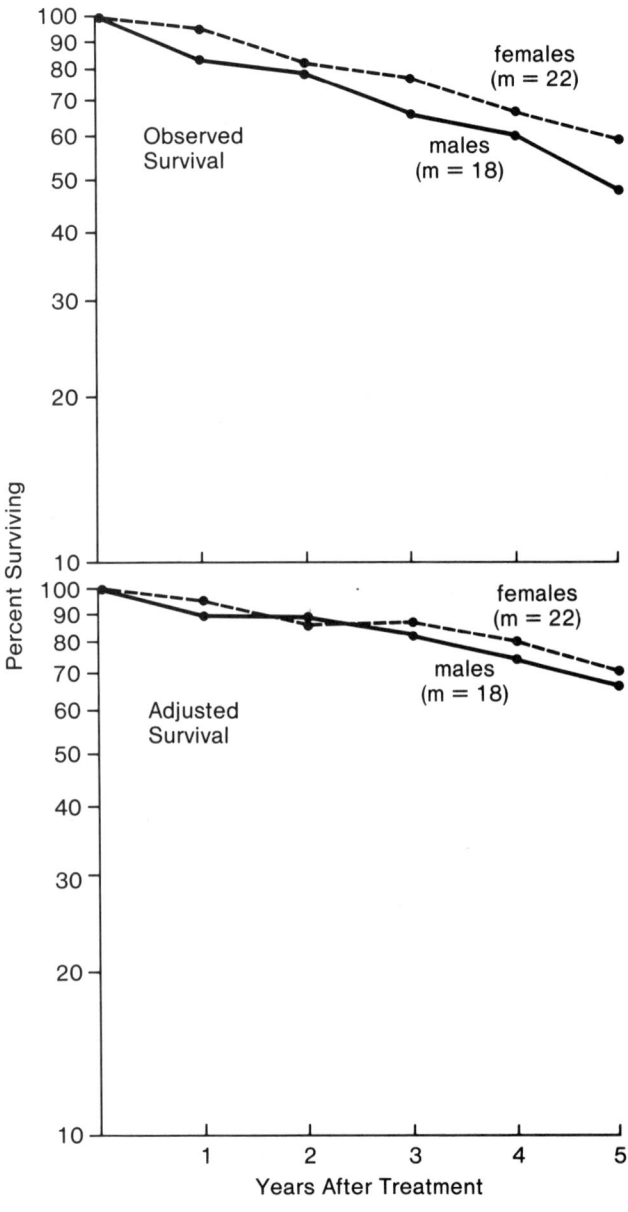

Fig. 2-5. Comparison of survival curves (logarithmic scale) for males and females with colon cancer: observed and adjusted survival rates

Table 2-4. Expected Probabilities for Surviving Five Years for U.S. Whites: 1950, 1955, 1960, 1965, 1970, 1975 and 1980

AGE IN YEARS (INCLUSIVE RANGE)	1950 (1948–1952)	1955 (1953–1957)	1960 (1958–1962)	1965 (1963–1967)	1970 (1968–1972)	1975 (1973–1977)	1980 (1978–1982)
Male							
<1	0.964	0.969	0.970	0.972	0.977	0.981	0.985
1 and 2	0.995	0.996	0.996	0.996	0.996	0.997	0.997
5 (3–7)	0.997	0.997	0.998	0.998	0.998	0.998	0.998
10 (8–12)	0.997	0.997	0.997	0.998	0.998	0.998	0.998
15 (13–17)	0.993	0.994	0.994	0.994	0.993	0.993	0.993
20 (18–22)	0.991	0.991	0.992	0.991	0.990	0.991	0.991
25 (23–27)	0.992	0.992	0.992	0.992	0.992	0.992	0.991
30 (28–32)	0.991	0.991	0.991	0.991	0.991	0.992	0.992
35 (33–37)	0.986	0.987	0.988	0.987	0.987	0.989	0.990
40 (38–42)	0.978	0.979	0.980	0.980	0.979	0.982	0.984
45 (43–47)	0.963	0.965	0.966	0.966	0.967	0.970	0.974
50 (48–52)	0.942	0.944	0.943	0.944	0.947	0.952	0.958
55 (53–57)	0.912	0.916	0.915	0.913	0.915	0.926	0.934
60 (58–62)	0.869	0.873	0.872	0.873	0.873	0.884	0.898
65 (63–67)	0.814	0.815	0.815	0.813	0.816	0.834	0.848
70 (68–72)	0.741	0.746	0.745	0.741	0.745	0.759	0.777
75 (73–77)	0.633	0.642	0.650	0.649	0.642	0.658	0.687
80 (78–82)	0.499	0.504	0.509	0.520	0.523	0.547	0.565
≥85 (83+)	0.350	0.349	0.349	0.350	0.379	0.421	0.426
Female							
<1	0.972	0.976	0.977	0.979	0.982	0.985	0.988
1 and 2	0.996	0.997	0.997	0.997	0.997	0.997	0.998
5 (3–7)	0.998	0.998	0.998	0.998	0.998	0.999	0.999
10 (8–12)	0.998	0.998	0.999	0.999	0.999	0.999	0.999
15 (13–17)	0.997	0.997	0.998	0.998	0.997	0.997	0.998
20 (18–22)	0.996	0.997	0.997	0.997	0.997	0.997	0.997
25 (23–27)	0.996	0.996	0.996	0.997	0.996	0.997	0.997
30 (28–32)	0.994	0.995	0.995	0.995	0.995	0.996	0.996
35 (33–37)	0.991	0.992	0.993	0.993	0.993	0.994	0.995
40 (38–42)	0.987	0.988	0.988	0.988	0.988	0.990	0.991
45 (43–47)	0.980	0.982	0.982	0.982	0.982	0.984	0.986
50 (48–52)	0.969	0.972	0.972	0.972	0.973	0.975	0.978
55 (53–57)	0.953	0.959	0.960	0.959	0.960	0.963	0.966
60 (58–62)	0.925	0.934	0.937	0.939	0.941	0.944	0.948
65 (63–67)	0.883	0.890	0.900	0.901	0.908	0.920	0.922
70 (68–72)	0.816	0.832	0.841	0.846	0.854	0.869	0.879
75 (73–77)	0.708	0.727	0.746	0.754	0.761	0.784	0.812
80 (78–82)	0.558	0.580	0.592	0.611	0.633	0.672	0.695
≥85 (83+)	0.406	0.394	0.400	0.405	0.472	0.512	0.542

(Demographic Analysis Section, National Cancer Institute, Bethesda, Maryland)

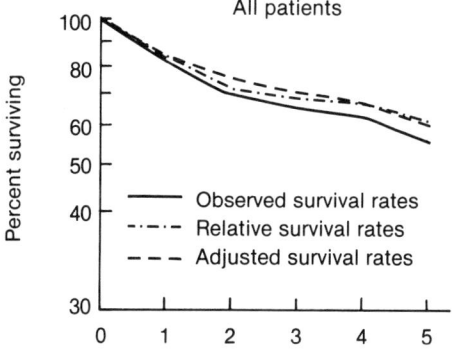

Fig. 2-6. Comparison of survival curves based on observed, adjusted, and relative rates (logarithmic scale)

survival curves are not always identical. In practice, if the series is not too small and the patients are roughly representative of the population of the United States (taking race, sex, and age into account), the relative survival rate provides a useful estimate of the probability of escaping death from the specific cancer under study. However, if reliable information on cause of death is available, it is preferable to use the adjusted rate. This is particularly true if the series is small or if the patients are largely drawn from a particular socioeconomic segment of the population.

In reporting on patient survival, the specific method used in calculating the rates must be indicated. The different types of rates described above

Table 2-5. Example of Kaplan-Meier Survival Calculations

TIME (MONTHS)	ALIVE	DIED	WITHDRAWN	PROPORTION DYING	PROPORTION SURVIVING	SURVIVAL RATE
1	5	1	0	0.200	0.800	0.800
4	4	1	0	0.250	0.750	0.600
7	3	1	0	0.333	0.667	0.400
10	2	1	0	0.500	0.500	0.200
19	1	1	0	1.000	0.000	0.000

are all useful, but rates computed by different methods are not directly comparable with each other. Thus, in comparing the survival of different patient groups, rates must be computed by the same method.

Calculation by the Kaplan-Meier Method. Another method of survival analysis that is widely used and for which computer programs are easily available is the Kaplan-Meier method (see bibliography entry 13). It is similar to the life-table method but also provides for calculating the proportion surviving to each point in time that a death occurs. The life-table and Kaplan-Meier methods give identical results in the absence of withdrawals.

As a simple introduction to Kaplan-Meier, consider five patients who died at 1, 4, 7, 10, and 19 months, respectively. The first survival proportion is calculated at 1 month, the time of the first death. Since 4 of the 5 patients survived beyond that point, the resulting proportion surviving to that time is 4 out of 5 or 0.80. Similarly at 4 months, the time of the second death, 3 out of the 4 (0.75) who survived the first month are still alive after 4 months. Thus, the cumulative 4-month survival rate is $0.80 \times 0.75 = 0.60$. The third interval of interest is from 4 to 7 months, the time of the third death. For the interval, the proportion surviving is 2/3 (0.67). Also from 7 to 10 months, the next interval of interest, the proportion surviving is 1/2 (0.50). Considering the last interval, 10 to 19 months, the proportion surviving is 0/1 (0.00). This is shown in Table 2-5. The 6-month and 1-year survival rates are 60% and 20%, respectively. This is because until a death occurs, the survival proportion last calculated remains in effect. This survival pattern is shown in Figure 2-7. Note that the survival curve proceeds in steps rather than as a sloped line.

In contrast to the life-table method, if a patient had been lost or withdrawn during an interval (*e.g.*, interval 5), that person's experience would have been included to the end of the last completed interval (ending at 4 months) and not entered into any of the subsequent calculations.

The Kaplan-Meier method applied to the data for our series of 40 stage II colon cancer cases (Table 2-1) is shown in Table 2-6. The 5-year survival rate is 0.529, which is very similar to the rate of 0.535 found by the life-table method. Figure 2-8 shows the comparison of survival curves based on life-table and Kaplan-Meier calculations on this series

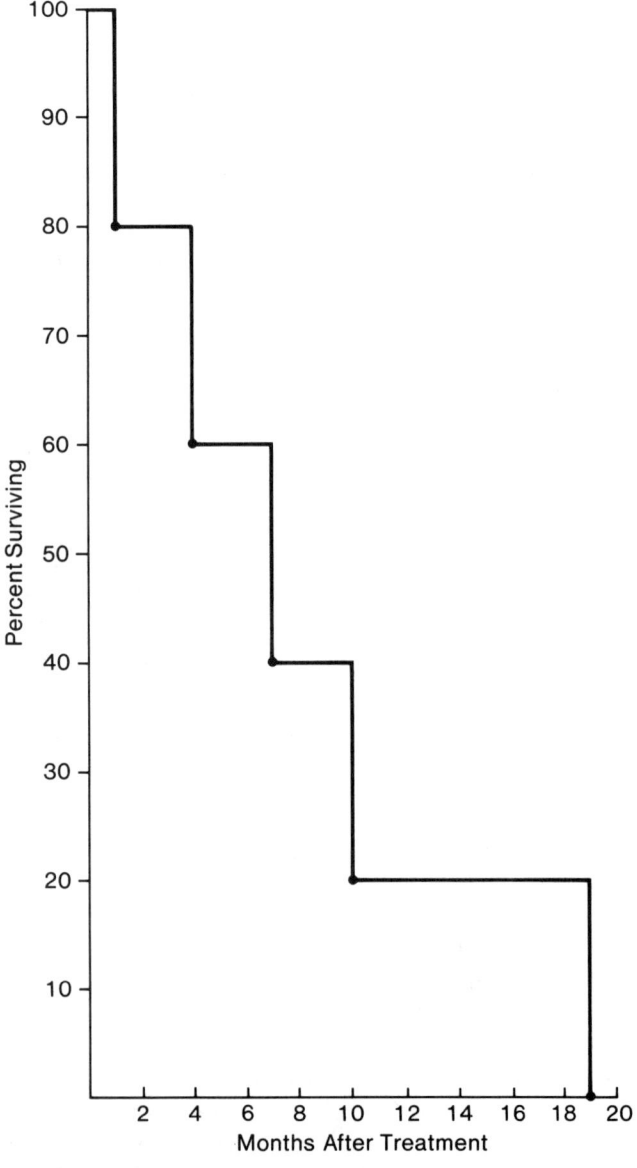

Fig. 2-7. Observed survival for five patients (data from Table 2-5), Kaplan–Meier method

Table 2-6. Calculation of Observed Survival by the Kaplan-Meier Method: 40 Stage II Colon Cancer Patients

TIME (MONTHS)	ENTERED ALIVE	DIED	WITHDRAWN	PROPORTION DYING	PROPORTION SURVIVING	SURVIVAL RATE
1	40	1	0	0.025	0.975	0.975
3	39	1	0	0.026	0.974	0.950
8	38	1	0	0.026	0.974	0.925
10	37	1	0	0.027	0.973	0.900
13	36	1	0	0.028	0.972	0.875
16	35	1	0	0.029	0.971	0.849
19	34	1	0	0.029	0.971	0.825
23	33	1	0	0.030	0.970	0.800
27	32	1	0	0.031	0.969	0.775
29	31	1	0	0.032	0.968	0.750
31	30	0	1			
34	29	0	1			
35	28	1	1	0.036	0.964	0.723
36	26	1	0	0.038	0.962	0.696
37	25	0	1			
40	24	0	1			
46	23	1	0	0.043	0.957	0.666
47	22	1	0	0.045	0.955	0.636
48	21	0	1			
51	20	0	1			
52	19	1	1	0.053	0.947	0.602
53	17	1	0	0.059	0.941	0.567
55	16	0	1			
56	15	1	0	0.067	0.933	0.529
≥60		3	11			

of 40 colon cancer patients. An adjusted rate can be calculated by the Kaplan-Meier method by handling noncancer deaths and withdrawals in a manner similar to that illustrated above for the life-table method.

A relative survival rate can also be calculated by using the observed rate derived by the Kaplan-Meier method and dividing it by the expected rate, as was done for the life-table method.

STANDARD ERROR OF A SURVIVAL RATE

A survival rate describes the experience of the specific group of patients from which it is computed. These results are frequently used to generalize to a larger population. The existence of population values is postulated and these values are estimated from the group under study, which thus represents a sample from the larger population. If a survival rate were calculated from a second sample taken from the same population, it is unlikely that the results would be exactly the same. The difference between the two results is called the *sampling variation* (chance variation or sampling error). The *standard error* is a measure of the extent to which sampling variation influences the computed survival rate. In repeated observations under the same conditions, the true or population survival rate will lie within the range of two standard errors on either side of the computed rate about 95 times in 100. This range is called the 95% confidence interval.

When the observed survival rate has been computed by the direct method, the standard error is computed from the formula

$$\sqrt{\frac{CP(1 - CP)}{n}}$$

in which CP is the survival rate and n is the number of patients at risk of death. In the illustration of the direct method, a 5-year survival rate of 52% (or p = 0.52) was obtained based on the experience of 27 patients.

Thus, the standard error is equal to 0.096 (square root of [0.52 × 0.48 ÷ 27]). To obtain the 95% confidence interval, twice the standard error (0.19) is subtracted from and then added to the survival rate. This means that the chances are about 95 in 100 that the true 5-year rate is between 0.33 and 0.71 for our example.

Standard Error of the Actuarial Survival Rate. To calculate the standard error of the 5-year survival rate when the actuarial method is used (see bibliography entries 6, 14, 16), two columns of figures may be added to Table 2-2 as shown in Table 2-7. The first additional column (column 9) is obtained by subtracting the values in column 3 from the

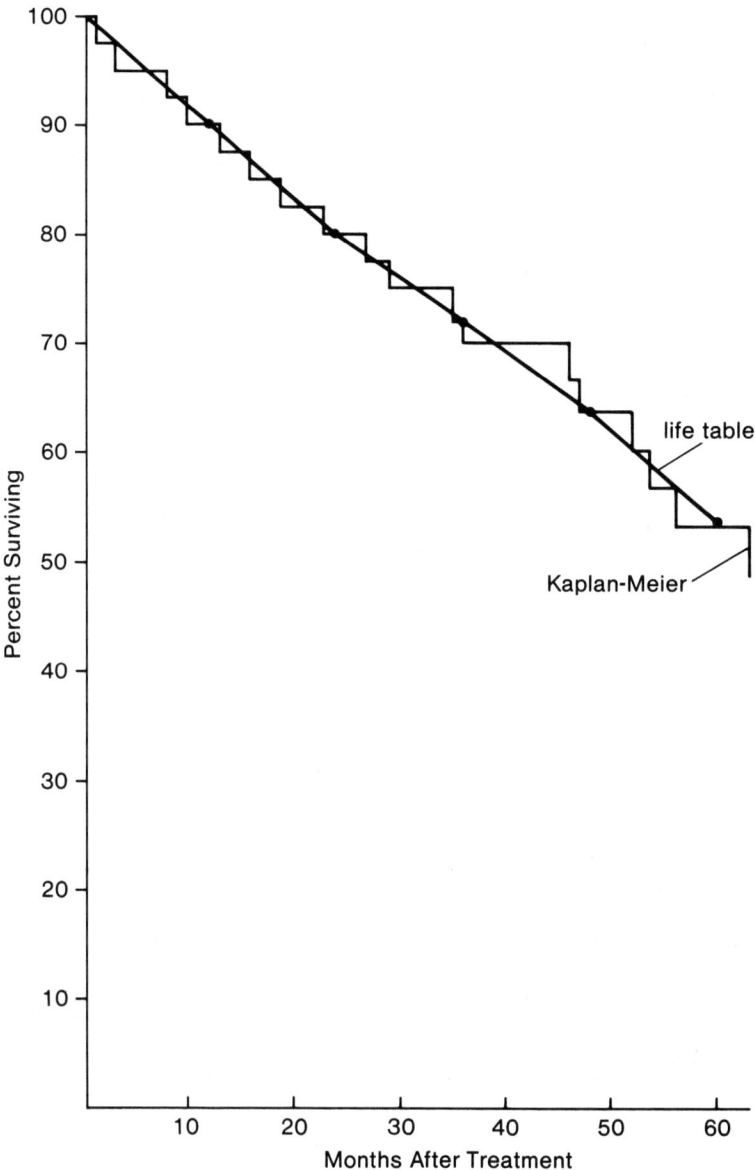

Fig. 2-8. Observed survival for life-table method versus Kaplan–Meier method calculations: 40 Stage II colon cancer patients

Table 2-7. Calculation of Standard Error of Survival Rate by Actuarial (Life-Table) Method

INTERVAL OF LAST OBSERVATION (YEARS) (1)	NO. ALIVE AT BEGINNING OF YEAR (2) l	NO. DYING DURING YEAR (3) d	NO. LAST SEEN ALIVE DURING YEAR (4) w	EFFECTIVE NO. EXPOSED TO RISK OF DYING (5) l'	PROPORTION DYING DURING YEAR (6) q	PROPORTION SURVIVING THE YEAR (7) p	PROP. SURV. FROM 1ST RX TO END OF INTERVAL (8) CP	ENTRY (5) MINUS ENTRY (3) (9)	ENTRY (6) DIVIDED BY ENTRY (9) (10)
0 — <1	40	4	0	40.0	0.100	0.900	0.900	36.0	.0028
1 — <2	36	4	0	36.0	0.111	0.889	0.800	32.0	.0035
2 — <3	32	3	3	30.5	0.098	0.902	0.722	27.5	.0036
3 — <4	26	3	2	25.0	0.120	0.880	0.635	22.0	.0055
4 — <5	21	3	4	19.0	0.158	0.842	0.535	16.0	.0099
5 or more	14	3	11						
Total		20	20						0.0253

Standard Error of 5-Year Survival Rate = 5-Year Survival Rate $\times \sqrt{\text{Total of Column (10)}}$
$= 0.535 \times \sqrt{0.0253} = 0.535 \times 0.1591 = 0.085$

values in column 5 of Table 2-2. The last column needed (column 10) is obtained by dividing the entries in column 6 by the corresponding figures in column 9. The sum of the figures in column 10 is also entered into the table and in this example equals 0.0253.

The standard error of the 5-year survival rate by the actuarial method is the calculated 5-year survival rate multiplied by the square root of the total of the entries in column 10 of Table 2-5, that is, $0.535 \times \sqrt{0.0253} = 0.085$. The approximate 95% confidence interval for the population 5-year survival rate is found, as shown earlier for the direct method, by adding and subtracting two times the standard error to and from the 5-year survival rate that has been calculated, that is, 0.535 plus and minus (2×0.085), which gives an interval from 0.36 to 0.70.

If the above computations seem to be too involved, an approximation to the standard error of the actuarial survival rate may be quickly obtained from published tables prepared by Ederer (see bibliography entry 7).

It is noteworthy that the standard error of the survival rate obtained by the actuarial method is smaller than the standard error of the survival rate calculated by the direct method (0.085 versus 0.096). This difference reflects the advantage in terms of statistical precision of using all available information, that is, including information on patients under observation for less than 5 years. The issue is discussed in detail by Cutler in bibliography entry 6.

The standard error of a survival rate obtained by the Kaplan-Meier method may be calculated as shown in bibliography entry 13.

Standard Error of Relative Survival Rate. The standard error of the relative survival rate is easily obtained by dividing the standard error of the observed survival rate (obtained by either the direct or actuarial method) by the expected survival rate. To illustrate these calculations, consider results for the 40 Stage II colon cancer patients: the expected 5-year survival rate was 0.781; the standard error of the observed survival rate was 0.085. Therefore, in this example the standard error of the 5-year relative survival rate is:

$$\frac{\text{Standard error of observed rate}}{\text{Expected survival rate}} = \frac{0.085}{0.781} = 0.109$$

The 95% confidence limits of the 5-year relative survival rate are therefore:

$$0.69 \pm 2 (0.109) = 0.47, 0.91$$

Comparison of Survival Rates in Two Patient Groups. In comparing survival rates of two patient groups, the statistical significance of the observed difference is of interest. The essential question is: What is the probability that the observed difference may have occurred by chance? The standard error of the survival rate provides a simple means for appraising this question. If the 95% confidence intervals of two survival rates do not overlap, the observed difference would be customarily considered as statistically significant, that is, unlikely to be due to chance.

Standard statistical texts describe the z-test, which provides a numeric estimate of the probability that a difference as large as that observed would have occurred if only chance were operating. The statistic z is calculated by the formula

$$z = \frac{|CP_1 - CP_2|}{\sqrt{(SE_1)^2 + (SE_2)^2}}$$

in which

1. CP_1 is the survival rate for group 1
2. CP_2 is the survival rate for group 2
3. $|CP_1 - CP_2|$ is the *absolute* value of the difference (i.e., the *magnitude* of the difference, whether positive or negative)
4. SE_1 is the standard error of CP_1
5. SE_2 is the standard error of CP_2

If $z \geq 1.96$, the probability that a difference as large as that observed occurred by chance is $\leq 5\%$. If $z \geq 2.56$, the probability is $\leq 1\%$. It is conventional in most (but not all) applications to regard as statistically significant a difference that would occur by chance with a probability of 5% or less.

For example, let us apply the z-test to the difference in observed 5-year survival rates by the actuarial method for the 18 males and 22 females among the 40 colon cancer patients, that is, let us test whether there is a statistically significant difference in survival of the males with colon cancer compared with the females.

Designate the 5-year survival rate for males by CP_1 and for females by CP_2. We find $CP_1 = 0.475$ and $CP_2 = 0.591$. Employing the method shown in Table 2-5, $SE_1 = 0.122$ and $SE_2 = 0.116$.

Then

$$z = \frac{|0.475 - 0.591|}{\sqrt{0.122^2 + 0.116^2}} = \frac{0.116}{0.168} = 0.69$$

The calculated z value is smaller than 1.96 and therefore not statistically significant at the 5% level. This result indicates that for a study of this size (18 males and 22 females) the difference in CPs (0.475

versus 0.591) is not large enough for us to reject chance or sampling variation as the cause.

In a study with more patients, the same size difference in survival rates as seen here would be less likely to be due to chance and might be statistically significant, that is, z might equal or exceed 1.96. In order for this to come about, the value of the denominator in the equation for z would have to decrease in value. The denominator,

$$\sqrt{(SE_1)^2 + (SE_2)^2}$$

is called the standard error of the difference in rates and tends to become smaller as study size increases. It should also be noted that superior survival of females with colon cancer compared with males has been observed in large series of patients with resultant significant z values.

Great care must be exercised in the interpretation of tests of statistical significance. For example, if differences exist in the patient and disease characteristics of two treatment groups, a statistically significant difference in survival results may primarily reflect differences in the two patient series rather than differences in efficacy of the treatment regimens. The more definitive approach to therapy evaluation requires a randomized clinical trial that helps to ensure comparability of the two treatment groups and their disease.

The methods of survival analysis presented in this chapter are appropriate for a single group of patients or may be applied to subgroups derived by cross-classifying patients with respect to several variables of interest. Multivariate models, although beyond the scope of this chapter, have now been extensively used to assess the relationship to survival time of a number of variables simultaneously. One of the most frequently used is the Cox proportional hazards model (see bibliography entry 5). Bibliography entry 12 is an excellent source for additional information on multivariate survival analysis.

BIBLIOGRAPHY

1. Berkson J, Gage RP: Calculation of survival rates for cancer. Proc Staff Meet Mayo Clin 25:270–286, 1950
2. Breslow N: A generalized Kruskal-Wallis test for comparing samples subject to unequal patterns of censoring. Biometrika 57:579–594, 1970
3. Chiang CL: A stochastic study of the life table and its applications. I. Probability distributions of the biometric functions. Biometrics 16:618–635, 1960
4. Chiang CL: The Life Table and Its Applications, p. 316. Malabar, FL, Robert E. Krieger Pub. Co., 1984
5. Cox DR: Regression models and life tables. J R Stat Soc B 34:187–220, 1972
6. Cutler SJ, Ederer F: Maximum utilization of the life table method in analyzing survival. J Chronic Dis 8:699–712, 1958
7. Ederer F: A simple method for determining standard errors of survival rates, with tables. J Chronic Dis 11:632–645, 1960
8. Ederer F, Axtell LM, Cutler SJ: The relative survival rate: A statistical methodology. Natl Cancer Inst Monogr 6:101–121, 1961
9. Gehan EA: A generalized Wilcoxon test for comparing arbitrarily single-censored samples. Biometrika 52:203–224, 1965
10. Gehan EA: Estimating survival functions from the life table. J Chronic Dis 21:629–644, 1969
11. Hankey BF, Myers MH: Evaluating differences in survival between two groups of patients. J Chronic Dis 24:523–531, 1971
12. Kalbfleisch JD, Prentice RL: The Statistical Analysis of Failure Time Data, p 321. New York, John Wiley and Sons, 1980
13. Kaplan EL, Meier P: Nonparametric estimation from incomplete observations. J Am Stat Assn 53:457–481, 1958
14. MacDonald EJ: Method of analysis for evaluation of treatment in cancer of the oropharynx. Radiology 78:783–788, 1962
15. Mantel N: Evaluation of survival data and two new rank order statistics arising in its consideration. Cancer Chemother Rep 50:163–170, 1966
16. Merrell M, Shulman LE: Determination of prognosis in chronic disease, illustrated by systemic lupus erythematosus. J Chronic Dis 1:12–32, 1955
17. Peto R, Pike MC, Armitage P et al: Design and analysis of randomized clinical trials requiring prolonged observation of each patient. II. Analysis and examples. Br J Cancer 35:1–35, 1977

PART II

STAGING OF CANCER AT SPECIFIC ANATOMIC SITES

HEAD AND NECK SITES

3

Lip and Oral Cavity

Cancers of the head and neck may arise on all lining membranes of the upper aerodigestive tract. The T classifications indicating the extent of the primary tumor are generally similar but differ in specific details for each site because of anatomic considerations. The N classification for cervical lymph node metastasis is uniform for all sites. The staging systems presented in this section are all clinical staging, based on the best possible estimate of the extent of the disease before first treatment. Although pathologic classification is possible, it is of less practical importance in the management of these tumors. However, when surgical treatment is carried out, cancer of the head and neck can be staged (pathologic stage) during this period of management using all information available from the resected specimen and from before treatment.

In reviewing these staging systems, task forces from the UICC and the AJCC made minor changes in the T classifications formerly in use. It was felt necessary, however, to make several major changes in the previous N classifications of cervical node metastasis. Bilateral cervical node metastases previously classified as N3 by the AJCC were changed to N2 as suggested by the UICC in view of their somewhat more favorable prognosis with current therapy. The term *fixed*, previously applied to cervical nodes in the N3 category by the UICC, was abandoned because the degree of fixation varies and is prone to subjective interpretation by different observers. It was replaced by the AJCC definition of N3 as a node 6 cm or more in greatest diameter. This is an objective measurement and most nodes this size would formerly have been considered fixed.

This section presents the staging classification for four major head and neck sites: the oral cavity, the pharynx (nasopharynx, oropharynx, hypopharynx), the larynx, and the paranasal sinuses.

ANATOMY

Primary Site. The oral cavity extends from the skin-vermilion junction of the lips to the junction of the hard and soft palate above and to the line of circumvallate papillae below and is divided into the following specific areas:

Lip (ICD-O 140). The lip begins at the junction of the vermilion border with the skin and includes only the vermilion surface or that portion of the lip that comes into contact with the opposing lip. It is well defined into an upper and lower lip joined at the commissures of the mouth.

Buccal Mucosa (ICD-O 145.0). This includes all the membrane lining of the inner surface of the cheeks and lips from the line of contact of the opposing lips to the line of attachment of mucosa of the alveolar ridge (upper and lower) and pterygomandibular raphe.

Lower Alveolar Ridge (ICD-O 143.1). This ridge includes the alveolar process of the mandible and its covering mucosa, which extends from the line of attachment of mucosa in the buccal gutter to the line of free mucosa of the floor of the mouth. Posteriorly it extends to the ascending ramus of the mandible.

Upper Alveolar Ridge (ICD-O 143.0). The upper ridge is the alveolar process of the maxilla and its covering mucosa, which extends from the line of attachment of mucosa in the upper gingival buccal gutter to the junction of the hard palate. Its posterior margin is the upper end of the pterygopalatine arch.

Retromolar Gingiva (Retromolar Trigone) (ICD-O 145.6). This is the attached mucosa overlying the ascending ramus of the mandible from the level of the posterior surface of the last molar tooth to the apex superiorly, adjacent to the tuberosity of the maxilla.

Floor of the Mouth (ICD-O 144). This is a semilunar space over the myelohyoid and hyoglossus muscles, extending from the inner surface of the lower alveolar ridge to the undersurface of the tongue. Its posterior boundary is the base of the anterior pillar of the tonsil. It is divided into two sides by the frenulum of the tongue and contains the ostia of the submaxillary and sublingual salivary glands.

Hard Palate (ICD-O 145.2). This is the semilunar area between the upper alveolar ridge and the mucous membrane covering the palatine process of the maxillary palatine bones. It extends from the inner surface of the superior alveolar ridge to the posterior edge of the palatine bone.

Anterior Two Thirds of the Tongue (Oral Tongue) (ICD-O 141.1–141.4). This is a freely mobile portion of the tongue that extends anteriorly from the line of circumvallate papillae to the undersurface of the tongue at the junction of the floor of the mouth. It is composed of four areas: the tip, the lateral borders, the dorsum, and the undersurface (nonvillous surface of the tongue). The undersurface of the tongue is considered as a separate category by the World Health Organization (WHO) (ICD-O 141.3).

Regional Lymph Nodes. The main routes of drainage are into the first station cervical lymph nodes, which are the jugulodigastric, jugulo-omohyoid, upper deep cervical, lower deep cervical, and submaxillary and submental lymph nodes. Some primary sites drain bilaterally.

In clinical evaluation, the actual size of the nodal mass should be measured, and allowance should be made for intervening soft tissues. It is recognized that most masses over 3 cm in diameter are not single nodes but are confluent nodes or tumor in soft tissues of the neck. There are three stages of clinically positive nodes: N1, N2, and N3. The use of subgroups a, b, and c is not required but is recommended. Midline nodes are considered homolateral nodes.

Metastatic Sites. Distant spread to the lungs is common; skeletal or hepatic metastases occur less often. Mediastinal lymph node metastases are considered distant metastases.

RULES FOR CLASSIFICATION

Clinical Staging. The assessment of the primary tumor is based upon inspection and palpation of the oral cavity and neck. Additional studies may include plain, tomographic, and contrast roentgenograms, particularly evaluating bone invasion of the mandible or upper alveoli. Examinations for distant metastases include chest film, blood chemistries, blood count, and other routine studies as indicated. The tumor must be confirmed histologically. All clinical and pathologic data available prior to first definitive treatment may be used for clinical staging.

Pathologic Staging. Complete resection of the primary site, radical nodal dissections, and pathologic examination of the resected specimens allow the use of this designation. Specimens that are resected after radiation or chemotherapy need to be especially noted.

Lip and Oral Cavity

DEFINITION OF TNM

Primary Tumor (T)

- TX Primary tumor cannot be assessed
- T0 No evidence of primary tumor
- Tis Carcinoma *in situ*
- T1 Tumor 2 cm or less in greatest dimension
- T2 Tumor more than 2 cm but not more than 4 cm in greatest dimension
- T3 Tumor more than 4 cm in greatest dimension
- T4 (lip) Tumor invades adjacent structures (*e.g.*, through cortical bone, tongue, skin of neck)
- T4 (oral cavity) Tumor invades adjacent structures (*e.g.*, through cortical bone, into deep [extrinsic] muscle of tongue, maxillary sinus, skin)

Regional Lymph Nodes (N)

- NX Regional lymph nodes cannot be assessed
- N0 No regional lymph node metastasis
- N1 Metastasis in a single ipsilateral lymph node, 3 cm or less in greatest dimension
- N2 Metastasis in a single ipsilateral lymph node, more than 3 cm but not more than 6 cm in greatest dimension; or in multiple ipsilateral lymph nodes, none more than 6 cm in greatest dimension; or in bilateral or contralateral lymph nodes, none more than 6 cm in greatest dimension
  - N2a Metastasis in single ipsilateral lymph node more than 3 cm but not more than 6 cm in greatest dimension
  - N2b Metastasis in multiple ipsilateral lymph nodes, none more than 6 cm in greatest dimension
  - N2c Metastasis in bilateral or contralateral lymph nodes, none more than 6 cm in greatest dimension
- N3 Metastasis in a lymph node more than 6 cm in greatest dimension

Distant Metastasis (M)

- MX Presence of distant metastasis cannot be assessed
- M0 No distant metastasis
- M1 Distant metastasis

STAGE GROUPING

Stage 0	Tis	N0	M0
Stage I	T1	N0	M0
Stage II	T2	N0	M0
Stage III	T3	N0	M0
	T1	N1	M0
	T2	N1	M0
	T3	N1	M0
Stage IV	T4	N0, N1	M0
	Any T	N2, N3	M0
	Any T	Any N	M1

DIFFERENCES BETWEEN THE 2ND AND 3RD EDITIONS

The definition of T4 has been made more specific for lip and oral cavity. The definitions of N2 and N3 have been modified.

HISTOPATHOLOGIC TYPE

The predominant cancer is squamous cell carcinoma; pathologic diagnosis is required to use this classification. Tumor grading is recommended using Broders' classification. Other tumors of glandular epithelium, odontogenic apparatus, lymphoid tissue, soft tissue, and bone and cartilage origin require special consideration and are not to be included. Reference to the WHO nomenclature is recommended. Although the grade of the tumor does not enter into staging of the tumor, it should be recorded.

HISTOPATHOLOGIC GRADE (G)

- GX Grade cannot be assessed
- G1 Well differentiated
- G2 Moderately well differentiated
- G3 Poorly differentiated
- G4 Undifferentiated

BIBLIOGRAPHY

1. Bloom ND, Spiro RH: Carcinoma of the cheek mucosa. Am J Surg 140:556–559, 1980
2. Evans JF, Shah VP: Epidermoid carcinoma of the palate. Am J Surg 142:451–455, 1981
3. Fayos JF, Lampe I: Treatment of squamous cell carcinoma of the tongue. Am J Surg 124:493–500, 1972
4. Feind CR, Cole RM: Cancer of the floor of the mouth and its lymphatic spread. Am J Surg 116:482–486, 1968
5. Flynn MB, Mullins FX, Moore C: Selection of treatment in squamous carcinoma of the floor of the mouth. Am J Surg 126:477–481, 1973

6. Guillamondegui OM, Oliver B, Hayden R: Cancer of the anterior floor of the mouth. Am J Surg 140:560–562, 1980
7. Harrold CC Jr: Management of cancer of the floor of the mouth. Am J Surg 122:487–493, 1971
8. Kalnins IK, Leonard AG, Sako K et al: Correlation between prognosis and degree of lymph node involvement in carcinoma of the oral cavity. Am J Surg 134:450–454, 1977
9. Marchetta FC, Sako K: Results of radical surgery for intraoral carcinoma related to tumor size. Am J Surg 112:554–557, 1966
10. Shah JP, Cendon RA, Farr HW et al: Carcinoma of the oral cavity: Factors affecting treatment failure at the primary site and neck. Am J Surg 132:504–507, 1976
11. Spiro RH, Alfonso AE, Farr HW et al: Cervical node metastasis from epidermoid carcinoma of the oral cavity: A critical assessment of current staging. Am J Surg 128:562–567, 1974
12. Spiro RH, Strong EW: Epidermoid carcinoma of the mobile tongue. Am J Surg 122:707–713, 1971

LIP AND ORAL CAVITY

Data Form for Cancer Staging

Patient identification
Name _____
Address _____
Hospital or clinic number _____
Age _____ Sex _____ Race _____

Institution identification
Hospital or clinic _____
Address _____

Oncology Record

Anatomic site of cancer _____
Histologic type _____
Grade (G) _____
Date of classification _____

Chronology of classification
(use separate form for each time staged)
[ ] Clinical (use all data prior to first treatment)
[ ] Pathologic (if definitively resected specimen available)

Definitions

Primary Tumor (T)
[ ] TX   Primary tumor cannot be assessed
[ ] T0   No evidence of primary tumor
[ ] Tis   Carcinoma *in situ*
[ ] T1   Tumor 2 cm or less in greatest dimension
[ ] T2   Tumor more than 2 cm but not more than 4 cm in greatest dimension
[ ] T3   Tumor more than 4 cm in greatest dimension
[ ] T4   (lip) Tumor invades adjacent structures, *e.g.*, through cortical bone, tongue, skin of neck
[ ] T4   (oral cavity) Tumor invades adjacent structures, *e.g.*, through cortical bone, into deep (extrinsic) muscle of tongue, maxillary sinus, skin

Lymph Node (N)
[ ] NX   Regional lymph nodes cannot be assessed
[ ] N0   No regional lymph node metastasis
[ ] N1   Metastasis in a single ipsilateral lymph node, 3 cm or less in greatest dimension
[ ] N2   Metastasis in a single ipsilateral lymph node, more than 3 cm but not more than 6 cm in greatest dimension, or multiple ipsilateral lymph nodes, none more than 6 cm in greatest dimension, or bilateral or contralateral lymph nodes, none more than 6 cm in greatest dimension
   [ ] N2a   Metastasis in a single ipsilateral lymph node more than 3 cm but not more than 6 cm in greatest dimension
   [ ] N2b   Metastasis in multiple ipsilateral lymph nodes, none more than 6 cm in greatest dimension
   [ ] N2c   Metastasis in bilateral or contralateral lymph nodes, none more than 6 cm in greatest dimension
[ ] N3   Metastasis in a lymph node more than 6 cm in greatest dimension

Distant Metastasis (M)
[ ] MX   Presence of distant metastasis cannot be assessed
[ ] M0   No distant metastasis
[ ] M1   Distant metastasis

Stage Grouping

[ ] 0	Tis	N0	M0
[ ] I	T1	N0	M0
[ ] II	T2	N0	M0
[ ] III	T3	N0	M0
	T1	N1	M0
	T2	N1	M0
	T3	N1	M0
[ ] IV	T4	N0	M0
	T4	N1	M0
	Any T	N2	M0
	Any T	N3	M0
	Any T	Any N	M1

Location of Tumor
[ ] Lips: Upper
       Lower
[ ] Buccal mucosa
[ ] Floor of mouth
[ ] Oral tongue
[ ] Hard palate
[ ] Gingivae: Upper
          Lower
          Retromolar trigone

Characteristics of Tumor
[ ] Exophytic
[ ] Superficial
[ ] Moderately infiltrating
[ ] Deeply infiltrating
[ ] Ulcerated
[ ] Extends to or overlies bone
[ ] Gross erosion of bone
[ ] Radiographic destruction of bone

Involvement of Neighboring Regions
[ ] Tonsillar pillar or soft palate
[ ] Nasal cavity or antrum
[ ] Nasopharynx
[ ] Pterygoid muscles
[ ] Soft tissues or skin of neck

Staged by _____ M.D.
_____ Registrar
Date _____

Illustrations

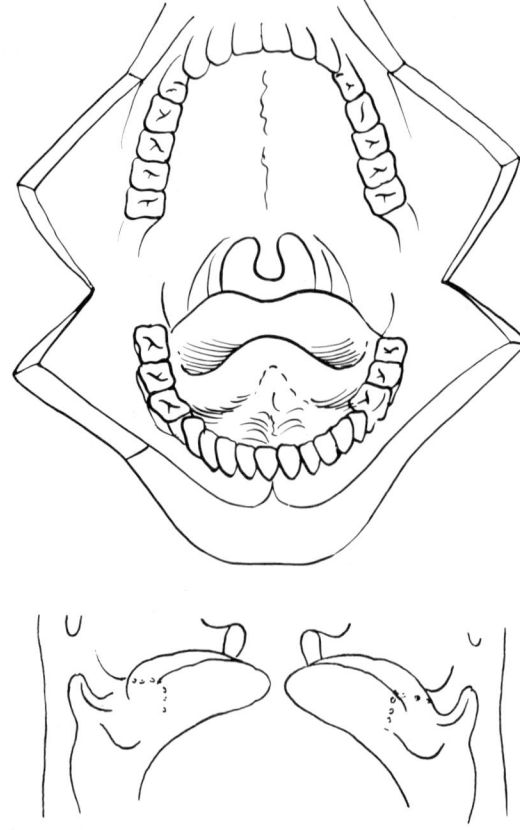

Tumor size: _____ cm

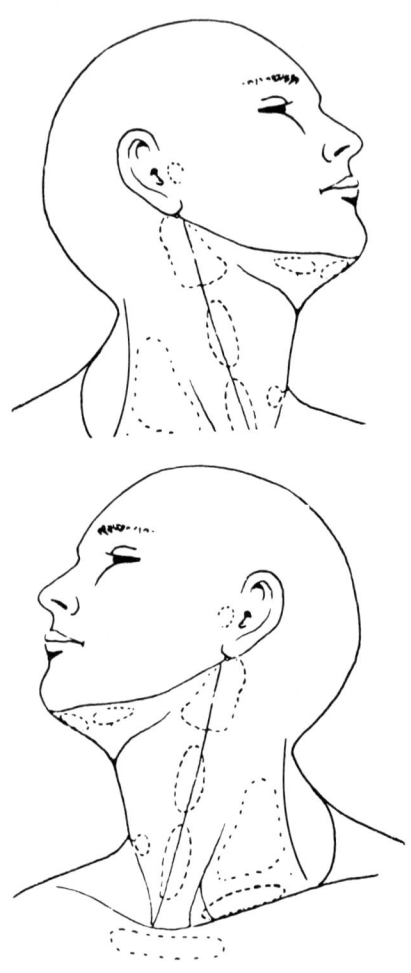

Indicate on diagram primary tumor and regional nodes involved.

Histopathologic Grade (G)

[ ] GX Grade cannot be assessed
[ ] G1 Well differentiated
[ ] G2 Moderately well differentiated
[ ] G3 Poorly differentiated
[ ] G4 Undifferentiated

Histopathologic Type

Predominant cancer is squamous cell carcinoma.

Sites of Distant Metastasis

Pulmonary	PUL
Osseous	OSS
Hepatic	HEP
Brain	BRA
Lymph nodes	LYM
Bone marrow	MAR
Pleura	PLE
Peritoneum	PER
Skin	SKI
Other	OTH

4

Pharynx (including base of tongue, soft palate, and uvula)

ANATOMY

Primary Sites and Subsites. The pharynx (including base of tongue, soft palate, and uvula) is divided into three regions: oropharynx; nasopharynx; and hypopharynx. Each region is further subdivided into specific sites that are summarized as follows:

Oropharynx (ICD-O 141.0; 145.3; 145.4; 146.1-146.3; 146.4; 146.6-146.7)

Anterior wall (glosso-epiglottic area)
   Tongue posterior to the vallate papillae
     (base of tongue or posterior third) (ICD-O 141.0)
   Vallecula (ICD-O 146.3)
Lateral wall (ICD-O 146.6)
   Tonsil (ICD-O 146.0)
   Tonsillar fossa (ICD-O 146.1) and faucial pillars (ICD-0 146.2)
   Glosso-tonsillar sulci (ICD-O 146.2)
Posterior wall (ICD-O 146.7)
Superior wall
   Inferior surface of soft palate (ICD-O 145.3)
   Uvula (ICD-O 145.4)

Nasopharynx (ICD-O 147)

Postero-superior wall, extends from the level of the junction of the hard and soft palates to the base of the skull (ICD-O 147.0, 1)
Lateral wall, including the fossa of Rosenmüller (ICD-O 147.2)
Inferior (anterior) wall, consists of the superior surface of the soft palate (ICD-O 147.3)

Note: The margin of the choanal orifices, including the posterior margin of the nasal septum, is included with the nasal fossa.

Hypopharynx (ICD-O 148)

Pharyngo-esophageal junction (postcricoid area) (ICD-O 148.0), extends from the level of the arytenoid cartilages and connecting folds to the inferior border of the cricoid cartilage

Pyriform sinus (ICD-O 148.1), extends from the pharyngo-epiglottic fold to the upper end of the esophagus, bounded laterally by the thyroid cartilage and medially by the surface of the aryepiglottic fold (ICD-O 148.2) and the arytenoid and cricoid cartilages

Posterior pharyngeal wall (ICD-O 148.3), extends from the level of the floor of the vallecula to the level of the crico-arytenoid joints

Regional Lymph Nodes. The main routes of drainage are into the first station cervical lymph nodes, which are the jugulodigastric, jugulo-omohyoid, upper deep cervical, lower deep cervical, and submaxillary and submental lymph nodes. Some primary sites drain bilaterally.

In clinical evaluation the actual size of the nodal mass should be measured, and allowance should be made for intervening soft tissues. It is recognized that most masses over 3 cm in diameter are not single nodes but are confluent nodes or tumor in soft tissues of the neck. There are three stages of clinically positive nodes: N1, N2, and N3. The use of subgroups a, b, and c is not required but is recommended. Midline nodes are considered homolateral nodes.

Metastatic Sites. Distant spread to the lungs is common; skeletal or hepatic metastases occur less often. Mediastinal lymph node metastases are considered distant metastases.

RULES FOR CLASSIFICATION

Clinical Staging. Clinical staging is generally employed for squamous cell carcinomas of the pharynx because many of these tumors are treated by nonsurgical methods. Assessment is based primarily on inspection by indirect mirror examination and by direct endoscopy. Palpation of sites (when feasible) and neck nodes is essential. Neurologic evaluation of all cranial nerves is required. A variety of imaging procedures, including tomograms, CT scans, and bone scans, are extremely useful in evaluating the extent of disease, particularly for locally advanced tumors. The tumor must be confirmed histologically, and any other data obtained by biopsies may be included.

Pathologic Staging. Pathologic staging requires the use of all information obtained in clinical staging in addition to histologic study of the surgically resected specimen. The surgeon's evaluation of gross unresected residual tumor must also be included.

DEFINITION OF TNM

Primary Tumor (T)

- TX Primary tumor cannot be assessed
- T0 No evidence of primary tumor
- Tis Carcinoma *in situ*

Oropharynx

- T1 Tumor 2 cm or less in greatest dimension
- T2 Tumor more than 2 cm but not more than 4 cm in greatest dimension
- T3 Tumor more than 4 cm in greatest dimension
- T4 Tumor invades adjacent structures (*e.g.,* through cortical bone, soft tissues of neck, deep (extrinsic) muscle of tongue)

Nasopharynx

- T1 Tumor limited to one subsite of nasopharynx (refer to text page 33)
- T2 Tumor invades more than one subsite of nasopharynx
- T3 Tumor invades nasal cavity and/or oropharynx
- T4 Tumor invades skull and/or cranial nerve(s)

Hypopharynx

- T1 Tumor limited to one subsite of hypopharynx (refer to text page 34)
- T2 Tumor invades more than one subsite of hypopharynx or an adjacent site, *without* fixation of hemilarynx
- T3 Tumor invades more than one subsite of hypopharynx or an adjacent site, *with* fixation of hemilarynx
- T4 Tumor invades adjacent structures (*e.g.,* cartilage or soft tissues of neck)

Regional Lymph Nodes (N)

- NX Regional lymph nodes cannot be assessed
- N0 No regional lymph node metastasis
- N1 Metastasis in a single ipsilateral lymph node, 3 cm or less in greatest dimension
- N2 Metastasis in a single ipsilateral lymph node, more than 3 cm but not more than 6 cm in greatest dimension, or in multiple ipsilateral lymph nodes, none more than 6 cm in greatest dimension, or in bilateral or contralateral lymph nodes, none more than 6 cm in greatest dimension

Pharynx (including base of tongue, soft palate, and uvula)

N2a Metastasis in a single ipsilateral lymph node more than 3 cm but not more than 6 cm in greatest dimension
N2b Metastasis in multiple ipsilateral lymph nodes, none more than 6 cm in greatest dimension
N2c Metastasis in bilateral or contralateral lymph nodes, none more than 6 cm in greatest dimension
N3 Metastasis in a lymph node more than 6 cm in greatest dimension

Distant Metastasis (M)

MX Presence of distant metastasis cannot be assessed
M0 No distant metastasis
M1 Distant metastasis

STAGE GROUPING

Stage	T	N	M
Stage 0	Tis	N0	M0
Stage I	T1	N0	M0
Stage II	T2	N0	M0
Stage III	T3	N0	M0
	T1	N1	M0
	T2	N1	M0
	T3	N1	M0
Stage IV	T4	N0, N1	M0
	Any T	N2, N3	M0
	Any T	Any N	M1

DIFFERENCES BETWEEN THE 2ND AND 3RD EDITIONS

The T definitions remain the same. The N definitions for N2 and N3 have been modified.

HISTOPATHOLOGIC TYPE

The predominant cancer is squamous cell carcinoma; pathologic diagnosis is required to use this classification. Other tumors of glandular epithelium, odontogenic apparatus origin, lymphoid tissue, soft tissue, and bone and cartilage origin require special consideration and are not to be included. Reference to the WHO nomenclature is recommended.

HISTOPATHOLOGIC GRADE (G)

GX Grade cannot be assessed
G1 Well differentiated
G2 Moderately well differentiated
G3 Poorly differentiated
G4 Undifferentiated

BIBLIOGRAPHY

1. Barkley HT Jr, Fletcher GT, Jesse RH et al: Management of cervical lymph node metastases in squamous carcinoma of the tonsillar fossa, base of tongue, supraglottic larynx and hypopharynx. Am J Surg 124: 462–467, 1972
2. Futrell JW, Bennett SH, Hoye RC et al: Predicting survival in cancer of the larynx or hypopharynx. Am J Surg 122:451–457, 1971
3. Garrett PG, Beale FA, Cummings BJ et al: Cancer of the tonsil: Results of radical radiation therapy with surgery in reserve. Am J Surg 146:432–435, 1983
4. Jesse RH, Sugarbaker EV: Squamous cell carcinoma of the oral pharynx: Why we fail. Am J Surg 132:435–439, 1976
5. Ring AH, Sako K, Razack MS et al: Nasopharyngeal carcinomas: Results of treatment over a 27 year period. Am J Surg 146:429–431, 1983
6. Silver AJ, Mawad ME, Hilal SK et al: Computed tomography of the nasopharynx and related spaces. Radiology 147:733–738, 1983

PHARYNX (INCLUDING BASE OF TONGUE, SOFT PALATE, AND UVULA)

Data Form for Cancer Staging

Patient identification
Name _____
Address _____
Hospital or clinic number _____
Age _____ Sex _____ Race _____

Institution identification
Hospital or clinic _____
Address _____

Oncology Record

Anatomic site of cancer _____
Histologic type _____
Grade (G) _____
Date of classification _____

Chronology of classification
 (use separate form for each time staged)
[ ] Clinical (use all data prior to first treatment)
[ ] Pathologic (if definitively resected specimen available)

Definitions

Primary Tumor (T)
[ ] TX Primary tumor cannot be assessed
[ ] T0 No evidence of primary tumor
[ ] Tis Carcinoma *in situ*

Oropharynx
[ ] T1 Tumor 2 cm or less in greatest dimension
[ ] T2 Tumor more than 2 cm but not more than 4 cm in greatest dimension
[ ] T3 Tumor more than 4 cm in greatest dimension
[ ] T4 Tumor invades adjacent structures, *e.g.*, through cortical bone, soft tissues of neck, deep (extrinsic) muscle of tongue

Nasopharynx
[ ] T1 Tumor limited to one subsite of nasopharynx
[ ] T2 Tumor invades more than one subsite of nasopharynx
[ ] T3 Tumor invades nasal cavity and/or oropharynx
[ ] T4 Tumor invades skull and/or cranial nerve(s)

Hypopharynx
[ ] T1 Tumor limited to one subsite of hypopharynx
[ ] T2 Tumor invades more than one subsite of hypopharynx or an adjacent site, without fixation of hemilarynx
[ ] T3 Tumor invades more than one subsite of hypopharynx or an adjacent site, with fixation of hemilarynx
[ ] T4 Tumor invades adjacent structures, *e.g.*, cartilage or soft tissues of neck

Lymph Node (N)
[ ] NX Regional lymph nodes cannot be assessed
[ ] N0 No regional lymph node metastasis
[ ] N1 Metastasis in a single ipsilateral lymph node, 3 cm or less in greatest dimension
[ ] N2 Metastasis in a single ipsilateral lymph node, more than 3 cm but not more than 6 cm in greatest dimension, or multiple ipsilateral lymph nodes, none more than 6 cm in greatest dimension, or bilateral or contralateral lymph nodes, none more than 6 cm in greatest dimension
  [ ] N2a Metastasis in a single ipsilateral lymph node more than 3 cm but not more than 6 cm in greatest dimension
  [ ] N2b Metastasis in multiple ipsilateral lymph nodes, none more than 6 cm in greatest dimension
  [ ] N2c Metastasis in bilateral or contralateral lymph nodes, none more than 6 cm in greatest dimension
[ ] N3 Metastasis in a lymph node more than 6 cm in greatest dimension

Distant Metastasis (M)
[ ] MX Presence of distant metastasis cannot be assessed
[ ] M0 No distant metastasis
[ ] M1 Distant metastasis

Stage Grouping

[ ] 0	Tis	N0	M0
[ ] I	T1	N0	M0
[ ] II	T2	N0	M0
[ ] III	T3	N0	M0
	T1	N1	M0
	T2	N1	M0
	T3	N1	M0
[ ] IV	T4	N0	M0
	T4	N1	M0
	Any T	N2	M0
	Any T	N3	M0
	Any T	Any N	M1

Histopathologic Grade (G)
[ ] GX Grade cannot be assessed
[ ] G1 Well differentiated
[ ] G2 Moderately well differentiated
[ ] G3 Poorly differentiated
[ ] G4 Undifferentiated

Location of Tumor

Oropharynx
[ ] Faucial arch
[ ] Tonsillar fossa, tonsil
[ ] Base of tongue
[ ] Pharyngeal wall

Nasopharynx
[ ] Posterosuperior wall
[ ] Lateral wall

Hypopharynx
[ ] Piriform fossa
[ ] Postcricoid area
[ ] Posterior wall

Staged by _____ M.D.
_____ Registrar
Date _____

American Joint Committee on Cancer—1988

Illustrations

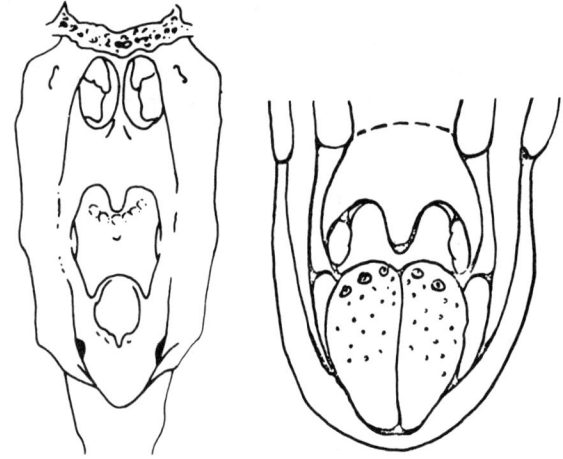

Size of primary tumor: _____ cm

Characteristics of Tumor

[ ] Superficial
[ ] Exophytic
[ ] Moderate infiltration
[ ] Deep infiltration

Histopathologic Type

Predominant cancer is squamous cell carcinoma.

Postsurgical Resection—Pathologic Residual Tumor (R)

Does not enter into staging but may be a factor in deciding further treatment

[ ] R0 No residual tumor
[ ] R1 Microscopic residual tumor
[ ] R2 Macroscopic residual tumor
     Specify _____

Sites of Distant Metastasis

Pulmonary	PUL
Osseous	OSS
Hepatic	HEP
Brain	BRA
Lymph nodes	LYM
Bone marrow	MAR
Pleura	PLE
Peritoneum	PER
Skin	SKI
Other	OTH

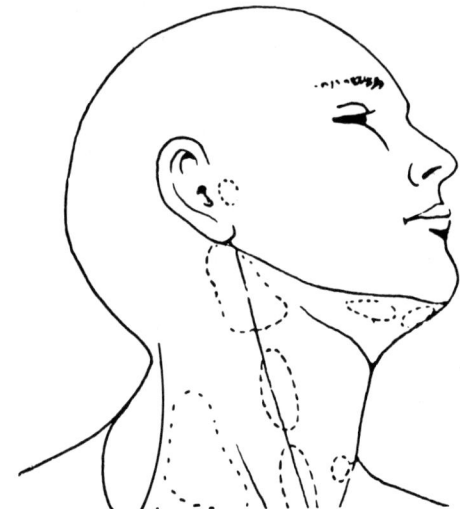
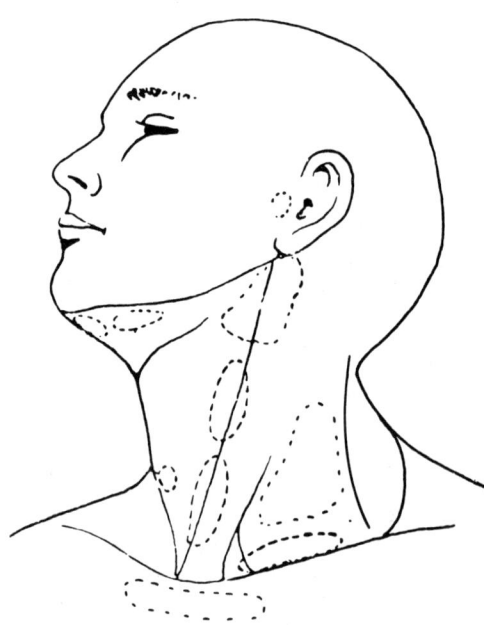

Regional lymph nodes; illustrate if metastatic.

5

Larynx

ANATOMY

Primary Site. The following anatomic definition of larynx allows classification of carcinomas arising in the encompassed mucous membranes but excludes cancers arising on the lateral or posterior pharyngeal wall, pyriform fossa, postcricoid area, and the base of tongue.

The anterior limit of the larynx is composed of the anterior or lingual surface of the suprahyoid epiglottis, the thyrohyoid membrane, the anterior commissure, and the anterior wall of the subglottic region, which is composed of the thyroid cartilage, the cricothyroid membrane, and the anterior arch of the cricoid cartilage.

The posterior and lateral limits include the arytenoepiglottic folds, the arytenoid region, the interarytenoid space, and the posterior surface of the subglottic space, represented by the mucous membrane covering the cricoid cartilage.

The superolateral limits are composed of the tip and the lateral borders of the epiglottis.

The inferior limits are made up of the plane passing through the inferior edge of the cricoid cartilage.

For purposes of this clinical-stage classification, the larynx is divided into three regions: supraglottis, glottis, and subglottis. The *supraglottis* is composed of the epiglottis (both its lingual and laryngeal aspects), arytenoepiglottic folds, arytenoids, and ventricular bands (false cords). The inferior boundary of the supraglottis is a horizontal plane passing through the apex of the ventricle. The *glottis* is composed of the true vocal cords, including the anterior and posterior commissures. The lower boundary is the horizontal plane, 1 cm below the apex of the ventricle. The *subglottis* is the region extending from the lower boundary of the glottis to the lower margin of the cricoid cartilage.

The division of the larynx is summarized in the following table:

Site	Subsite
Supraglottis (ICD-O 161.1)	Ventricular bands (false cords)
	Arytenoids
	Epiglottis (both lingual and laryngeal aspects)
	Suprahyoid epiglottis
	Infrahyoid epiglottis
	Arytenoepiglottic folds
Glottis (ICD-O 161.0)	True vocal cords including anterior and posterior commissures
Subglottis (ICD-O 161.2)	Subglottis

Regional Lymph Nodes. The main routes of drainage are into the first station cervical lymph nodes, which are the jugulodigastric, jugulo-omohyoid, upper deep cervical, lower deep cervical, and submaxillary and submental lymph nodes. Some primary sites drain bilaterally.

In clinical evaluation the actual size of the nodal mass should be measured, and allowance should be made for intervening soft tissues. It is recognized that most masses over 3 cm in diameter are not single nodes but are confluent nodes or tumor in soft tissues of the neck. There are three stages of clinically positive nodes: N1, N2, and N3. The use of subgroups a, b, and c is not required but is recommended. Midline nodes are considered homolateral nodes.

Metastatic Sites. Distant spread to the lungs is common; skeletal or hepatic metastases occur less often. Mediastinal lymph node metastases are considered distant metastases.

RULES FOR CLASSIFICATION

Clinical Staging. The assessment of the larynx is accomplished primarily by inspection, using both indirect mirror examination and direct laryngoscopy. A variety of imaging procedures are valuable in evaluating the extent of disease, particularly for advanced tumors. These include laryngeal tomograms, CT scans, and MRI scans. Diagnostic ultrasound may help detect destruction of laryngeal cartilages. Palpation of neck nodes to evaluate laryngeal fremitus is essential. The tumor must be confirmed histologically, and any other data obtained by biopsies may be included.

Pathologic Staging. All information used in clinical staging and in histologic studies of the surgically resected specimen is used for pathologic staging. The surgeon's evaluation of gross unresected residual tumor must also be included.

DEFINITION OF TNM

Primary Tumor (T)

TX Primary tumor cannot be assessed
T0 No evidence of primary tumor
Tis Carcinoma *in situ*

Supraglottis

T1 Tumor limited to one subsite of supraglottis with normal vocal cord mobility (refer to text page 40)
T2 Tumor invades more than one subsite of supraglottis or glottis, with normal vocal cord mobility
T3 Tumor limited to larynx with vocal cord fixation and/or invades postcricoid area, medial wall of pyriform sinus, or pre-epiglottic tissues
T4 Tumor invades through thyroid cartilage, and/or extends to other tissues beyond the larynx (*e.g.*, to oropharynx, soft tissues of neck)

Glottis

T1 Tumor limited to vocal cord(s) (may involve anterior or posterior commissures) with normal mobility
  T1a Tumor limited to one vocal cord
  T1b Tumor involves both vocal cords
T2 Tumor extends to supraglottis and/or subglottis, and/or with impaired vocal cord mobility
T3 Tumor limited to the larynx with vocal cord fixation
T4 Tumor invades through thyroid cartilage and/or extends to other tissues beyond the larynx (*e.g.*, oropharynx, soft tissues of neck)

Subglottis

T1 Tumor limited to the subglottis
T2 Tumor extends to vocal cord(s) with normal or impaired mobility
T3 Tumor limited to larynx with vocal cord fixation
T4 Tumor invades through cricoid or thyroid cartilage and/or extends to other tissues beyond the larynx (*e.g.*, oropharynx, soft tissues of neck)

Regional Lymph Nodes (N)

NX Regional lymph nodes cannot be assessed
N0 No regional lymph node metastasis
N1 Metastasis in a single ipsilateral lymph node, 3 cm or less in greatest dimension
N2 Metastasis in a single ipsilateral lymph node, more than 3 cm but not more than 6 cm in

greatest dimension, or in multiple ipsilateral lymph nodes, none more than 6 cm in greatest dimension, or in bilateral or contralateral lymph nodes, none more than 6 cm in greatest dimension

- N2a Metastasis in a single ipsilateral lymph node more than 3 cm but not more than 6 cm in greatest dimension
- N2b Metastasis in multiple ipsilateral lymph nodes, none more than 6 cm in greatest dimension
- N2c Metastasis in bilateral or contralateral lymph nodes, none more than 6 cm in greatest dimension

N3 Metastasis in a lymph node more than 6 cm in greatest dimension

Distant Metastasis (M)

MX Presence of distant metastasis cannot be assessed
M0 No distant metastasis
M1 Distant metastasis

STAGE GROUPING

Stage 0	Tis	N0	M0
Stage I	T1	N0	M0
Stage II	T2	N0	M0
Stage III	T3	N0	M0
	T1	N1	M0
	T2	N1	M0
	T3	N1	M0
Stage IV	T4	N0, N1	M0
	Any T	N2, N3	M0
	Any T	Any N	M1

DIFFERENCES BETWEEN THE 2ND AND 3RD EDITIONS

The T definitions remain essentially the same. The definitions of N2 and N3 have been modified.

HISTOPATHOLOGIC TYPE

The predominant cancer is squamous cell carcinoma; pathologic diagnosis is required to use this classification. Tumor grading is recommended using Broders' classification. Other tumors of glandular epithelium, odontogenic apparatus origin, lymphoid tissue, soft tissue, and bone and cartilage origin require special consideration and are not to be included. Reference to the WHO nomenclature is recommended.

HISTOPATHOLOGIC GRADE (G)

GX Grade cannot be assessed
G1 Well differentiated
G2 Moderately well differentiated
G3 Poorly differentiated
G4 Undifferentiated

BIBLIOGRAPHY

1. Flynn MB, Jesse RH, Lindberg RT: Surgery and irradiation in the treatment of squamous cell cancer of the supraglottic larynx. Am J Surg 124:477–481, 1972
2. Futrell JW, Bennett SH, Hoye RC et al: Predicting survival in cancer of the larynx or hypopharynx. Am J Surg 122:451–457, 1971
3. Harris HS, Watson FR, Spratt JS Jr: Carcinoma of the larynx. Am J Surg 118:676–684, 1969
4. Powell RW, Redd BL, Wilkins SA: An evaluation of treatment of cancer of the larynx. Am J Surg 10:635–643, 1965
5. Shah JP, Tollefson HR: Epidermoid carcinoma of the supraglottic larynx: Role of neck dissection in initial surgical treatment. Am J Surg 128:494–499, 1974
6. Shaha AR and Shah JP: Carcinoma of the supraglottic larynx. Am J Surg 144:456–458, 1982
7. Wang CC, Schultz MD, Miller D: Combined radiation therapy and surgery for carcinoma of the supraglottis and pyriform sinus. Am J Surg 124:551–554, 1972

LARYNX

Data Form for Cancer Staging

Patient identification
Name _____
Address _____
Hospital or clinic number _____
Age _____ Sex _____ Race _____

Institution identification
Hospital or clinic _____
Address _____

Oncology Record

Anatomic site of cancer _____
Histologic type _____
Grade (G) _____
Date of classification _____

Chronology of classification
(use separate form for each time staged)
[ ] Clinical (use all data prior to first treatment)
[ ] Pathologic (if definitively resected specimen available)

Definitions

Primary Tumor (T)
[ ] TX Primary tumor cannot be assessed
[ ] T0 No evidence of primary tumor
[ ] Tis Carcinoma *in situ*

Supraglottis
[ ] T1 Tumor limited to one subsite of supraglottis with normal vocal cord mobility
[ ] T2 Tumor invades more than one subsite of supraglottis or glottis, with normal vocal cord mobility
[ ] T3 Tumor limited to larynx with vocal cord fixation and/or invades postcricoid area, medial wall of piriform sinus, or pre-epiglottic tissues
[ ] T4 Tumor invades through thyroid cartilage, and/or extends to other tissues beyond the larynx, *e.g.*, to oropharynx, soft tissues of neck.

Glottis
[ ] T1 Tumor limited to vocal cord(s) (may involve anterior or posterior commissures) with normal mobility
  [ ] T1a Tumor limited to one vocal cord
  [ ] T1b Tumor involves both vocal cords
[ ] T2 Tumor extends to supraglottis and/or subglottis, and/or with impaired vocal cord mobility
[ ] T3 Tumor limited to the larynx with vocal cord fixation
[ ] T4 Tumor invades through thyroid cartilage and/or extends to other tissues beyond the larynx, *e.g.*, oropharynx, soft tissues of neck

Subglottis
[ ] T1 Tumor limited to the subglottis
[ ] T2 Tumor extends to vocal cord(s) with normal or impaired mobility
[ ] T3 Tumor limited to larynx with vocal cord fixation
[ ] T4 Tumor invades through cricoid or thyroid cartilage and/or extends to other tissues beyond the larynx, *e.g.*, oropharynx, soft tissues of neck

Lymph Node (N)
[ ] NX Regional lymph nodes cannot be assessed
[ ] N0 No regional lymph node metastasis
[ ] N1 Metastasis in a single ipsilateral lymph node, 3 cm or less in greatest dimension
[ ] N2 Metastasis in a single ipsilateral lymph node, more than 3 cm but not more than 6 cm in greatest dimension, or multiple ipsilateral lymph nodes, none more than 6 cm in greatest dimension or bilateral or contralateral lymph nodes, none more than 6 cm in greatest dimension
  [ ] N2a Metastasis in a single ipsilateral lymph node more than 3 cm but not more than 6 cm in greatest dimension
  [ ] N2b Metastasis in multiple ipsilateral lymph nodes, none more than 6 cm in greatest dimension
  [ ] N2c Metastasis in bilateral or contralateral lymph nodes, none more than 6 cm in greatest dimension
[ ] N3 Metastasis in a lymph node more than 6 cm in greatest dimension

Distant Metastasis (M)
[ ] MX Presence of distant metastasis cannot be assessed
[ ] M0 No distant metastasis
[ ] M1 Distant metastasis

Stage Grouping

[ ] 0	Tis	N0	M0
[ ] I.	T1	N0	M0
[ ] II	T2	N0	M0
[ ] III	T3	N0	M0
	T1	N1	M0
	T2	N1	M0
	T3	N1	M0
[ ] IV	T4	N0	M0
	T4	N1	M0
	Any T	N2	M0
	Any T	N3	M0
	Any T	Any N	M1

Sites of Distant Metastasis

Pulmonary	PUL
Osseous	OSS
Hepatic	HEP
Brain	BRA
Lymph nodes	LYM
Bone marrow	MAR
Pleura	PLE
Peritoneum	PER
Skin	SKI
Other	OTH

Histopathologic Type

The predominant cancer is squamous cell carcinoma.

Histopathologic Grade (G)

[ ] GX Grade cannot be assessed
[ ] G1 Well differentiated
[ ] G2 Moderately well differentiated
[ ] G3 Poorly differentiated
[ ] G4 Undifferentiated

Staged by _____ M.D.
_____ Registrar
Date _____

Illustrations

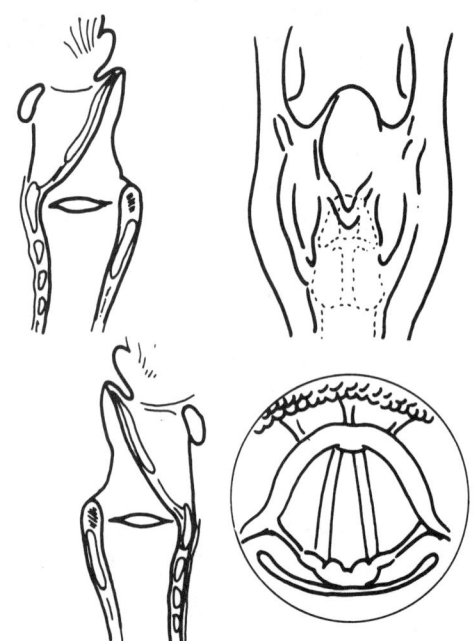

Indicate size and location of primary tumor.

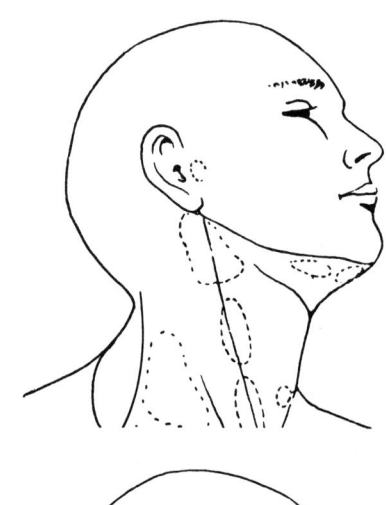

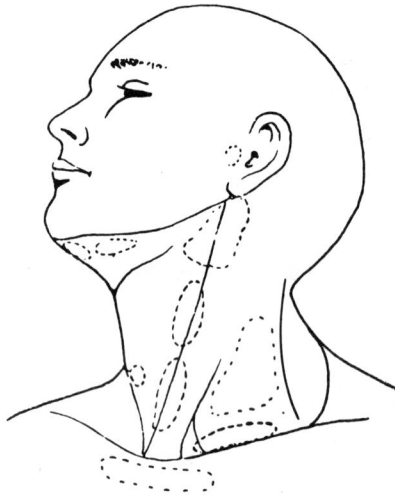

Indicate on diagram primary tumor and regional nodes involved.

Maxillary Sinus

ANATOMY

Primary Site. Cancer of the maxillary sinus (ICD-O 160.2) is the most common of the paranasal sinus cancers; it is the only site to which the following classification applies. The ethmoid sinuses and nasal cavity may ultimately be defined similarly with further study. Tumors of the sphenoid and frontal sinuses are so rare as not to warrant staging.

Ohngren's line, a theoretic plane joining the medial canthus of the eye with the angle of the mandible, may be used to divide the maxillary antrum into the anteroinferior portion (the infrastructure) and the superoposterior portion (the suprastructure).

Regional Lymph Nodes. The main routes of drainage are into the first station cervical lymph nodes, which are the jugulodigastric, jugulo-omohyoid, upper deep cervical, lower deep cervical, and submaxillary and submental lymph nodes. Some primary sites drain bilaterally.

In clinical evaluation the actual size of the nodal mass should be measured, and allowance should be made for intervening soft tissues. It is recognized that most masses over 3 cm in diameter are not single nodes but are confluent nodes or tumor in soft tissues of the neck. There are three stages of clinically positive nodes: N1, N2, and N3. The use of subgroups a, b, and c is not required but is recommended. Midline nodes are considered homolateral nodes.

Metastatic Sites. Distant spread to lungs is most common; occasionally there is spread to bone and remote lymph nodes.

RULES FOR CLASSIFICATION

Clinical Staging. The assessment of primary maxillary antrum tumors is based on inspection, palpation, including examination of the orbit, nasal and oral cavities, and nasopharynx, and neurologic evaluation of the cranial nerves. Radiographic studies include plain films and tomograms for evaluation of bone destruction. Neck nodes are assessed by palpation. Examinations for distant metastases include chest film, blood chemistries, blood count, and other routine studies as indicated.

Pathologic Staging. Complete resection of primary sites and major nodal dissections allow the use of this designation. Specimens that are resected after radiation or chemotherapy need to be noted especially.

DEFINITION OF TNM

Primary Tumor (T)

TX Primary tumor cannot be assessed
T0 No evidence of primary tumor
Tis Carcinoma *in situ*
T1 Tumor limited to the antral mucosa with no erosion or destruction of bone
T2 Tumor with erosion or destruction of the infrastructure (see anatomic division, above), including the hard palate and/or the middle nasal meatus
T3 Tumor invades any of the following: skin of cheek, posterior wall of maxillary sinus, floor or medial wall of orbit, anterior ethmoid sinus
T4 Tumor invades orbital contents and/or any of the following: cribriform plate, posterior ethmoid or sphenoid sinuses, nasopharynx, soft palate, pterygomaxillary or temporal fossae or base of skull

Regional Lymph Nodes (N)

NX Regional lymph nodes cannot be assessed
N0 No regional lymph node metastasis
N1 Metastasis in a single ipsilateral lymph node, 3 cm or less in greatest dimension
N2 Metastasis in a single ipsilateral lymph node, more than 3 cm but not more than 6 cm in greatest dimension, or in multiple ipsilateral lymph nodes, none more than 6 cm in greatest dimension, or in bilateral or contralateral lymph nodes, none more than 6 cm in greatest dimension
  N2a Metastasis in a single ipsilateral lymph node more than 3 cm but not more than 6 cm in greatest dimension
  N2b Metastasis in multiple ipsilateral lymph nodes, none more than 6 cm in greatest dimension
  N2c Metastasis in bilateral or contralateral lymph nodes, none more than 6 cm in greatest dimension
N3 Metastasis in a lymph node more than 6 cm in greatest dimension

Distant Metastasis (M)

MX Presence of distant metastases cannot be assessed
M0 No distant metastasis
M1 Distant metastasis

STAGE GROUPING

Stage 0	Tis	N0	M0
Stage I	T1	N0	M0
Stage II	T2	N0	M0
Stage III	T3	N0	M0
	T1	N1	M0
	T2	N1	M0
	T3	N1	M0
Stage IV	T4	N0, N1	M0
	Any T	N2, N3	M0
	Any T	Any N	M1

DIFFERENCES BETWEEN THE 2ND AND 3RD EDITIONS

In the 1988 edition the definitions of the primary tumor (T) have been more clearly defined in four categories. The lymph node (N) categories have been brought into conformity with the N definitions as at other head and neck sites.

HISTOPATHOLOGIC TYPE

The predominant cancer is squamous cell carcinoma; pathologic diagnosis is required to use this classification. Tumor grading is recommended using Broders' classification. Other tumors of glandular epithelium, odontogenic apparatus, lymphoid tissue, soft tissue, and bone and cartilage origin require special consideration and are not to be included. Reference to the WHO nomenclature is recommended.

HISTOPATHOLOGIC GRADE (G)

GX Grade cannot be assessed
G1 Well differentiated
G2 Moderately well differentiated
G3 Poorly differentiated
G4 Undifferentiated

BIBLIOGRAPHY

1. Goepfert H, Jesse RH, Lindberg RD: Arterial infusion and radiation therapy in the treatment of advanced cancer of the nasal cavity and perinasal sinuses. Am J Surg 126:464–468, 1973
2. Jesse RH: Preoperative versus postoperative radiation in the treatment of squamous carcinoma of the perinasal sinuses. Am J Surg 110:552–556, 1965
3. Sisson GA, Johnson NE, Ammiri CS: Cancer of the maxillary sinus: Clinical classification and management. Ann Otol Rhinol Laryngol 72:1050–1059, 1963

MAXILLARY SINUS

Data Form for Cancer Staging

Patient identification
Name _____
Address _____
Hospital or clinic number _____
Age _____ Sex _____ Race _____

Institution identification
Hospital or clinic _____
Address _____

Oncology Record

Anatomic site of cancer _____
Histologic type _____
Grade (G) _____
Date of classification _____

Chronology of classification
 (use separate form for each time staged)
[ ] Clinical (use all data prior to first treatment)
[ ] Pathologic (if definitively resected specimen available)

Definitions

Primary Tumor (T)

[ ] TX Primary tumor cannot be assessed
[ ] T0 No evidence of primary tumor
[ ] Tis Carcinoma *in situ*
[ ] T1 Tumor limited to the antral mucosa with no erosion or destruction of bone
[ ] T2 Tumor with erosion or destruction of the infrastructure including the hard palate and/or the middle nasal meatus
[ ] T3 Tumor invades any of the following: skin of cheek, posterior wall of the maxillary sinus, floor or medial wall of orbit, anterior ethmoid sinus
[ ] T4 Tumor invades orbital contents and/or any of the following: cribriform plate, posterior ethmoid or sphenoid sinuses, nasopharynx, soft palate, pterygomaxillary or temporal fossae or base of skull

Lymph Node (N)

[ ] NX Regional lymph nodes cannot be assessed
[ ] N0 No regional lymph node metastasis
[ ] N1 Metastasis in a single ipsilateral lymph node, 3 cm or less in greatest dimension
[ ] N2 Metastasis in a single ipsilateral lymph node, more than 3 cm but not more than 6 cm in greatest dimension, or multiple ipsilateral lymph nodes, none more than 6 cm in greatest dimension, or bilateral or contralateral lymph nodes, none more than 6 cm in greatest dimension
  [ ] N2a Metastasis in a single ipsilateral lymph node more than 3 cm but not more than 6 cm in greatest dimension
  [ ] N2b Metastasis in multiple ipsilateral lymph nodes, none more than 6 cm in greatest dimension
  [ ] N2c Metastasis in bilateral or contralateral lymph nodes, none more than 6 cm in greatest dimension
[ ] N3 Metastasis in a lymph node more than 6 cm in greatest dimension

Distant Metastasis (M)

[ ] MX Presence of distant metastasis cannot be assessed
[ ] M0 No distant metastasis
[ ] M1 Distant metastasis

Stage Grouping

[ ]	0	Tis	N0	M0
[ ]	I	T1	N0	M0
[ ]	II	T2	N0	M0
[ ]	III	T3	N0	M0
		T1	N1	M0
		T2	N1	M0
		T3	N1	M0
[ ]	IV	T4	N0	M0
		T4	N1	M0
		Any T	N2	M0
		Any T	N3	M0
		Any T	Any N	M1

Illustrations

Indicate on diagram primary tumor and regional nodes involved.

Staged by _____ M.D.
_____ Registrar
Date _____

Location of Tumor

[ ] Antrum
    [ ] Infrastructure
    [ ] Suprastructure
    [ ] Both
[ ] Nasal Cavity
    [ ] Septum
    [ ] Root
    [ ] Lateral wall
    [ ] Floor
[ ] Ethmoid
    [ ] Anterior
    [ ] Posterior
[ ] Sphenoid
[ ] Frontal

Histopathologic Type

Predominant cancer is squamous cell or undifferentiated carcinoma. Adenocarcinoma and other cellular types also occur.

Histopathologic Grade (G)

[ ] GX Grade cannot be assessed
[ ] G1 Well differentiated
[ ] G2 Moderately well differentiated
[ ] G3 Poorly differentiated
[ ] G4 Undifferentiated

Sites of Distant Metastasis

Pulmonary PUL
Osseous OSS
Hepatic HEP
Brain BRA
Lymph nodes LYM
Bone marrow MAR
Pleura PLE
Peritoneum PER
Skin SKI
Other OTH

7 Salivary Glands (including parotid, submaxillary, and sublingual)

This staging system is based on an extensive retrospective study of malignant tumors of the major salivary glands collected from eleven participating United States and Canadian institutions. Statistical analysis of the data revealed that numerous factors affected patient survival, including the histologic diagnosis, cellular differentiation of the tumor, its site, size, degree of fixation, or local extension, and nerve involvement. The status of regional lymph nodes and of distant metastases were also of major significance. The classification here proposed involves only four clinical variables: tumor size, local extension of the tumor, the palpability and suspicion of nodes, and the presence or absence of distant metastasis. It offers a simple but effective and accurate method of evaluating the stage of salivary gland cancer.

ANATOMY

Primary Site. The major salivary glands include the parotid (ICD-O 142.0), submaxillary (ICD-O 142.1), and sublingual (ICD-O 142.2) glands. Tumors arising in minor salivary glands (mucus-secreting glands in the lining membrane of the upper aerodigestive tract) are not included in this staging system.

Regional Lymph Nodes. The first station nodes are immediately adjacent to the salivary glands and include parotid, submaxillary, and submental lymph nodes. The first station also includes the deep cervical lymph nodes. Specifically the regional nodes are:

Parotid gland only—intraparotid, infra-auricular, preauricular
Submandibular gland only—submandibular (submaxillary), upper cervical (including cervical, NOS), submental-internal (upper deep) jugular: subdigastric.

Other lymph node metastases are distant metastases.

Metastatic Sites. Distant spread is most frequently to the lungs.

RULES FOR CLASSIFICATION

Clinical Staging. The assessment of primary tumor includes inspection and palpation and neurologic evaluation of the seventh cranial or other nerves. Radiologic studies may include films of the mandible and possibly sialograms.

Pathologic Staging. The surgical pathology report and all other available data should be used to assign a pathologic classification to those patients who have a resection of the cancer.

DEFINITION OF TNM

Primary Tumor (T)

- TX Primary tumor cannot be assessed
- T0 No evidence of primary tumor
- T1 Tumor 2 cm or less in greatest dimension
- T2 Tumor more than 2 cm but not more than 4 cm in greatest dimension
- T3 Tumor more than 4 cm but not more than 6 cm in greatest dimension
- T4 Tumor more than 6 cm in greatest dimension

Note: All categories are subdivided: (a) no local extension; (b) local extension. Local extension is clinical or macroscopic evidence of invasion of skin, soft tissues, bone, or nerve. Microscopic evidence alone is not local extension for classification purposes.

Regional Lymph Nodes (N)

- NX Regional lymph nodes cannot be assessed
- N0 No regional lymph node metastasis
- N1 Metastasis in a single ipsilateral lymph node, 3 cm or less in greatest dimension
- N2 Metastasis in a single ipsilateral lymph node, more than 3 cm but not more than 6 cm in greatest dimension, or in multiple ipsilateral lymph nodes, none more than 6 cm in greatest dimension, or in bilateral or contralateral lymph nodes, none more than 6 cm in greatest dimension
  - N2a Metastasis in a single ipsilateral lymph node more than 3 cm but not more than 6 cm in greatest dimension
  - N2b Metastasis in multiple ipsilateral lymph nodes, none more than 6 cm in greatest dimension
  - N2c Metastasis in bilateral or contralateral lymph nodes, none more than 6 cm in greatest dimension
- N3 Metastasis in a lymph node more than 6 cm in greatest dimension

Distant Metastasis (M)

- MX Presence of distant metastasis cannot be assessed
- M0 No distant metastases
- M1 Distant metastasis

STAGE GROUPING

Stage	T	N	M
Stage I	T1a	N0	M0
	T2a	N0	M0
Stage II	T1b	N0	M0
	T2b	N0	M0
	T3a	N0	M0
Stage III	T3b	N0	M0
	T4a	N0	M0
	Any T (except T4b)	N1	M0
Stage IV	T4b	Any N	M0
	Any T	N2, N3	M0
	Any T	Any N	M1

DIFFERENCES BETWEEN THE 2ND AND 3RD EDITIONS

The UICC and the AJCC agreed to some significant changes in the staging of salivary gland neoplasms. In the former staging scheme, "significant local extension" of any salivary gland cancer automatically placed it in a T4b category. Review of survival data has revealed that local extension is far less ominous in smaller tumors than in larger ones. In this revised staging system, the presence or absence of local extension is indicated as a suffix to each T category representing the size of the primary tumor. Arrangement of tumors in this revised system correlates far more closely with observed 5-year survivals.

HISTOPATHOLOGIC TYPE

The histologic classification recommended is a modification of the WHO classification of salivary gland tumors. The major malignant varieties include the following:

Acinic cell carcinoma
Adenoid cystic carcinoma (cylindroma)
Adenocarcinoma
Squamous cell carcinoma
Carcinoma in pleomorphic adenoma (malignant mixed tumor)

Salivary Glands (including parotid, submaxillary, and sublingual)

Mucoepidermoid carcinoma
   Well differentiated (low grade)
   Poorly differentiated (high grade)
Other

HISTOPATHOLOGIC GRADE (G)

GX Grade cannot be assessed
G1 Well differentiated
G2 Moderately well differentiated
G3 Poorly differentiated
G4 Undifferentiated

SALIVARY GLANDS (INCLUDING PAROTID, SUBMAXILLARY, AND SUBLINGUAL)

Data Form for Cancer Staging

Patient identification
Name _____
Address _____
Hospital or clinic number _____
Age _____ Sex _____ Race _____

Institution identification
Hospital or clinic _____
Address _____

Oncology Record

Anatomic site of cancer _____
Histologic type _____
Grade (G) _____
Date of classification _____

Chronology of classification
  (use separate form for each time staged)
[ ] Clinical (use all data prior to first treatment)
[ ] Pathologic (if definitively resected specimen available)

Definitions

Primary Tumor (T)

[ ] TX Primary tumor cannot be assessed
[ ] T0 No evidence of primary tumor
[ ] T1 Tumor 2 cm or less in greatest dimension
[ ] T2 Tumor more than 2 cm but not more than 4 cm in greatest dimension
[ ] T3 Tumor more than 4 cm but not more than 6 cm in greatest dimension
[ ] T4 Tumor more than 6 cm in greatest dimension

Note: All categories are subdivided: (a) no local extension; (b) local extension. Local extension is clinical or macroscopic evidence of invasion of skin, soft tissues, bone, or nerve. Microscopic evidence alone is not local extension for classification purposes.

Stage Grouping

[ ]	I	T1a	N0	M0
		T2a	N0	M0
[ ]	II	T1b	N0	M0
		T2b	N0	M0
		T3a	N0	M0
[ ]	III	T3b	N0	M0
		T4a	N0	M0
		Any T	N1	M0
		(except T4b)		
[ ]	IV	T4b	Any N	M0
		Any T	N2	M0
		Any T	N3	M0
		Any T	Any N	M1

Lymph Node (N)

[ ] NX Regional lymph nodes cannot be assessed
[ ] N0 No regional lymph node metastasis
[ ] N1 Metastasis in a single ipsilateral lymph node, 3 cm or less in greatest dimension
[ ] N2 Metastasis in a single ipsilateral lymph node, more than 3 cm but not more than 6 cm in greatest dimension, or in multiple ipsilateral lymph nodes, none more than 6 cm in greatest dimension, or in bilateral or in contralateral lymph nodes, none more than 6 cm in greatest dimension
  [ ] N2a Metastasis in a single ipsilateral lymph node more than 3 cm but not more than 6 cm in greatest dimension
  [ ] N2b Metastasis in multiple ipsilateral lymph nodes, none more than 6 cm in greatest dimension
  [ ] N2c Metastasis in bilateral or contralateral lymph nodes, none more than 6 cm in greatest dimension
[ ] N3 Metastasis in a lymph node more than 6 cm in greatest dimension

Distant Metastasis (M)

[ ] MX Presence of distant metastasis cannot be assessed
[ ] M0 No distant metastasis
[ ] M1 Distant metastasis

Illustration

Parotid gland
Sublingual gland
Submaxillary gland

Indicate on diagram primary tumor and regional nodes involved.

Staged by _____ M.D.
_____ Registrar
Date _____

Histopathologic Grade (G)

[ ] GX   Grade cannot be assessed
[ ] G1   Well differentiated
[ ] G2   Moderately well differentiated
[ ] G3   Poorly differentiated
[ ] G4   Undifferentiated

Histopathologic Type

The histologic classification recommended is a modification of the WHO classification of salivary gland tumors. The major malignant varieties include the following:

Acinic cell carcinoma
Adenoid cystic carcinoma (cylindroma)
Adenocarcinoma
Squamous cell carcinoma
Carcinoma in pleomorphic adenoma (malignant mixed tumor)
Mucoepidermoid carcinoma
   Well differentiated (low grade)
   Poorly differentiated (high grade)
Other

8 Thyroid Gland

The following staging system for cancer of the thyroid gland was developed after an analysis of more than 1000 case protocols. Although staging for cancers in other head and neck sites is based entirely on the anatomic extent of disease, it is not possible to follow this pattern for the unique group of malignant tumors that arise in the thyroid. Both the histologic diagnosis and the age of the patient are of such importance in the behavior and prognosis of thyroid cancer that these factors have to be accounted for in any staging system.

ANATOMY

Primary Site. The thyroid gland (ICD-O 193) ordinarily is composed of a right and a left lobe lying adjacent and lateral to the upper trachea and esophagus. An isthmus connects the two lobes and in some cases a pyramidal lobe is present extending upward anterior to the thyroid cartilage.

Regional Lymph Nodes. Lymphatic drainage from the thyroid gland is in several directions: to the tracheoesophageal nodes bilaterally, to upper anterior mediastinal nodes, to the delphian node overlying the thyroid cartilage. Regional nodes include anterior deep cervical: pretracheal, laterotracheal (recurrent laryngeal nerve chain), internal (upper deep jugular, subdigastric and suprahyoid), retropharyngeal, anterior mediastinal and upper cervical (including cervical not otherwise specified).

Metastatic Sites. Distant spread occurs by contiguous lymphatic or hematogenous routes, for example, to lungs and bones, but many other sites may be involved. Metastases to submandibular and submental nodes are considered distant spread.

RULES FOR CLASSIFICATION

Clinical Staging. The assessment of a thyroid tumor depends on inspection and palpation of the thyroid gland and regional lymph nodes in the neck. Indirect laryngoscopy to evaluate vocal cord motion is important. A variety of imaging procedures can provide additional useful information. These include radioisotope thyroid scans, CT scans, MRI scans, and ultrasound examinations. The diagnosis of thyroid cancer must be confirmed by needle biopsy or open biopsy of the tumor. Further information for clinical staging may be obtained by biopsy of lymph nodes or other areas of suspected local or distant spread. All information available prior to first treatment should be used.

Pathologic Staging. All available clinical data are combined with pathologic study of the surgically resected specimen for pathologic staging. The surgeon's evaluation of gross unresected residual tumor must be included.

DEFINITION OF TNM
Primary Tumor (T)

Note: All categories may be subdivided: (a) solitary tumor, (b) multifocal tumor (the largest determines the classification).

- TX Primary tumor cannot be assessed
- T0 No evidence of primary tumor
- T1 Tumor 1 cm or less in greatest dimension limited to the thyroid
- T2 Tumor more than 1 cm but not more than 4 cm in greatest dimension limited to the thyroid
- T3 Tumor more than 4 cm in greatest dimension limited to the thyroid
- T4 Tumor of any size extending beyond the thyroid capsule

Regional Lymph Nodes (N)

Regional lymph nodes are the cervical and upper mediastinal lymph nodes.

- NX Regional lymph nodes cannot be assessed
- N0 No regional lymph node metastasis
- N1 Regional lymph node metastasis
  - N1a Metastasis in ipsilateral cervical lymph node(s)
  - N1b Metastasis in bilateral, midline, or contralateral cervical or mediastinal lymph node(s)

Distant Metastasis (M)

- MX Presence of distant metastasis cannot be assessed
- M0 No distant metastasis
- M1 Distant metastasis

STAGE GROUPING

Separate stage groupings are recommended for papillary and follicular, medullary, and undifferentiated.

Papillary or Follicular

	UNDER 45 YEARS	45 YEARS AND OLDER
Stage I	Any T, Any N, M0	T1, N0, M0
Stage II	Any T, Any N, M1	T2, N0, M0
		T3, N0, M0
Stage III		T4, N0, M0
		Any T, N1, M0
Stage IV		Any T, Any N, M1

Medullary

Stage I	T1	N0	M0
Stage II	T2	N0	M0
	T3	N0	M0
	T4	N0	M0
Stage III	Any T	N1	M0
Stage IV	Any T	Any N	M1

Undifferentiated

All cases are stage IV.

Stage IV	Any T	Any N	Any M

DIFFERENCES BETWEEN THE 2ND AND 3RD EDITIONS

A primary difference between the second edition of the *Manual* and the present recommendations is using 4 cm as a dividing measurement in the definitions of T2 and T3 and not considering an age division for medullary and undifferentiated cancers.

HISTOPATHOLOGIC TYPE

The World Health Organization (WHO) classification of thyroid cancer should be used, including at least the four major types and "unclassified":

Papillary carcinoma (with or without follicular foci)
Follicular carcinoma (extent of invasion of tumor capsule should be noted)
Medullary carcinoma
Undifferentiated (anaplastic) carcinoma
Unclassified malignant tumor

HISTOPATHOLOGIC GRADE (G)

- GX Grade cannot be assessed
- G1 Well differentiated
- G2 Moderately well differentiated

Thyroid Gland

G3 Poorly differentiated
G4 Undifferentiated

BIBLIOGRAPHY

1. Bengtsson A, Malmaeus J, Grimelius L, et al: Measurement of nuclear DNA content in thyroid diagnosis. World J Surg 8:481–486, 1984
2. Cady B, Sedgwick CE, Meissner WA et al: Changing clinical, pathologic, therapeutic and survival patterns in differentiated thyroid carcinoma. Ann Surg 184:541–553, 1976
3. Cohn K, Blackdahl M, Forsslund G et al: Prognostic value of nuclear DNA content in papillary thyroid carcinoma. World J Surg 8:474–480, 1984
4. Franssila KO: Prognosis in thyroid carcinoma. Cancer 36:1138–1146, 1975
5. Halnan KE: Influence of age and sex on incidence and prognosis of thyroid cancer: Three hundred forty-four cases followed for ten years. Cancer 19:1534–1536, 1966
6. Hedinger C, Sobin LH: Histological Typing of Thyroid Tumours. International Histological Classification of Tumours, No. 11, World Health Organization, Geneva, 1974
7. Heitz P, Moser H, Staub JJ: Thyroid cancer: A study of 573 thyroid tumors and 161 autopsy cases observed over a thirty-year period. Cancer 37:2329–2337, 1976
8. Mazzaferri E, Young R: Papillary thyroid carcinoma. A ten year report of the impact of therapy in five hundred and seventy six patients. Am J Med 70:511–517, 1981
9. Russell MA, Gilbert EF, Jaeschke WF: Prognostic features of thyroid cancer: A long-term followup of 68 cases. Cancer 36:553–559, 1975
10. Woolner LB, Beahrs OH, Black BM et al: Thyroid carcinoma: General considerations and follow-up data on 1181 cases. In Thyroid Neoplasia, Proceedings of the 2nd Imperial Cancer Research Fund Symposium, pp 51–79. London, Academic Press, 1968

THYROID GLAND

Data Form for Cancer Staging

Patient identification
Name _____
Address _____
Hospital or clinic number _____
Age _____ Sex _____ Race _____

Institution identification
Hospital or clinic _____
Address _____

Oncology Record

Anatomic site of cancer _____
Histologic type _____
Grade (G) _____
Date of classification _____

Chronology of classification
(use separate form for each time staged)
[ ] Clinical (use all data prior to first treatment)
[ ] Pathologic (if definitively resected specimen available)

Definitions

Primary Tumor (T)
All categories may be subdivided: (a) solitary; (b) multifocal—measure the largest for classification
[ ] TX Primary tumor cannot be assessed
[ ] T0 No evidence of primary tumor
[ ] T1 Tumor 1 cm or less in greatest dimension limited to the thyroid
[ ] T2 Tumor more than 1 cm but not more than 4 cm
[ ] T3 Tumor more than 4 cm in greatest dimension limited to the thyroid
[ ] T4 Tumor of any size extending beyond the thyroid capsule

Lymph Node (N)
Regional nodes are the cervical and upper mediastinal lymph nodes
[ ] NX Regional lymph nodes cannot be assessed
[ ] N0 No regional lymph node metastasis
[ ] N1 Regional lymph node metastasis
  [ ] N1a Metastasis in ipsilateral cervical lymph nodes
  [ ] N1b Metastasis in bilateral, midline, or contralateral cervical or mediastinal lymph nodes

Distant Metastases (M)
[ ] MX Presence of distant metastasis cannot be assessed
[ ] M0 No distant metastasis
[ ] M1 Distant metastasis
        Specify

Nodal involvement
Cervical unilateral _____
Cervical bilateral _____
Delphian _____
Mediastinal _____

Indicate on diagram primary tumor and regional nodes involved.

Stage Grouping

Separate stage groupings are recommended for papillary and follicular, medullary, and undifferentiated

Papillary or Follicular

Under 45 Years
[ ] Stage I   Any T, Any N, M0
[ ] Stage II   Any T, Any N, M1

45 Years and Over
[ ] Stage I   T1, N0, M0
[ ] Stage II   T2, N0, M0
               T3, N0, M0
[ ] Stage III T4, N0, M0
               Any T, N1, M0
[ ] Stage IV   Any T, Any N, M1

Medullary
[ ] Stage I   T1   N0   M0
[ ] Stage II   T2   N0   M0
               T3   N0   M0
               T4   N0   M0
[ ] Stage III Any T   N1   M0
[ ] Stage IV   Any T   Any N   M1

Undifferentiated
All cases are Stage IV
[ ] Stage IV   Any T   Any N   Any M

Histopathologic Grade (G)

[ ] GX Grade cannot be assessed
[ ] G1 Well differentiated
[ ] G2 Moderately well differentiated
[ ] G3 Poorly differentiated
[ ] G4 Undifferentiated

Staged by _____ M.D.
_____ Registrar
Date _____

Illustrations

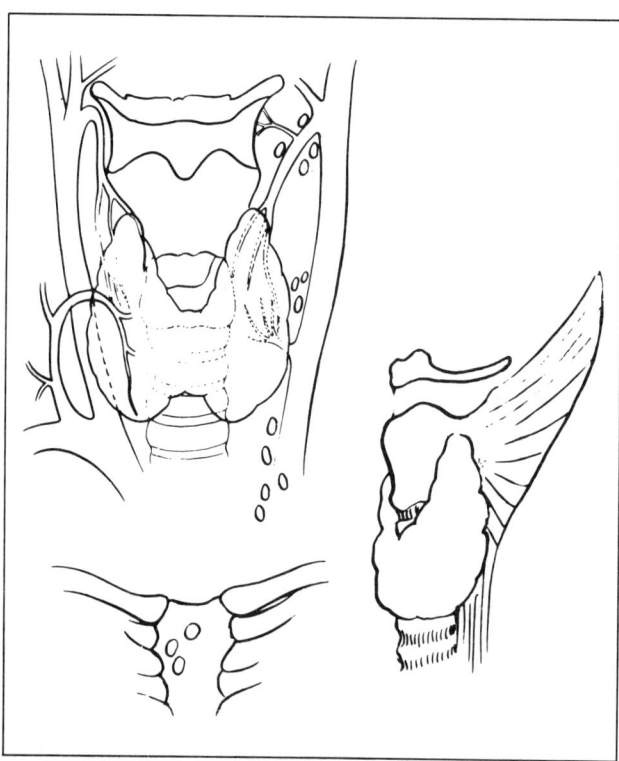

Tumor size ___ cm (greatest diameter). Indicate node(s) considered metastatic.

Histopathologic Type

The World Health Organization (WHO) classification of thyroid cancer should be used, including at least the four major types:

Papillary carcinoma (with or without follicular foci)
Follicular carcinoma (extent of invasion of tumor capsule should be noted)
Medullary carcinoma
Undifferentiated (anaplastic) carcinoma
Unclassified malignant tumor

Sites of Distant Metastasis

Pulmonary	PUL
Osseous	OSS
Hepatic	HEP
Brain	BRA
Lymph nodes	LYM
Bone marrow	MAR
Pleura	PLE
Peritoneum	PER
Skin	SKI
Other	OTH

DIGESTIVE SYSTEM SITES

9

Esophagus

Occurring more often in males, cancers of the esophagus are relatively uncommon in the United States, accounting for only 4% of all cancers. Predisposing factors are thought to include a high alcohol intake and heavy use of tobacco. Esophageal cancers are more common in some other countries, for example, in China, than in North America. The disease may be difficult to diagnose in its early stages. Most cancers arise in the middle or lower third of the esophagus. Squamous cell carcinomas comprise 98% of all the cancers. These tumors may extend over wide areas of the mucosal surface. Adenocarcinomas, which comprise the remaining 2%, are usually found in the distal esophagus. Dysphagia is the most common clinical symptom.

ANATOMY

Primary Site. Beginning at the hypopharynx, the esophagus lies posterior to the trachea and the heart, passing through the posterior mediastinum and entering the stomach through an opening in the diaphragm called the hiatus.

Histologically, the esophagus has four layers—mucosa, submucosa or lamina propria, muscle coat or muscularis propria, and adventitia. There is no serosa.

For purposes of classification, staging, and reporting of cancer, the esophagus is divided into four regions. Because the behavior of esophageal cancer and its treatment vary with the anatomic divisions, these regions should be recorded and reported separately. The location of the esophageal lesions is often measured from the incisors (front teeth).

Cervical esophagus (ICD-O 150.0)
  The cervical esophagus begins at the lower border of the cricoid cartilage and ends at the thoracic inlet (the suprasternal notch), approximately 18 cm from the upper incisor teeth.
Intrathoracic esophagus (ICD-O 150.1–150.5)
  The upper thoracic portion (ICD-O 150.3) extends from the thoracic inlet to the level of the tracheal bifurcation, approximately 24 cm from the upper incisor teeth.
  The mid-thoracic portion (ICD-O 150.4) is the proximal half of the esophagus between the tracheal bifurcation and the esophago-gastric junction. The lower level is approximately 32 cm from the upper incisor teeth.
  The lower thoracic portion (ICD-O 150.5), 8 cm in length (includes the abdominal esophagus, ICD-O 150.2), is the distal half of the esophagus between the tracheal bifurcation and the esophago-gastric junction, approximately 40 cm from the upper incisor teeth.

Regional Lymph Nodes. The regional lymph nodes are:

Cervical esophagus: The cervical nodes including the supraclavicular lymph nodes
Intrathoracic esophagus: The mediastinal and perigastric lymph nodes, excluding the celiac nodes

Involvement of more distant nodes is considered distant metastasis.

Specific regional lymph nodes are listed as follows:

Cervical esophagus
  superior mediastinal
  internal jugular
  upper cervical
  cervical, NOS
  periesophageal
  supraclavicular
Intrathoracic esophagus—upper, middle
  internal jugular
  tracheobronchial
  peritracheal
  perigastric
  carinal
  hilar (pulmonary roots)
  posterior mediastinal
  periesophageal
Intrathoracic esophagus—lower
  left gastric
  cardiac
  perigastric, NOS
  posterior mediastinal
  nodes of lesser curvature of stomach

In the cervical esophagus, any lymph node involvement other than that of the cervical or supraclavicular lymph nodes is considered distant metastasis. For the thoracic esophagus any cervical, supraclavicular, scalene, or abdominal lymph nodes are considered distant metastatic sites. For the lower esophagus, the abdominal nodes listed above are considered regional; all others are distant.

Metastatic Sites. The liver, lungs, pleura, and kidneys are the most common sites of distant metastases. Occasionally, the tumor may extend directly into the mediastinum before distant spread is evident.

RULES FOR CLASSIFICATION

Clinical Staging. Clinical staging is based on the anatomical extent of the primary tumor that can be ascertained by examination before treatment. Such an examination may include physical examination, medical history, biopsy, routine laboratory studies, endoscopic examinations and imaging.

Pathologic Staging. Pathologic staging is based on surgical exploration and on the examination of the surgically resected esophagus and associated lymph nodes. Direct extension of the tumor to adjacent structures and the presence of distant metastases should be carefully documented. A single classification is used for all regions of the esophagus. It serves both clinical and pathologic staging. Involvement of the adjacent structures depends on the location of the primary tumor. These structures should be specified when involved with tumor.

DEFINITION OF TNM
Primary Tumor (T)

TX Primary tumor cannot be assessed
T0 No evidence of primary tumor
Tis Carcinoma *in situ*
T1 Tumor invades lamina propria or submucosa
T2 Tumor invades muscularis propria
T3 Tumor invades adventitia
T4 Tumor invades adjacent structures

Regional Lymph Nodes (N)

NX Regional lymph nodes cannot be assessed
N0 No regional lymph node metastasis
N1 Regional lymph node metastasis

Distant Metastasis (M)

MX Presence of distant metastasis cannot be assessed

Esophagus

M0 No distant metastasis
M1 Distant metastasis

STAGE GROUPING

Stage 0	Tis	N0	M0
Stage I	T1	N0	M0
Stage IIA	T2	N0	M0
	T3	N0	M0
Stage IIB	T1	N1	M0
	T2	N1	M0
Stage III	T3	N1	M0
	T4	Any N	M0
Stage IV	Any T	Any N	M1

DIFFERENCES BETWEEN THE 2ND AND 3RD EDITIONS

In the previous AJCC classification of 1983, invasion of the adjacent structures was classified as T3; now it is T4. In the new system, Stage II is subdivided into Stage IIA and Stage IIB for finer discrimination. This subdivision is based on lymph node involvement. Also, the number of lymph node categories has been reduced from five to three. The separate classifications for clinical and pathologic staging have been merged and a single TNM classification is now used.

HISTOPATHOLOGIC TYPE

The staging classification applies to all squamous cell carcinomas, which are most common, and to the adenocarcinomas. Other histologic types are reported separately.

HISTOPATHOLOGIC GRADE (G)

GX Grade cannot be assessed
G1 Well differentiated
G2 Moderately well differentiated
G3 Poorly differentiated
G4 Undifferentiated

BIBLIOGRAPHY

1. Appelqvist P: Carcinoma of the oesophagus and gastric cardia: A retrospective study based on statistical and clinical material from Finland. Acta Chir Scand (Suppl) 430:1–92, 1972
2. Bergman F: Cancer of the esophagus: A histological study of development and local spread of 10 cases of squamous cell carcinoma in the lower third of oesophagus. Acta Chir Scand 117:356–365, 1959
3. Fu-Sheng L, Ling L, and Song-Liang Q: Clinical and Pathological Characteristics of Early Oesophageal Cancer. Clinics in Oncology 1, No. 2: 539–557, 1982
4. Merendino KA, Mark VH: An analysis of 100 cases of squamous-cell carcinoma of the esophagus. Surg Gynecol Obstet 94:110–114, 1952
5. Skinner DB, Ferguson MK, Little AG: Selection of operation for esophageal cancer based on staging. Ann Surg 204:391–400, 1986
6. Turnbull ADM, Goodner JT: Primary adenocarcinoma of the esophagus. Cancer 22:915–918, 1968

ESOPHAGUS

Data Form for Cancer Staging

Patient identification
Name _____
Address _____
Hospital or clinic number _____
Age _____ Sex _____ Race _____

Institution identification
Hospital or clinic _____
Address _____

Oncology Record

Anatomic site of cancer _____
Histologic type _____
Grade (G) _____
Date of classification _____

Chronology of classification
(use separate form for each time staged)
[ ] Clinical (use all data prior to first treatment)
[ ] Pathologic (if definitively resected specimen available)

Definitions

Primary Tumor (T)
[ ] TX   Primary tumor cannot be assessed
[ ] T0   No evidence of primary tumor
[ ] Tis Carcinoma *in situ*
[ ] T1   Tumor invades lamina propria or submucosa
[ ] T2   Tumor invades muscularis propria
[ ] T3   Tumor invades adventitia
[ ] T4   Tumor invades adjacent structures

Lymph Node (N)
[ ] NX Regional lymph nodes cannot be assessed
[ ] N0 No regional lymph node metastasis
[ ] N1 Regional lymph node metastasis

Distant Metastasis (M)
[ ] MX Presence of distant metastasis cannot be assessed
[ ] M0 No distant metastasis
[ ] M1 Distant metastasis

Stage Grouping

[ ]	0	Tis	N0	M0
[ ]	I	T1	N0	M0
[ ]	IIA	T2	N0	M0
		T3	N0	M0
[ ]	IIB	T1	N1	M0
		T2	N1	M0
[ ]	III	T3	N1	M0
		T4	Any N	M0
[ ]	IV	Any T	Any N	M1

Histopathologic Grade (G)

[ ] GX Grade cannot be assessed
[ ] G1 Well differentiated
[ ] G2 Moderately well differentiated
[ ] G3 Poorly differentiated
[ ] G4 Undifferentiated

Histopathologic Type

The staging classification applies to all squamous cell carcinomas, which are most common, and to the adenocarcinomas. Other histologic types are reported separately.

Illustration

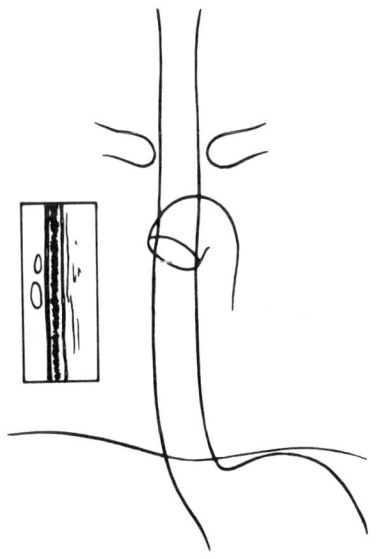

Length of tumor: _____ cm

Indicate on diagram primary tumor and regional nodes involved.

Sites of Distant Metastasis

Pulmonary	PUL
Osseous	OSS
Hepatic	HEP
Brain	BRA
Lymph nodes	LYM
Bone marrow	MAR
Pleura	PLE
Peritoneum	PER
Skin	SKI
Other	OTH

Staged by _____ M.D.
_____ Registrar
Date _____

American Joint Committee on Cancer—1988

10 Stomach

As in most hollow organs, the prognosis of carcinomas of the stomach depends on the extent of penetration of the wall by the tumor and involvement of adjacent organs. Size, location, and the histologic type of cancer have not been found to be useful for estimating prognosis. The overall prognosis for carcinomas of the stomach is poor. For reasons unknown, the incidence of stomach cancer has been declining since 1930 in most of the developed countries. Chronic atrophic gastritis is a predisposing factor. Nearly all carcinomas arise from the mucus-secreting cells of the gastric crypts.

ANATOMY

Primary Site. The stomach (ICD-O 151) is the first division of the abdominal alimentary tract. Its first part is the esophagogastric junction, which is immediately below the diaphragm and often called the cardia. The upper part of the stomach is the fundus, and the lower part is the antrum. The pylorus is continuous with the duodenum. The shorter right border is the lesser curvature and the longer border on the left is the greater curvature. The wall of the stomach has three layers: an inner mucosal and submucosal layer, a smooth muscle layer, and an outer serosal or visceral peritoneal surface.

For staging purposes, the stomach is divided into three anatomic regions:

Upper third: Includes the cardiac area (151.0) and fundus (151.3)

Middle third: Includes the bulk of the corpus (151.4)

Lower third: Includes the antral area (151.2) and pylorus (151.1)

In order to delimit these regions, the lesser (ICD-O 151.5) and greater (ICD-O 151.6) curvatures are divided at two equidistant points and these are joined.

Regional Lymph Nodes. The regional lymph nodes are as follows.

Inferior (right) gastric:
    Greater curvature
    Greater omental
    Gastroduodenal
    Gastrocolic
    Gastroepiploic, right, or NOS
    Gastrohepatic
    Pyloric, including subpyloric and infrapyloric
    Pancreaticoduodenal

Splenic:
    Gastroepiploic, left
    Pancreaticolienal
    Peripancreatic
    Splenic hilar

Superior (left) gastric:
    Lesser curvature
    Lesser omental
    Gastropancreatic, left
    Gastric, left
    Paracardial; cardial
    Cardioesophageal

Perigastric, NOS
Celiac
Hepatic

All other lymph nodes are considered distant. They include:

Retropancreatic
Hepatoduodenal
Aortic
Portal
Retroperitoneal
Mesenteric

Metastatic Sites. Distant spread to the liver, lungs, and supraclavicular lymph nodes is common, although widespread visceral involvement can also occur. Frequently there is direct extension to the liver, the transverse colon, the pancreas, or the diaphragm.

RULES FOR CLASSIFICATION

Clinical Staging. Designated as cTNM, clinical staging is based on evidence acquired before definitive treatment is instituted. It includes physical examination, imaging, endoscopy, biopsy, and other findings. All cases must be confirmed histologically.

Pathologic Staging. Pathologic staging depends on data acquired clinically along with results of surgical exploration and examination of the resected specimen or biopsy. Pathologic assessment of the regional lymph nodes entails removal of nodes adequate to validate the absence of metastasis and to evaluate the highest pN category. If there is doubt concerning the correct T, N, or M assignment, the lower (less advanced) category should be selected. This also will reflect in the stage grouping.

DEFINITION OF TNM

Primary Tumor (T)

TX Primary tumor cannot be assessed
T0 No evidence of primary tumor
Tis Carcinoma *in situ*: intraepithelial tumor without invasion of the lamina propria
T1 Tumor invades lamina propria or submucosa
T2 Tumor invades the muscularis propria or the subserosa*
T3 Tumor penetrates the serosa (visceral peritoneum) without invasion of adjacent structures†, ‡
T4 Tumor invades adjacent structures†, ‡

Note: A tumor may penetrate the muscularis propria with extension into the gastrocolic or gastrohepatic ligaments or into the greater or lesser omentum without perforation of the visceral peritoneum covering these structures. In this case, the tumor is classified T2. If there is perforation of the visceral peritoneum covering the gastric ligaments or omenta, the tumor should be classified T3.

†*The adjacent structures of the stomach are the spleen, transverse colon, liver, diaphragm, pancreas, abdominal wall, adrenal gland, kidney, small intestine, and retroperitoneum.*

‡*Intramural extension to the duodenum or esophagus is classified by the depth of greatest invasion in any of these sites, including stomach.*

Regional Lymph Nodes (N)

NX Regional lymph node(s) cannot be assessed
N0 No regional lymph node metastasis

N1 Metastasis in perigastric lymph node(s) within 3 cm of the edge of the primary tumor

N2 Metastasis in perigastric lymph node(s) more than 3 cm from the edge of the primary tumor, or in lymph nodes along the left gastric, common hepatic, splenic, or celiac arteries

Distant Metastasis (M)

MX Presence of distant metastasis cannot be assessed

M0 No distant metastasis

M1 Distant metastasis

STAGE GROUPING

Stage	T	N	M
Stage 0	Tis	N0	M0
Stage IA	T1	N0	M0
Stage IB	T1	N1	M0
	T2	N0	M0
Stage II	T1	N2	M0
	T2	N1	M0
	T3	N0	M0
Stage IIIA	T2	N2	M0
	T3	N1	M0
	T4	N0	M0
Stage IIIB	T3	N2	M0
	T4	N1	M0
Stage IV	T4	N2	M0
	Any T	Any N	M1

DIFFERENCES BETWEEN THE 2ND AND 3RD EDITIONS

The T4 category has been simplified and is no longer divided into a and b. The N categories have been reduced from five to four. Many abdominal lymph nodes listed in the previous N3 category are now considered distant sites and should be recorded as M1. These include the para-aortic, hepato-duodenal, retropancreatic, and mesenteric nodes. In the new system there are seven stage groupings for finer discrimination. Stage I and Stage III have been subdivided into A and B groupings.

HISTOPATHOLOGIC TYPE

The staging recommendations apply only to carcinomas and not to other histologic types such as lymphomas or sarcomas. Adenocarcinomas should be divided into the following subtypes and recorded:

Intestinal
Diffuse
Mixed

The prognosis is worse for the diffuse type.

HISTOPATHOLOGIC GRADE (G)

GX Grade cannot be assessed
G1 Well differentiated
G2 Moderately well differentiated
G3 Poorly differentiated
G4 Undifferentiated

BIBLIOGRAPHY

1. Coller FA, Kay EB, MacIntyre RS: Regional lymphatic metastases of carcinoma of the stomach. Arch Surg 43:748–761, 1941
2. Cook AO, Levine BA, Sirinek KR et al: Evaluation of gastric adenocarcinoma: Abdominal computed tomography does not replace celiotomy. Arch Surg 121:603–606, 1986
3. Dupont JB Jr, Lee JR, Burton GR et al: Adenocarcinoma of the stomach: Review of 1,497 cases. Cancer 41:941–947, 1978
4. Eker R, Efskind J: The pathology and prognosis of gastric carcinoma. Acta Chir Scand (Suppl) 264:1–182, 1960
5. Horn RC Jr: Carcinoma of the stomach: Autopsy findings in untreated cases. Gastroenterology 29:515–525, 1955
6. Kennedy BJ: TNM classification of stomach cancer. Cancer 26:971–983, 1970
7. Lauren P: The two histological main types of gastric carcinoma. Acta Pathol Microbiol Scand 64:31–49, 1965
8. Ming SC: *Tumors of the Esophagus and Stomach.* Atlas of Tumor Pathology, Second Series, Fascicle 7. Washington, DC: Armed Forces Institute of Pathology, 1973
9. Possik RA, Franco EL, Pires DR et al: Sensitivity, specificity, and predictive value of laparoscopy for the staging for gastric cancer and for the detection of liver metastases. Cancer 58:1–6, 1986
10. Saario I, Schroder T, Talppanen EM et al: Factors influencing 5-year survival in gastric malignancies after total gastrectomy. Annales Chirurgiae et Gynaecologiae (Helsinki) 75:23–27, 1986
11. Serlin O, Keehn RJ, Higgins GA et al: Factors related to survival following resection for gastric carcinoma: Analysis of 903 cases. Cancer 40:1318–1329, 1977
12. Sunderland DA, McNeer G, Ortega LS et al: The lymphatic spread of gastric cancer. Cancer 6:987–996, 1953
13. Zinninger MM, Colling WT: Extension of carcinomas of the stomach into the duodenum and esophagus. Ann Surg 130:557–566, 1949

STOMACH

Data Form for Cancer Staging

Patient identification
Name _____
Address _____
Hospital or clinic number _____
Age _____ Sex _____ Race _____

Institution identification
Hospital or clinic _____
Address _____

Oncology Record

Anatomic site of cancer _____
Histologic type _____
Grade (G) _____
Date of classification _____

Chronology of classification
  (use separate form for each time staged)
[ ] Clinical (use all data prior to first treatment)
[ ] Pathologic (if definitively resected specimen available)

Definitions

Primary Tumor (T)

[ ] TX Primary tumor cannot be assessed
[ ] T0 No evidence of primary tumor
[ ] Tis Carcinoma *in situ:* intraepithelial tumor without invasion of lamina propria
[ ] T1 Tumor invades lamina propria or submucosa
[ ] T2 Tumor invades muscularis propria or subserosa
[ ] T3 Tumor penetrates serosa (visceral peritoneum) without invasion of adjacent structures
[ ] T4 Tumor invades adjacent structures

Lymph Node (N)

[ ] NX Regional lymph node(s) cannot be assessed
[ ] N0 No regional lymph node metastasis
[ ] N1 Metastasis in perigastric lymph node(s) within 3 cm of edge of primary tumor
[ ] N2 Metastasis in perigastric lymph node(s) more than 3 cm from edge of primary tumor, or in lymph nodes along left gastric, common hepatic, splenic, or celiac arteries.

Distant Metastasis (M)

[ ] MX Presence of distant metastasis cannot be assessed
[ ] M0 No distant metastasis
[ ] M1 Distant metastasis

Histopathologic Grade (G)

[ ] GX Grade cannot be assessed
[ ] G1 Well differentiated
[ ] G2 Moderately well differentiated
[ ] G3 Poorly differentiated
[ ] G4 Undifferentiated

Histopathologic Type

The staging recommendations apply only to carcinomas and not to other histologic types such as lymphomas or sarcomas. Adenocarcinomas should be divided into the following subtypes and recorded.

a. Intestinal
b. Diffuse
c. Mixed

The prognosis is worse for the diffuse type.

Illustration

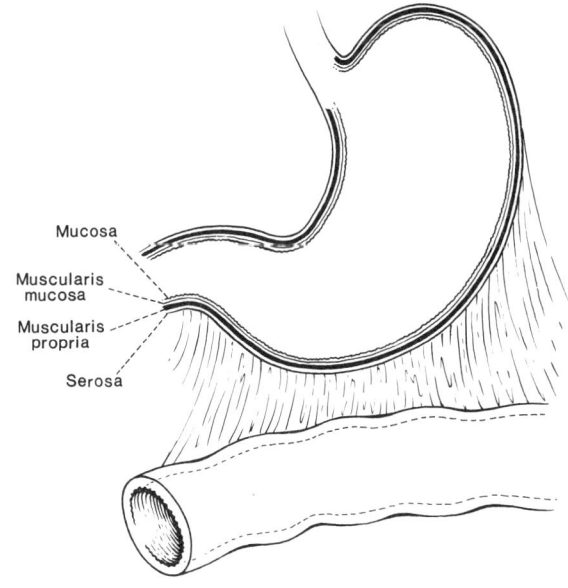

Indicate on diagram primary tumor and regional nodes involved.

Staged by _____ M.D.
_____ Registrar
Date _____

Stage Grouping

[ ] 0	Tis	N0	M0
[ ] IA	T1	N0	M0
[ ] IB	T1	N1	M0
	T2	N0	M0
[ ] II	T1	N2	M0
	T2	N1	M0
	T3	N0	M0
[ ] IIIA	T2	N2	M0
	T3	N1	M0
	T4	N0	M0
[ ] IIIB	T3	N2	M0
	T4	N1	M0
[ ] IV	T4	N2	M0
	Any T	Any N	M1

Sites of Distant Metastasis

Pulmonary	PUL
Osseous	OSS
Hepatic	HEP
Brain	BRA
Lymph nodes	LYM
Bone marrow	MAR
Pleura	PLE
Peritoneum	PER
Skin	SKI
Other	OTH

Colon and Rectum

11

The TNM classification for cancers of the colon and rectum has been modified to correspond directly with the Dukes' classification, which is often used for estimating the prognosis of colorectal cancers. By using the detail provided by the TNM combinations within each stage grouping, more information about the status of the cancer can be described. Furthermore, cases staged according to the new system can be compared with cases previously staged by the Dukes' system.

As in other sites, staging of the primary cancers of the colon or rectum depends on the extent of the tumor. Important determinants for staging include the depth of tumor penetration into the wall of the intestine, the number of regional lymph nodes involved, and the presence or absence of distant metastasis. Other prognostic variables that are important but do not enter into the TNM classification are the histologic type, differentiation, invasion of blood vessels or lymphatic channels, and complications such as fistula formation.

The classification can be used for both clinical and pathologic staging. Most cancers of the colon and rectum, however, are staged pathologically, after examination of the resected specimen. This system of staging applies to all carcinomas arising in the colon or rectum. It does not apply to sarcomas, lymphomas, or carcinoids.

ANATOMY

Primary Site. The colon extends from the terminal ileum to the anal canal. Excluding the rectum, the colon is divided into four parts: the right or ascending colon, the middle or transverse colon, the left or descending colon, and the sigmoid colon. The sigmoid is continuous with the rectum, which terminates in the anal canal. Except for the distal 10 cm of the rectum, the entire colon and proximal rectum are covered with peritoneum.

The cecum is a large pouch that forms the proximal segment of the right colon. It usually measures 6 cm by 9 cm and is covered with peritoneum. The ascending colon measures from 15 to 20 cm in length and is located retroperitoneally. Connecting the ascending colon to the transverse colon is the hepatic flexure, which lies under the right lobe of the liver near the duodenum.

The transverse colon lies more anteriorly than the other divisions of the colon. As a result, tumors can be more readily palpated through the anterior abdominal wall. It is supported by the transverse mesocolon, which is attached to the pancreas. Anteriorly, its serosa is continuous with the gastrocolic ligament. The transverse colon is connected to the descending colon by the splenic flexure, which is located near the spleen, tail of pancreas, and left kidney. The descending colon, which measures from 10 to 15 cm in length, is also located retroperitoneally. The descending colon becomes the sigmoid at the origin of the mesosigmoid. The sigmoid loop extends from the medial border of the left posterior major psoas muscle to the rectum, which begins at the termination of the mesosigmoid.

The rectum, which is normally 12 cm in length, extends from a point opposite the third sacral vertebra to the apex of the prostate gland in the male and to the apex of the perineal body in the female, that is, to a point 4 cm anterior to the tip of the coccyx. It is often defined, arbitrarily, as the distal 10 cm of the large intestine as measured from the anal verge with the sigmoidoscope. The rectosigmoid segment is usually 10 to 15 cm from the anal mucocutaneous junction. The rectum has no epiploic appendages, haustrations, or taeniae coli. It is covered by peritoneum in front and on both sides in its upper third and on the anterior wall only in its middle third. The peritoneum is reflected laterally from the rectum to form the perirectal fossa and anteriorly the uterine or rectovesical fold. There is no peritoneal covering in the lower third, which is often known as the rectal ampulla. The anal canal, which measures 4 to 5 cm in length, courses downward and backward from the apex of the prostate gland or from the perineal body to the anal verge.

Regional Lymph Nodes. In staging, the status of the lymph nodes at the base of the mesocolon should be recorded—especially those proximal to the origins of the ileocolic, right colic, middle colic, and inferior mesenteric arteries. Regional nodes are as follows: those along the course of the major vessels supplying the colon, those following the vascular arcades of the marginal artery, and those in close proximity to the colon, that is, located along the mesocolic border of the colon, and often in the epiploic appendages.

The regional lymph nodes are the pericolic and perirectal nodes and those located along the ileocolic, right colic, middle colic, left colic, inferior mesenteric artery, and superior (rectal) hemorrhoidal arteries.

The regional lymph nodes for each segment of the colon are:

SEGMENT	REGIONAL LYMPH NODES
Cecum (ICD-O 153.4) and appendix (ICD-O 153.5)	Anterior cecal, posterior cecal, ileocolic, right colic
Ascending colon (ICD-O 153.6)	Ileocolic, right colic, middle colic
Hepatic flexure (ICD-O 153.0)	Middle colic, right colic
Transverse colon (ICD-O 153.1)	Middle colic
Splenic flexure (ICD-O 153.7)	Middle colic, left colic, inferior mesenteric
Descending colon (ICD-O 153.2)	Left colic, inferior mesenteric, sigmoid
Sigmoid colon (ICD-O 153.3)	Inferior mesenteric, superior rectal, superior hemorrhoidal, sigmoidal, sigmoid mesenteric
Rectosigmoid (ICD-O 154.0)	Perirectal, left colic, sigmoid mesenteric, sigmoidal, inferior mesenteric, superior rectal, superior hemorrhoidal, middle hemorrhoidal
Rectum (ICD-O 154.1)	Perirectal, sigmoid mesenteric, inferior mesenteric, lateral sacral, presacral, internal iliac, sacral promontory (Gerota's), superior hemorrhoidal, inferior hemorrhoidal

Metastatic Sites. Carcinomas of the colon and rectum can spread to almost any organ. The most common sites of spread are the liver and lungs. Tumor can also spread to local structures after growing through the wall of the bowel. Extension to other segments of the colon may occur.

RULES FOR CLASSIFICATION

Clinical Staging. Clinical assessment is based on medical history, physical examination, routine and special roentgenograms, including barium enema, sigmoidoscopy, colonoscopy (with biopsy when

Colon and Rectum

possible), and special examinations used to demonstrate the presence of extracolonic metastasis, for example, chest films, liver function tests, and liver scans.

Pathologic Staging. Staging of colorectal cancers is usually done after pathologic examination of the resected specimen and surgical exploration of the abdomen. Important for estimating prognosis is the depth of tumor penetration into the wall of the colon or rectum. *In situ* carcinomas, Tis, are noninvasive cancers arising in either flat mucosa or in polyps. If a tumor invades the stalk of the polyp, then it is classified as T1. In some cases in which tumor is resected for palliation only, lymph nodes may not be present or may be few in number. Evaluation of the number and location of involved lymph nodes is critical.

DEFINITION OF TNM

The same classification is used for both clinical and pathologic staging.

Primary Tumor (T)

TX Primary tumor cannot be assessed
T0 No evidence of primary tumor
Tis Carcinoma *in situ*
T1 Tumor invades submucosa
T2 Tumor invades muscularis propria
T3 Tumor invades through the muscularis propria into the subserosa, or into nonperitonealized pericolic or perirectal tissues.
T4 Tumor perforates the visceral peritoneum, or directly invades other organs or structures.*

*Note: Direct invasion of other organs or structures includes invasion of other segments of colorectum by way of serosa (e.g., invasion of the sigmoid colon by a carcinoma of the cecum).

Regional Lymph Nodes (N)

NX Regional lymph nodes cannot be assessed
N0 No regional lymph node metastasis
N1 Metastasis in 1 to 3 pericolic or perirectal lymph nodes
N2 Metastasis in 4 or more pericolic or perirectal lymph nodes
N3 Metastasis in any lymph node along the course of a named vascular trunk

Distant Metastasis (M)

MX Presence of distant metastasis cannot be assessed
M0 No distant metastasis
M1 Distant metastasis

STAGE GROUPING

				DUKES
Stage 0	Tis	N0	M0	
Stage I	T1	N0	M0	A
	T2	N0	M0	A
Stage II	T3	N0	M0	B
	T4	N0	M0	B
Stage III	Any T	N1	M0	C
	Any T	N2, N3	M0	C
Stage IV	Any T	Any N	M1	

Note: Dukes' B is a composite of better (T3, N0, M0) and worse (T4, N0, M0) prognostic groups as is Dukes' C (Any T, N1, M0) and (Any T, N2, N3, M0).

DIFFERENCES BETWEEN THE 2ND AND 3RD EDITIONS

The differences between the previous (1983) and the new staging systems for carcinomas of the colon and rectum are extensive. In this edition of the *Manual*, the definitions for Tis, T1, and T2 have been shortened and simplified. T2a and T2b, which were used in the 1983 edition, are not included in this edition. T2 now refers to invasion of the muscularis propria for both colon and rectum. The definition for T3 has been simplified to accommodate the different anatomic structures of the colon and the rectum.

The N definitions have also been changed. In this edition, N1 refers to 1 to 3 involved lymph nodes, and N2 refers to 4 or more involved nodes. In the 1983 edition N2 referred to the regional nodes involved that extended to the line of resection or ligature around the blood vessels. In this edition the definition of N3 has been changed from lymph nodes whose location was not identified to those along the course of a major, named vascular trunk.

Stage I is no longer subdivided into A and B categories. Stage II now includes T3, N0, M0 and T4, N0, M0. In the previous edition T4, N0, M0 was assigned to Stage III.

Histopathologic Type

This staging classification applies to all carcinomas that arise in the colon and rectum.

Histopathologic Grade (G)

GX Grade cannot be assessed
G1 Well differentiated
G2 Moderately well differentiated
G3 Poorly differentiated
G4 Undifferentiated

BIBLIOGRAPHY

1. Astler VB, Coller FA: The prognostic significance of direct extension of carcinoma of the colon and rectum. Ann Surg 139:846–852, 1954
2. Beart RW Jr, van Heerden JA, Beahrs OH: Evolution in the pathologic staging of carcinoma of the colon. Surg Gynecol Obstet 146:257–259, 1978
3. Butch RJ, Stark DD, Wittenberg J et al: Staging rectal cancer by MR and CT. Am J Roentgenol 146:1155–1160, 1986
4. Chapins PH, Fisher R, Dent DF et al: The relationship between different staging methods and survival in colorectal carcinoma. Dis Colon Rectum 28:158–161, 1985
5. Dukes CE: The classification of cancer of the rectum. J Pathol Bacteriol 35:322–332, 1932
6. Dukes CE: Cancer of the rectum: An analysis of 1000 cases. J Pathol Bacteriol 50:527–539, 1940
7. Dukes CE, Bussey HJR: The spread of rectal cancer and its effect on prognosis. Br J Cancer 12:309–320, 1958
8. Gabriel WB, Dukes CE, Bussey HJR: Lymphatic spread in cancer of the rectum. Br J Surg 23:395–399; 412–413, 1935
9. Goligher JC: The Dukes' A, B, and C categorization of the extent of spread of carcinomas of the rectum. Surg Gynecol Obstet 143:793–794, 1976
10. Grinnell RS: The grading and prognosis of carcinoma of the colon and rectum. Ann Surg 109:500–533, 1939
11. Grinnell RS: The spread of carcinoma of the colon and rectum. Cancer 3:641–652, 1950
12. Newland RC, Chapins PH, Pheils MT et al: The relationship of survival to staging and grading of colorectal carcinoma: A prospective study of 503 cases. Cancer 47:1424–1429, 1981
13. Qizilbash AH: Pathologic studies in colorectal cancer: A guide to the surgical pathology examination of colorectal specimens and review of features of prognostic significance. Pathol Annu 17 (part 1):1–46, 1982
14. Rubio CA, Emas S, Nylander G: A critical reappraisal of Dukes' classification. Surg Gynecol Obstet 145:682–684, 1977
15. Shepard JM, Jones JSP: Adenocarcinoma of the large bowel. Br J Cancer 25:680–690, 1971
16. Steinberg SM, Barkin JS, Kaplan RS et al: Prognostic indicators of colon tumors: The gastrointestinal tumor study group experience. Cancer 57:1866–1870, 1986
17. Williams NS, Durdey P, Qwihe P et al: Pre-operative staging of rectal neoplasm and its impact on clinical management. Br J Surg 72:868–874, 1985
18. Wolmark N, Fisher ER, Wieand HS et al: The relationship of depth of penetration and tumor size to the number of positive nodes in Dukes' C colorectal cancer. Cancer 53:2707–2712, 1984
19. Wolmark N, Fisher B, Wieand HS: The prognostic value of the modifications of the Dukes' C class of colorectal cancer: An analysis of the NSABP clinical trials. Ann Surg 203:115–122, 1986
20. Wood DA: Tumors of the Intestines. In Atlas of Tumor Pathology, Section VI, Fascicle 22. Washington DC, Armed Forces Institute of Pathology under the auspices of the National Academy of Sciences, 1967
21. Wood DA: Clinical staging and end results classification: TNM system of clinical classification as applicable to carcinoma of the colon and rectum. Cancer 28:109–114, 1971
22. Wood DA, Robbins GF, Zippin C et al: Staging of cancer of the colon and rectum. Cancer 43:961–968, 1979

COLON AND RECTUM

Data Form for Cancer Staging

Patient identification
Name _____
Address _____
Hospital or clinic number _____
Age _____ Sex _____ Race _____

Institution identification
Hospital or clinic _____
Address _____

Oncology Record

Anatomic site of cancer _____
Histologic type _____
Grade (G) _____
Date of classification _____

Chronology of classification
(use separate form for each time staged)
[ ] Clinical (use all data prior to first treatment)
[ ] Pathologic (if definitively resected specimen available)

Definitions

Primary Tumor (T)
[ ] TX Primary tumor cannot be assessed
[ ] T0 No evidence of primary tumor
[ ] Tis Carcinoma in situ *mucosa only*
[ ] T1 Tumor invades submucosa
[ ] T2 Tumor invades muscularis propria
[ ] T3 Tumor invades through muscularis propria into subserosa, or into nonperitonealized pericolic or perirectal tissues
[ ] T4 Tumor perforates visceral peritoneum, or directly invades other organs or structures

Lymph Node (N)
[ ] NX Regional lymph nodes cannot be assessed
[ ] N0 No regional lymph node metastasis
[ ] N1 Metastasis in 1 to 3 pericolic or perirectal lymph nodes
[ ] N2 Metastasis in 4 or more pericolic or perirectal lymph nodes
[ ] N3 Metastasis in any lymph node along course of a major named vascular trunk

Distant Metastasis (M)
[ ] MX Presence of distant metastasis cannot be assessed
[ ] M0 No distant metastasis
[ ] M1 Distant metastasis

Histopathologic Grade (G)
[ ] GX Grade cannot be assessed
[ ] G1 Well differentiated
[ ] G2 Moderately well differentiated
[ ] G3 Poorly differentiated
[ ] G4 Undifferentiated

Histopathologic Type

This staging classification applies to all carcinomas that arise in the colon and rectum.

Sites of Distant Metastasis

Pulmonary	PUL
Osseous	OSS
Hepatic	HEP
Brain	BRA
Lymph nodes	LYM
Bone marrow	MAR
Pleura	PLE
Peritoneum	PER
Skin	SKI
Other	OTH

Stage Grouping

[ ] 0	Tis	N0	M0
[ ] I	T1	N0	M0
	T2	N0	M0
[ ] II	T3	N0	M0
	T4	N0	M0
[ ] III	Any T	N1	M0
	Any T	N2	M0
	Any T	N3	M0
[ ] IV	Any T	Any N	M1

Staged by _____ M.D.
_____ Registrar
Date _____

Illustrations

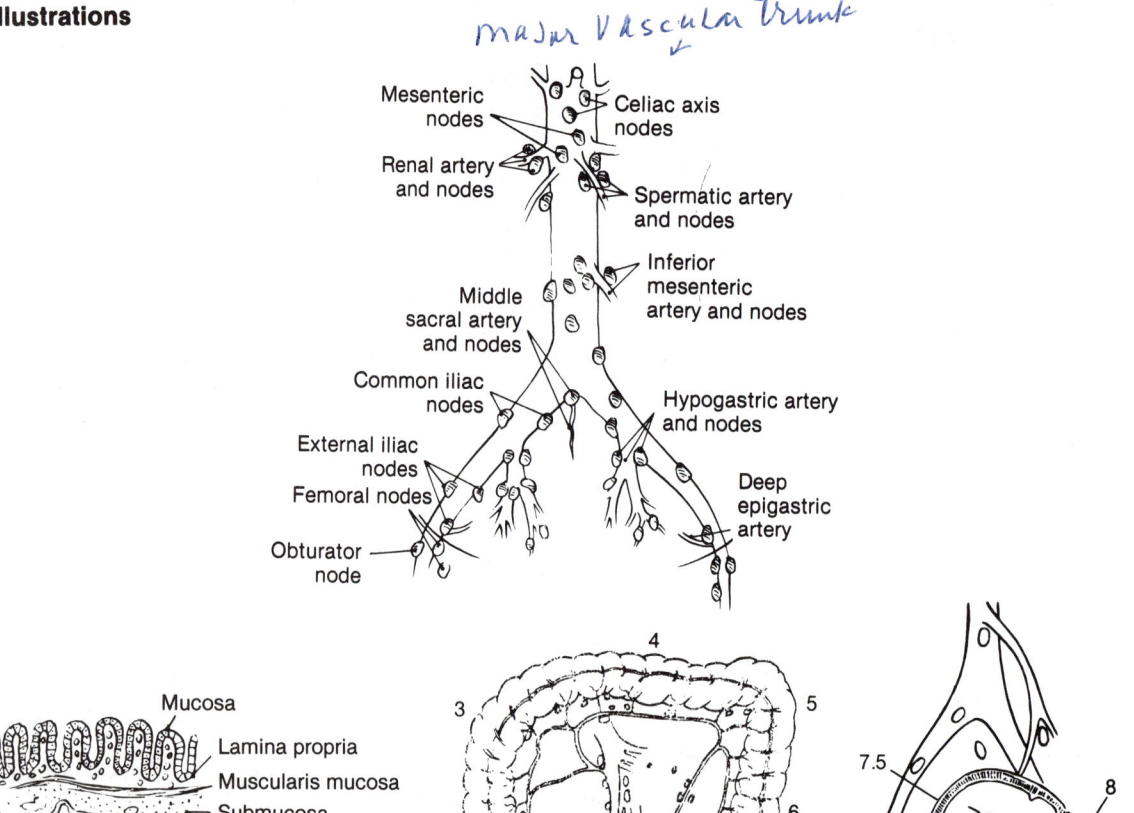

For anatomic areas corresponding to numbers, see list above.
Indicate on diagram primary and regional nodes involved.

Anatomic Areas of Colon and Rectum

1. Cecum
2. Ascending colon
3. Hepatic flexure
4. Transverse colon
5. Splenic flexure
6. Descending colon
7. Sigmoid
7.5. Rectosigmoid
8. Rectum
9. Anal canal

12

Anal Canal

There are two staging systems for cancers of the anus, one for the anal canal and the other for the anal margin. The separation is important because it affects prognosis and treatment. The staging classification for the anus is new and was not published in previous editions of the *Manual*.

Cancers of the anal canal are staged clinically according to the size and extent of the primary tumor. Thus, patients with cancer of the canal can be classified at the time of presentation by inspection of the lesion and palpation of adjacent structures, including regional lymph nodes. Although additional information concerning depth of penetration can often be provided by the pathologist after resection, in many cases, especially those treated with radiation, the depth of invasion cannot be assessed. As a result, only a single staging system is recommended. Radiation and chemotherapy not only destroy tumor cells but also cause inflammatory changes and edema, which makes it difficult for the pathologist to assess the true depth of invasion.

Cancers that arise at the anal margin, that is, the junction of the hair-bearing skin with the mucous membrane of the anal canal, or below, are staged according to the system used for skin cancers (see page 133).

ANATOMY

Primary Site. The anatomic limits of the anal canal (ICD-O 154.2) are defined as follows for staging purposes: The anal canal extends from the rectum to the perianal skin and is lined by the mucous membrane overlying the internal sphincter, including the transitional epithelium and dentate line, to the junction with the hair-bearing skin.

Regional Lymph Nodes. The regional lymph nodes are the perirectal, internal iliac, and inguinal lymph nodes.

Regional nodal groups include:

anorectal
perirectal
superficial inguinal
internal iliac
hypogastric
femoral
lateral sacral

All other nodal groups represent sites of distant metastasis. The sites of regional node involvement are explained by lymphatic drainage, which may go in either of two directions: above to the rectal ampulla and below to the perineum. Tumors that arise in the anal canal usually spread initially to the anorectal and perirectal nodes, and those that arise at the anal margin spread to the superficial inguinal nodes.

Metastatic Sites. Cancers of the anus can metastasize to most organs, especially the liver and lungs. Involvement of the abdominal cavity is not unusual.

RULES FOR CLASSIFICATION

The staging system does not preclude the surgeon from recording the depth of penetration or extension of tumor based on information provided by the pathologist or radiologist. This information, however, does not enter into the staging classification.

The primary tumor is staged according to its size and local extension as determined by clinical or pathologic examination. For most of the histologic types, the diameter of the tumor correlates with the depth of penetration. Extension of tumor to the anorectal, perirectal, superficial inguinal nodes, femoral nodes, and adjacent structures can usually be assessed by palpation. Tumor can extend to the rectal mucosa or submucosa, subcutaneous perianal tissue, perianal skin, ischiorectal fat, and/or local skeletal muscles, such as the external anal sphincter, levator ani, and coccygeus muscles. Tumor can also invade the perineum, vulva, prostate gland, urinary bladder, urethra, vagina, cervix uteri, corpus uteri, pelvic peritoneum, and broad ligaments.

Spread to other nodal groups, such as inferior mesenteric, can often be suspected by computed tomography or magnetic nuclear imaging.

Clinical Staging. Anal cancers are staged primarily by inspection and palpation. Imaging may help define extent of tumor. There is no pathologic staging in the classification.

DEFINITION OF TNM

Anal Canal

The following is the TNM classification for the staging of cancers that arise in the anal canal only. Cancers that arise at the anal margin are staged according to cancers of the skin.

Primary Tumor (T)

TX Primary tumor cannot be assessed
T0 No evidence of primary tumor
Tis Carcinoma *in situ*
T1 Tumor 2 cm or less in greatest dimension
T2 Tumor more than 2 cm but not more than 5 cm in greatest dimension
T3 Tumor more than 5 cm in greatest dimension
T4 Tumor of any size invades adjacent organ(s), *e.g.*, vagina, urethra, bladder (involvement of the sphincter muscle(s) *alone* is not classified as T4)

Note: The adjacent organs involved with tumor should be specified.

Regional Lymph Nodes (N)

NX Regional lymph nodes cannot be assessed
N0 No regional lymph node metastasis
N1 Metastasis in perirectal lymph node(s)
N2 Metastasis in unilateral internal iliac and/or inguinal lymph node(s)
N3 Metastasis in perirectal and inguinal lymph nodes and/or bilateral internal iliac and/or inguinal lymph nodes

Distant Metastasis (M)

MX Presence of distant metastasis cannot be assessed
M0 No distant metastasis
M1 Distant metastasis

STAGE GROUPING

Stage	T	N	M
Stage 0	Tis	N0	M0
Stage I	T1	N0	M0
Stage II	T2	N0	M0
	T3	N0	M0
Stage IIIA	T4	N0	M0
	T1	N1	M0
	T2	N1	M0
	T3	N1	M0
Stage IIIB	T4	N1	M0
	Any T	N2, N3	M0
Stage IV	Any T	Any N	M1

Anal Canal

DIFFERENCES BETWEEN THE 2ND AND 3RD EDITIONS

This is a new TNM classification.

HISTOPATHOLOGIC TYPE

The staging system applies to all carcinomas arising in the anal canal, including carcinomas that arise within an anorectal fistula. Melanomas are excluded.

HISTOPATHOLOGIC GRADE

GX Grade cannot be assessed
G1 Well differentiated
G2 Moderately well differentiated
G3 Poorly differentiated
G4 Undifferentiated

BIBLIOGRAPHY

1. Boman BM, Moertel CG, O'Connell MJ et al: Carcinoma of the anal canal: A clinical and pathologic study of 188 cases. Cancer 54:114–125, 1984
2. Cummings B, Keane T, Thomas G et al: Results and toxicity of the treatment of anal canal carcinoma by radiation therapy or radiation therapy and chemotherapy. Cancer 54:2062–2068, 1984
3. Dillard BM, Spratt JS Jr, Ackerman LV et al: Epidermoid cancer of anal margin and canal. Arch Surg 86:772–776, 1963
4. Flam MS, John M, Lovalvo LJ et al: Definitive nonsurgical therapy of epithelial malignancies of the anal canal. Cancer 51:1378–1387, 1983
5. Gabriel WB: Squamous cell carcinoma of the anus and anal canal. Proceedings of the Royal Society of Medicine 34 (Part 1):139–157, 1941
6. Greenall MJ, Quan SHQ, Stearns MW et al: Epidermoid cancer of the anal margin. Am J Surg 149:95–101, 1985
7. Keyes EL: Squamous cell carcinoma of the lower rectum and anus. Ann Surg 106:1046–1058, 1937
8. Morson BC: The pathology and results of treatment of squamous cell carcinoma of the anal canal and anal margin. Journal of the Royal Society of Medicine 53:416–420, 1960
9. Nigro ND: An evaluation of combined therapy for squamous cell cancer of the anal canal. Dis Colon Rectum 27:763–766, 1984
10. Nigro ND: Treatment of squamous cell cancer of the anus. Cancer Treat Res 18:221–242, 1984
11. Paradis P, Douglass HO Jr, Holyoke ED: The clinical implications of a staging system for carcinoma of the anus. Surg Gynecol Obstet 141:411–416, 1975
12. Salmon RJ, Fenton J, Asselain B et al: Treatment of epidermoid anal canal cancer. Am J Surg 147:43–47, 1984
13. Salmon RJ, Zafrani B, Labib A et al: Prognosis of cloacogenic and squamous cancers of the anal canal. Dis Colon Rectum 29:336–340, 1986
14. Schraut WH, Wang CH, Dawson PJ et al.: Depth of invasion, location, and size of cancer of the anus dictate operative treatment. Cancer 51:1291–1296, 1983
15. Shank B: Treatment of anal canal carcinoma. Cancer (Suppl) 55:2156–2162, 1985
16. Spratt JS, ed: Neoplasms of the Colon, Rectum, and Anus. Philadelphia, WB Saunders Co., 1984.
17. Wittoesch JH, Woolner LB, Jackman RJ: Basal cell epithelioma and basaloid lesions of the anus. Surg Gynecol Obstet 104:75–80, 1957

ANAL CANAL

Data Form for Cancer Staging

Patient identification
Name _____
Address _____
Hospital or clinic number _____
Age _____ Sex _____ Race _____

Institution identification
Hospital or clinic _____
Address _____

Oncology Record

Anatomic site of cancer _____
Histologic type _____
Grade (G) _____
Date of classification _____

Chronology of classification
(use separate form for each time staged)
[ ] Clinical (use all data prior to first treatment)
[ ] Pathologic (if definitively resected specimen available)

Definitions

Primary Tumor (T)
[ ] TX Primary tumor cannot be assessed
[ ] T0 No evidence of primary tumor
[ ] Tis Carcinoma in situ
[ ] T1 Tumor 2 cm or less in greatest dimension
[ ] T2 Tumor more than 2 cm but not more than 5 cm in greatest dimension
[ ] T3 Tumor more than 5 cm in greatest dimension
[ ] T4 Tumor of any size invades adjacent organ(s): vagina, urethra, bladder (involvement of sphincter muscle(s) *alone* is not classified as T4

Lymph Node (N)
[ ] NX Regional lymph nodes cannot be assessed
[ ] N0 No regional lymph node metastasis
[ ] N1 Metastasis in perirectal lymph node(s)
[ ] N2 Metastasis in unilateral internal iliac and/or inguinal lymph node(s)
[ ] N3 Metastasis in perirectal and inguinal lymph nodes and/or bilateral internal iliac and/or inguinal lymph nodes

Distant Metastasis (M)
[ ] MX Presence of distant metastasis cannot be assessed
[ ] M0 No distant metastasis
[ ] M1 Distant metastasis

Stage Grouping

[ ] 0	Tis	N0	M0
[ ] I	T1	N0	M0
[ ] II	T2	N0	M0
	T3	N0	M0
[ ] IIIA	T4	N0	M0
	T1	N1	M0
	T2	N1	M0
	T3	N1	M0
[ ] IIIB	T4	N1	M0
	Any T	N2	M0
	Any T	N3	M0
[ ] IV	Any T	Any N	M1

Histopathologic Type

The staging system applies to all carcinomas arising in the anal canal, including carcinomas that arise within an anorectal fistula. Melanomas are excluded.

Histopathologic Grade (G)

[ ] GX Grade cannot be assessed
[ ] G1 Well differentiated
[ ] G2 Moderately well differentiated
[ ] G3 Poorly differentiated
[ ] G4 Undifferentiated

Sites of Distant Metastasis

Pulmonary   PUL
Osseous   OSS
Hepatic   HEP
Brain   BRA
Lymph nodes LYM
Bone marrow MAR
Pleura   PLE
Peritoneum   PER
Skin   SKI
Other   OTH

Illustration

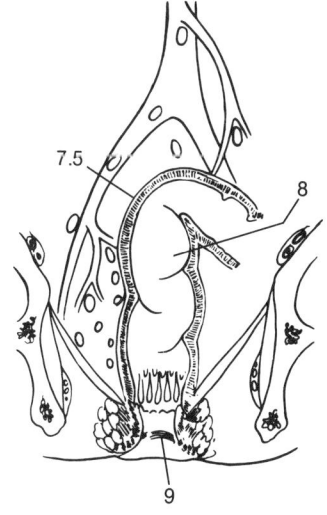

Indicate on diagram primary tumor and regional nodes involved.

Staged by _____ M.D.
_____ Registrar
Date _____

American Joint Committee on Cancer—1988

13

Liver (including intrahepatic bile ducts)

The liver (including intrahepatic bile ducts), the largest parenchymatous organ in the body, is often the site of metastatic cancer, usually from malignant tumors that arise in abdominal viscera, such as in the colon. Primary cancers of the liver are uncommon in the United States, although common in many other countries. Fewer than 300 cases are diagnosed in the United States every year. The liver gives rise to several distinctive malignant tumors that are derived from its various components. These include hepatocellular carcinomas that arise from the hepatocytes, cholangiocarcinomas or intrahepatic bile duct carcinomas that arise from the bile ducts, and various sarcomas that arise from the mesenchymal elements. Hepatocellular carcinomas are often associated with pre-existing liver disease, usually cirrhosis, which may dominate the clinical picture. The liver has a dual blood supply: the hepatic artery, which branches from the celiac artery, and the portal vein, which drains the intestine. Blood from the liver passes through the hepatic vein and enters the inferior vena cava. Hepatocellular carcinomas have a proclivity to invade blood vessels, a fact that is considered in the staging classification.

ANATOMY

Histologically, the liver is divided into lobules. Between the lobules are the portal areas that contain the intrahepatic (ICD-O 155.1) bile ducts.

Primary Site. The liver (ICD-O 155.0) is located in the right upper abdominal cavity below the right leaf of the diaphragm. It extends from the fifth rib and midclavicular line on the left side to the inferior costal margin and midaxillary line on the right side. Covered by a smooth reddish brown capsule, the organ is divided into right and left lobes, the former being much larger. Two smaller lobes, the quadrate and the caudate, are subdivisions of the undersurface of the right lobe. Separated by the gallbladder fossa, the quadrate is on the left and the caudate is on the right. Between the left and right lobes is the porta hepatis through which pass the hepatic artery and its major branches, the portal vein, the extrahepatic bile ducts and lymphatic vessels.

Note: For classification, the plane projecting between the bed of the gallbladder and the inferior vena cava divides the liver into two lobes.

Regional Lymph Nodes. The regional lymph nodes are the hilar (*i.e.*, those in the hepatoduodenal ligament: hepatic and periportal nodes). Any lymph node involvement beyond these nodes is considered distant metastasis for staging purposes and should be coded as M1.

Metastatic Sites. Hepatocellular carcinomas can spread to almost every organ in the body. The most common sites of metastatic spread are to the lungs and to bone. Extension often occurs into the diaphragm.

RULES FOR CLASSIFICATION

T categories are based on the observation of single versus multiple tumor nodules, the size of the largest nodule (2 cm is the discriminating limit), and vascular invasion. The staging system does not deal with etiologic mechanisms such as whether multiple nodules represent multiple, independent primary tumors or intra-hepatic metastasis from a single primary hepatic carcinoma.

Because of the tendency for vascular invasion, imaging of the liver is important for staging primary hepatocellular carcinomas, unless distant metastasis can be demonstrated at the time of diagnosis.

Clinical Staging. Staging depends on some type of imaging procedure to demonstrate the size of the primary tumor and vascular invasion. Surgical exploration is usually not carried out because the chance for complete resection is not great.

DEFINITION OF TNM

Primary Tumor (T)

TX Primary tumor cannot be assessed
T0 No evidence of primary tumor
T1 Solitary tumor 2 cm or less in greatest dimension without vascular invasion
T2 Solitary tumor 2 cm or less in greatest dimension with vascular invasion, *or*
    Multiple tumors limited to one lobe, none more than 2 cm in greatest dimension without vascular invasion, *or*
    A solitary tumor more than 2 cm in greatest dimension without vascular invasion
T3 Solitary tumor more than 2 cm in greatest dimension with vascular invasion, *or*
    Multiple tumors limited to one lobe, none more than 2 cm in greatest dimension, with vascular invasion, *or*
    Multiple tumors limited to one lobe, any more than 2 cm in greatest dimension, with or without vascular invasion
T4 Multiple tumors in more than one lobe *or* Tumor(s) involve(s) a major branch of portal or hepatic vein(s)

Regional Lymph Nodes (N)

NX Regional lymph nodes cannot be assessed
N0 No regional lymph node metastasis
N1 Regional lymph node metastasis

Distant Metastasis (M)

MX Presence of distant metastasis cannot be assessed
M0 No distant metastasis
M1 Distant metastasis

STAGE GROUPING

Stage I	T1	N0	M0
Stage II	T2	N0	M0
Stage III	T1	N1	M0
	T2	N1	M0
	T3	N0, N1	M0
Stage IVA	T4	Any N	M0
Stage IVB	Any T	Any N	M1

DIFFERENCES BETWEEN THE 2ND AND 3RD EDITIONS

This staging classification is a radical change from that published in the 1983 *Manual.* Cirrhosis is no longer considered in the staging classification. Vascular invasion, size, and number of lesions are the important elements in the new system.

HISTOPATHOLOGIC TYPE

The staging system applies to all primary carcinomas of the liver. These include hepatomas or hepatocellular carcinomas and intrahepatic bile duct carcinomas or cholangiocarcinomas, and mixed types. (Hepatomas are by far the most common.) The classification does not apply to sarcomas.

Liver (including intrahepatic bile ducts)

HISTOPATHOLOGIC GRADE (G)

GX Grade cannot be assessed
G1 Well differentiated
G2 Moderately well differentiated
G3 Poorly differentiated
G4 Undifferentiated

BIBLIOGRAPHY

1. Adson MA, Beart RW: Elective hepatic resections. Surg Clin North Am 57:339–360, 1977
2. Bartok I, Remenar E, Toth J et al: Clinico-pathological studies of liver cirrhosis and hepatocellular carcinoma in a general hospital. Hum Pathol 12:794–803, 1981
3. Chuong JJ, Livstone EM, Barwick KW: The histopathologic and clinical indicators of prognosis in hepatoma. J Clin Gastroenterol 4:547–552, 1982
4. Okuda K, Peters RL (eds): Hepatocellular Carcinoma, New York, Wiley Publications, 1976
5. Schaff Z, Lapis K, Henson DE: Liver. In Henson DE, Albores-Saavedra J (eds): The Pathology of Incipient Neoplasia. Philadelphia, WB Saunders, 1986
6. Warvi WN: Primary neoplasms of the liver. Archives of Pathology and Laboratory Medicine 37:367–382, 1944

LIVER (INCLUDING INTRAHEPATIC BILE DUCTS)

Data Form for Cancer Staging

Patient identification
Name _____
Address _____
Hospital or clinic number _____
Age _____ Sex _____ Race _____

Institution identification
Hospital or clinic _____
Address _____

Oncology Record

Anatomic site of cancer _____
Histologic type _____
Grade (G) _____
Date of classification _____

Chronology of classification
(use separate form for each time staged)
[ ] Clinical (use all data prior to first treatment)
[ ] Pathologic (if definitively resected specimen available)

Definitions

Primary Tumor (T)

[ ] TX   Primary tumor cannot be assessed
[ ] T0   No evidence of primary tumor
[ ] T1   Solitary tumor 2 cm or less in greatest dimension without vascular invasion
[ ] T2   Solitary tumor 2 cm or less in greatest dimension with vascular invasion, or
[ ]   Multiple tumors limited to one lobe none more than 2 cm in greatest dimension without vascular invasion, or
[ ]   A solitary tumor more than 2 cm in greatest dimension without vascular invasion
[ ] T3   Solitary tumor more than 2 cm in greatest dimension with vascular invasion, or
[ ]   Multiple tumors limited to one lobe, none more than 2 cm in greatest dimension, with vascular invasion, or
[ ]   Multiple tumors limited to one lobe, any more than 2 cm in greatest dimension, with or without vascular invasion
[ ] T4   Multiple tumors in more than one lobe or
[ ]   Tumor(s) involve(s) a major branch of portal or hepatic vein(s)

Lymph Node (N)

[ ] NX   Regional lymph nodes cannot be assessed
[ ] N0   No regional lymph node metastasis
[ ] N1   Regional lymph node metastasis

Distant Metastasis (M)

[ ] MX   Presence of distant metastasis cannot be assessed
[ ] M0   No distant metastasis
[ ] M1   Distant metastasis

Histopathologic Grade (G)

[ ] GX   Grade cannot be assessed
[ ] G1   Well differentiated
[ ] G2   Moderately well differentiated
[ ] G3   Poorly differentiated
[ ] G4   Undifferentiated

Illustration

Indicate on diagram primary tumor and regional nodes involved.

Histopathologic Type

The staging system applies to all primary carcinomas of the liver. These include hepatomas or hepatocellular carcinomas and intrahepatic bile duct carcinomas or cholangiocarcinomas and mixed types. Hepatomas are by far the most common. There is also a mixed type that is found in the liver. The classification does not apply to sarcomas.

Stage Grouping

	T	N	M
[ ] I	T1	N0	M0
[ ] II	T2	N0	M0
[ ] III	T1	N1	M0
	T2	N1	M0
	T3	N0	M0
	T3	N1	M0
[ ] IVA	T4	Any N	M0
[ ] IVB	Any T	Any N	M1

Staged by _____ M.D.
_____ Registrar
Date _____

American Joint Committee on Cancer—1988

Sites of Distant Metastasis

Pulmonary	PUL
Osseous	OSS
Hepatic	HEP
Brain	BRA
Lymph nodes	LYM
Bone marrow	MAR
Pleura	PLE
Peritoneum	PER
Skin	SKI
Other	OTH

14

Gallbladder

Cancers of the gallbladder are staged according to their level of penetration into the wall and involvement of one or more adjacent organs. Spread of cancer to the liver, which is found in 70% of patients at the time of surgical evaluation, is regarded as regional metastasis, although tumors that have invaded more than 2 cm usually cannot be resected. Malignant tumors of the gallbladder are insidious in their spread, often metastasizing early before a diagnosis is made. This proclivity for early spread before the appearance of signs and symptoms includes all types of malignant tumors known to occur in the gallbladder with the possible exception of papillary carcinoma. Tumors can also perforate the wall of the gallbladder and cause intra-abdominal metastases, carcinomatosis, and ascites. Unfortunately, because gallbladder cancer is relatively uncommon and usually diagnosed late, physicians have tended to ignore anatomic staging, even though its importance for survival, management, and prognosis has been emphasized. Many cases are not suspected clinically and first are discovered at laparotomy or incidentally by the pathologist.

ANATOMY

Primary Site. The gallbladder (ICD-O 156.0) is a pear-shaped saccular organ located under the liver in the gallbladder fossa. It has three parts: a fundus, a body, and a neck that tapers into the cystic duct. The wall of the gallbladder is much thinner than that of the intestine, lacking a thick circular and transverse muscle. The wall has a mucosa, that is, an epithelial lining, and lamina propria, a smooth muscle layer, which is analogous to the muscularis mucosa of the small intestine, perimuscular connective tissue, and serosa. There is no submucosa. Along the attachment to the hepatic surface, no serosa exists, and the perimuscular connective tissue is continuous with the interlobular connective tissue of the liver.

Regional Lymph Nodes. The regional lymph nodes include the following:

Cystic duct
Pericholedochal
Hilar
Celiac
Node of foramen of Winslow
Periduodenal
Periportal
Peripancreatic
Superior mesenteric

Peripancreatic nodes near the body and tail of the pancreas are considered sites of distant metastasis.

Metastatic Sites. Cancers of the gallbladder usually spread to the lungs, pleura, and diaphragm, and intra-abdominally, although any site can be involved.

RULES FOR CLASSIFICATION

Gallbladder cancers are staged primarily on the basis of surgical exploration. Many *in situ* and early stage carcinomas are not recognized grossly and can only be staged pathologically after a histologic diagnosis has been made following examination of the resected specimen.

The staging classification is based on the depth of tumor penetration into the wall, invasion into the liver, and the number of organs adjacent to the gallbladder that are involved with regional spread of the tumor.

Pathologic Staging. Staging is based on imaging, surgical exploration, which is most important, and/or examination of the resected specimen. Involvement of the liver should be confirmed histologically, especially if a hepatic resection is planned. Complete resection of the cancer is not possible in many cases.

DEFINITION OF TNM
Primary Tumor (T)

TX Primary tumor cannot be assessed
T0 No evidence of primary tumor
Tis Carcinoma *in situ*
T1 Tumor invades mucosa or muscle layer
    T1a Tumor invades mucosa
    T1b Tumor invades muscle layer
T2 Tumor invades perimuscular connective tissue; no extension beyond serosa or into liver
T3 Tumor invades beyond serosa or into one adjacent organ, or both (extension 2 cm or less into liver)
T4 Tumor extends more than 2 cm into liver, and/or into two or more adjacent organs (stomach, duodenum, colon, pancreas, omentum, extrahepatic bile ducts, any involvement of liver)

Regional Lymph Nodes (N)

NX Regional lymph nodes cannot be assessed
N0 No regional lymph node metastasis
N1 Regional lymph node metastasis
    N1a Metastasis in cystic duct, pericholedochal, and/or hilar lymph nodes (*i.e.*, in the hepatoduodenal ligament)
    N1b Metastasis in peripancreatic (head only), periduodenal, periportal, celiac, and/or superior mesenteric lymph nodes

Distant Metastasis (M)

MX Presence of distant metastasis cannot be assessed
M0 No distant metastasis
M1 Distant metastasis

STAGE GROUPING

Stage 0	Tis	N0	M0
Stage I	T1	N0	M0
Stage II	T2	N0	M0
Stage III	T1	N1	M0
	T2	N1	M0
	T3	Any N	M0
Stage IV	T4	Any N	M0
	Any T	Any N	M1

DIFFERENCES BETWEEN THE 2ND AND 3RD EDITIONS

The staging classification in this edition is essentially the same as that published in the 1983 edition of the *Manual*, except for the division of the lymph nodes into N1a and N1b, and the separation of the T1 category into T1a and T1b.

Histopathologic Type

The staging system applies to all primary carcinomas and adenocarcinomas, which include the following types. Other types of malignant tumors are rare in the gallbladder. It is important to record the histologic type because some have a better prognosis than others. Papillary carcinomas have the best prognosis.

Well differentiated
Papillary

Gallbladder

Intestinal type
Pleomorphic giant cell
Poorly differentiated, small cell
Signet ring cell
Clear cell
Colloid
Adenocarcinoma with choriocarcinoma-like areas
Squamous cell
Adenosquamous
Oat cell (small cell)

Histopathologic Grade (G)

GX Grade cannot be assessed
G1 Well differentiated
G2 Moderately well differentiated
G3 Poorly differentiated
G4 Undifferentiated

BIBLIOGRAPHY

1. Albores-Saavedra J, Cruz-Ortiz H, Alcantara-Vazquez A et al: Unusual types of gallbladder carcinoma. Arch Pathol Lab Med 105:287–293, 1981
2. Albores-Saavedra J, Henson DE: Extrahepatic biliary system. In Henson and Albores-Saavedra (eds): The Pathology of Incipient Neoplasia. Philadelphia, WB Saunders, 1986
3. Albores-Saavedra J, Henson DE: Tumors of the gallbladder and extrahepatic bile ducts. Atlas of Tumor Pathology, Fascicle 22, Second Series, Washington, DC, Armed Forces Institute of Pathology, 1986
4. Bergdahl L: Gallbladder carcinoma first diagnosed at microscopic examination of gallbladder removed for presumed benign disease. Ann Surg 191:19–22, 1980
5. Bivins BA, Meeker WR Jr, Griffen WO Jr: Importance of histologic classification of carcinoma of the gallbladder. Ann Surg 41:121–124, 1975
6. Fahim RB, McDonald JR, Richards JC et al: Carcinoma of the gallbladder: A study of its modes of spread. Ann Surg 156:114–124, 1962
7. Lurie BB, Loewenstein MS, Zamcheck N: Elevated carcinoembryonic antigen levels and biliary tract obstruction. JAMA 233:326–330, 1975
8. Nevin JE, Moran TJ, Day S et al: Carcinoma of the gallbladder: Staging, treatment, and prognosis. Cancer 37:141–148, 1976
9. Perpetuo MMO, Valdivieso M, Heilbrun LK et al: Natural history study of gallbladder cancer. Cancer 42:330–335, 1978
10. Richard PF, Cantin J: Primary carcinoma of the gallbladder: Study of 108 cases. Can J Surg 19:27–32, 1976
11. Wanebo HJ, Castle WN, Fechner R: Is carcinoma of the gallbladder a curable lesion? Ann Surg 195:624–630, 1982

GALLBLADDER

Data Form for Cancer Staging

Patient identification
Name _____
Address _____
Hospital or clinic number _____
Age _____ Sex _____ Race _____

Institution identification
Hospital or clinic _____
Address _____

Oncology Record

Anatomic site of cancer _____
Histologic type _____
Grade (G) _____
Date of classification _____

Chronology of classification
 (use separate form for each time staged)
[ ] Clinical (use all data prior to first treatment)
[ ] Pathologic (if definitively resected specimen available)

Definitions

Primary Tumor (T)

[ ] TX Primary tumor cannot be assessed
[ ] T0 No evidence of primary tumor
[ ] Tis Carcinoma in situ
[ ] T1 Tumor invades mucosa or muscle layer
  [ ] T1a Tumor invades mucosa
  [ ] T1b Tumor invades muscle layer
[ ] T2 Tumor invades perimuscular connective tissue; no extension beyond serosa or into liver
[ ] T3 Tumor invades beyond serosa or into one adjacent organ, or both (extension 2 cm or less into liver)
[ ] T4 Tumor extends more than 2 cm into liver, and/or into two or more adjacent organs (stomach, duodenum, colon, pancreas, omentum, extrahepatic bile ducts, any involvement of liver)

Lymph Node (N)

[ ] NX Regional lymph nodes cannot be assessed
[ ] N0 No regional lymph node metastasis
[ ] N1 Regional lymph node metastasis
  [ ] N1a Metastasis in cystic duct, pericholedochal, and/or hilar lymph nodes, i.e., in hepatoduodenal ligament
  [ ] N1b Metastasis in peripancreatic (head only), periduodenal, periportal, celiac, and/or superior mesenteric lymph nodes

Distant Metastasis (M)

[ ] MX Presence of distant metastasis cannot be assessed
[ ] M0 No distant metastasis
[ ] M1 Distant metastasis

Stage Grouping

[ ] 0	Tis	N0	M0
[ ] I	T1	N0	M0
[ ] II	T2	N0	M0
[ ] III	T1	N1	M0
	T2	N1	M0
	T3	Any N	M0
[ ] IV	T4	Any N	M0
	Any T	Any N	M1

Histopathologic Type

The staging system applies to all primary carcinomas and adenocarcinomas, which include the following types. Other types of malignant tumors are rare in the gallbladder. It is important to record the histologic type because some have a better prognosis than others. Papillary carcinomas have the best prognosis.

Well differentiated
Papillary
Intestinal type
Pleomorphic giant cell
Poorly differentiated, small cell
Signet ring cell
Clear cell
Colloid
Adenocarcinoma with choriocarcinoma-like areas
Squamous cell
Adenosquamous
Oat cell (small cell)

Histopathologic Grade (G)

[ ] GX Grade cannot be assessed
[ ] G1 Well differentiated
[ ] G2 Moderately well differentiated
[ ] G3 Poorly differentiated
[ ] G4 Undifferentiated

Illustration

Indicate on diagram primary tumor and regional nodes involved.

Staged by _____ M.D.
_____ Registrar
Date _____

Sites of Distant Metastasis

Pulmonary	PUL
Osseous	OSS
Hepatic	HEP
Brain	BRA
Lymph nodes	LYM
Bone marrow	MAR
Pleura	PLE
Peritoneum	PER
Skin	SKI
Other	OTH

15

Extrahepatic Bile Ducts

Malignant tumors can develop in any segment of the extrahepatic bile ducts. Nearly 50% are found in the upper third, 25% in the middle third, and 19% in the lower third. In nearly 10% of all cases, the ducts are diffusely involved. Tumors that arise near the hilum of the liver are most difficult to resect. As a result, they have the worst prognosis. All malignant tumors invariably cause partial or complete obstruction of the extrahepatic bile ducts and proximal distention. Clinical symptoms often occur while the tumor is relatively small, before widespread dissemination. This staging classification applies only to cancers arising in the extrahepatic bile ducts and does not include those arising in the ampulla of Vater or in the pancreatic ducts. Malignant epithelial tumors that arise in the right or left hepatic ducts are often referred to as *hilar carcinomas of the liver.*

ANATOMY

Primary Site. Emerging from the transverse fissure of the liver are the right and left hepatic bile ducts (ICD-O 156.1), which join to form the common hepatic duct. The cystic duct, which connects to the gallbladder, joins the common hepatic duct to form the common bile duct, which passes behind the first part of the duodenum and then traverses the head of the pancreas until it opens into the second part of the duodenum at the ampulla of Vater. The bile ducts are lined by a single layer of tall columnar cells. The mucosa usually forms irregular pleats or small folds that run longitudinally. The wall of the bile duct has a layer of subepithelial connective tissue and muscle fibers.

Regional Lymph Nodes. The regional nodes are essentially the same as for the gallbladder, but also include those located near the duodenum and head of the pancreas. They include the following:

Cystic node
Superior mesenteric
Periduodenal
Node on the anterior border of the foramen of Winslow
Superior retropancreaticoduodenal
Posterior pancreaticoduodenal
Peripancreatic
Periportal
Pericholedochal
Celiac

Any lymph node involvement beyond these nodes is considered distant metastasis for staging purposes and should be coded M1.

Metastatic Sites. Carcinomas can extend to the liver, pancreas, ampulla of Vater, duodenum, colon, omentum, stomach, or gallbladder. Tumors arising in the right or left hepatic ducts usually extend proximally into the liver or distal to the common hepatic duct. Neoplasms from the cystic duct invade the gallbladder and/or the common bile duct. Carcinomas that arise in the distal segment of the common duct can spread to the pancreas, duodenum, stomach, colon, or omentum. Distant metastases usually occur late in the course of the disease, most often to the lungs.

RULES FOR CLASSIFICATION

Most cancers are staged following surgery and pathologic examination of the resected specimen. Evaluation of the extent of disease at laparotomy is most important for staging.

Clinical Staging. See Pathologic Staging.

Pathologic Staging. Staging depends on imaging, which often defines the limits of the tumor, and surgical exploration with pathologic examination of the resected specimen. It may be difficult to completely resect the primary tumor in many cases.

DEFINITION OF TNM

Primary Tumor (T)

TX Primary tumor cannot be assessed
T0 No evidence of primary tumor
Tis Carcinoma *in situ*
T1 Tumor invades mucosa or muscle layer
    T1a Tumor invades mucosa
    T1b Tumor invades muscle layer
T2 Tumor invades perimuscular connective tissue
T3 Tumor invades adjacent structures: liver, pancreas, duodenum, gallbladder, colon, stomach

Regional Lymph Nodes (N)

NX Regional lymph nodes cannot be assessed
N0 No regional lymph node metastasis
N1 Regional lymph node metastasis
    N1a Metastasis in cystic duct, pericholedochal and/or hilar lymph nodes (*i.e.*, in the hepatoduodenal ligament)
    N1b Metastasis in peripancreatic (head only), periduodenal, periportal, celiac, and/or superior mesenteric lymph nodes

Distant Metastasis (M)

MX Presence of distant metastasis cannot be assessed
M0 No distant metastasis
M1 Distant metastasis

STAGE GROUPING

Stage	T	N	M
Stage 0	Tis	N0	M0
Stage I	T1	N0	M0
Stage II	T2	N0	M0
Stage III	T1	N1	M0
	T2	N1	M0
Stage IVA	T3	Any N	M0
Stage IVB	Any T	Any N	M1

DIFFERENCES BETWEEN THE 2ND AND 3RD EDITIONS

The new classification simplifies the T categories, having only 3 instead of the previous 4. Also, for greater precision in classification, T1 has been subdivided into T1a and T1b and N1 has been separated into N1a and N1b.

HISTOPATHOLOGIC TYPE

The staging system applies to all primary carcinomas that arise in the extrahepatic bile ducts. Histologically, these are the same as those found in the gallbladder. Other types of malignant tumors are exceedingly rare.

SITE-SPECIFIC INFORMATION

Recording the location of the primary tumor is important for prognosis. However, it is often difficult to establish with certainty the origin of these tumors when the pathologic process is far advanced.

Location of tumor ( ) Upper third
( ) Middle third
( ) Lower third
( ) Diffuse

HISTOPATHOLOGIC GRADE (G)

GX Grade cannot be assessed
G1 Well differentiated
G2 Moderately well differentiated
G3 Poorly differentiated
G4 Undifferentiated

BIBLIOGRAPHY

1. Albores-Saavedra J, Henson DE: Tumors of the Gallbladder and Extrahepatic Bile Ducts. Atlas of Tumor Pathology, Fascicle 22, Second Series. Washington, DC, Armed Forces Institute of Pathology, 1986
2. Braasch JW, Warren KW, Kune GA: Malignant neoplasms of the bile ducts. Surg Clin North Am 47: 627–638, 1967
3. Krain LS: Gallbladder and extrahepatic bile duct carcinoma. Geriatrics 27:111–117, 1972
4. Longmire WP Jr, McArthur MS, Bastounis EA et al: Carcinoma of the extrahepatic biliary tract. Ann Surg 178:333–343, 1973
5. Tompkins RK, Thomas D, Wile A et al: Prognostic factors in bile duct carcinoma. Ann Surg 194:447–455, 1981
6. Wanebo JH, Grimes OF: Cancer of the bile duct: The occult malignancy. Am J Surg 130:262–268, 1975

EXTRAHEPATIC BILE DUCTS

Data Form for Cancer Staging

Patient identification
Name _____
Address _____
Hospital or clinic number _____
Age _____ Sex _____ Race _____

Institution identification
Hospital or clinic _____
Address _____

Oncology Record

Anatomic site of cancer _____
Histologic type _____
Grade (G) _____
Date of classification _____

Chronology of classification
 (use separate form for each time staged)
[ ] Clinical (use all data prior to first treatment)
[ ] Pathologic (if definitively resected specimen available)

Definitions

Primary Tumor (T)
[ ] TX Primary tumor cannot be assessed
[ ] T0 No evidence of primary tumor
[ ] Tis Carcinoma *in situ*
[ ] T1 Tumor invades mucosa or muscle layer
  [ ] T1a Tumor invades mucosa
  [ ] T1b Tumor invades muscle layer
[ ] T2 Tumor invades perimuscular connective tissue
[ ] T3 Tumor invades adjacent structure(s), liver, pancreas, duodenum, gallbladder, colon, and/or stomach

Lymph Node (N)
[ ] NX Regional lymph nodes cannot be assessed
[ ] N0 No regional lymph node metastasis
[ ] N1 Regional lymph node metastasis
  [ ] N1a Metastasis in cystic duct, pericholedochal and/or hilar lymph nodes
  [ ] N1b Metastasis in peripancreatic (head only), periduodenal, periportal, celiac, and/or superior mesenteric lymph nodes

Distant Metastasis (M)
[ ] MX Presence of distant metastasis cannot be assessed
[ ] M0 No distant metastasis
[ ] M1 Distant metastasis

Stage Grouping

[ ] 0	Tis	N0	M0
[ ] I	T1	N0	M0
[ ] II	T2	N0	M0
[ ] III	T1	N1	M0
	T2	N1	M0
[ ] IVA	T3	Any N	M0
[ ] IVB	Any T	Any N	M1

Histopathologic Grade (G)

[ ] GX Grade cannot be assessed
[ ] G1 Well differentiated
[ ] G2 Moderately well differentiated
[ ] G3 Poorly differentiated
[ ] G4 Undifferentiated

Illustration

Upper third
Middle third
Lower third
Diffuse

Indicate on diagram primary tumor and regional nodes involved.

Histopathologic Type

The staging system applies to all primary carcinomas and adenocarcinomas, which include the following types. Other types of malignant tumors are rare in the gallbladder. It is important to record the histologic type because some have a better prognosis than others. Papillary carcinomas have the best prognosis.

Well differentiated
Papillary
Intestinal type
Pleomorphic giant cell
Poorly differentiated, small cell
Signet ring cell
Clear cell
Colloid
Adenocarcinoma with choriocarcinoma-like areas
Squamous cell
Adenosquamous
Oat cell (small cell)

Staged by _____ M.D.
_____ Registrar
Date _____

Sites of Distant Metastasis

Pulmonary	PUL
Osseous	OSS
Hepatic	HEP
Brain	BRA
Lymph nodes	LYM
Bone marrow	MAR
Pleura	PLE
Peritoneum	PER
Skin	SKI
Other	OTH

16

Ampulla of Vater

The importance of the ampulla of Vater is in its strategic location. Most tumors that arise in this small structure will obstruct the common bile duct, causing severe jaundice. Clinically, cancers of the ampulla may be difficult to differentiate from those arising in the head of the pancreas or even in the distal segment of the common bile duct, especially if they become large and bulky. Primary cancers of the ampulla are not common, although they comprise a high proportion of the malignant tumors found in the duodenum.

ANATOMY

Primary Site. A small dilated duct, less than 1.5 cm in length, the ampulla (ICD-O 156.2) is formed in most individuals by the union of the terminal segments of the pancreatic and common bile ducts. In 25% of individuals, however, the ampulla is the termination of the common duct only, the pancreatic duct having its own entrance into the duodenum, adjacent to the ampulla. In these individuals, the ampulla may be difficult to define or even nonexistent. The ampulla opens into the duodenum, usually on the posterior-medial wall, through a small mucosal elevation—the duodenal papilla, which is also called the papilla of Vater. The ampulla is lined by tall columnar epithelium similar to that found along the common bile duct. Although carcinomas can arise in either the ampulla or on the papilla, they most commonly arise near the junction of the mucosa of the ampulla with that of the papilla. Nearly all cancers that arise in this area are well-differentiated adenocarcinomas. They may have a variety of designations, for example: carcinoma of the ampulla of Vater; carcinoma of the periampullary portion of the duodenum; or carcinoma of the peripapillary portion of the duodenum.

Regional Lymph Nodes. The regional lymph nodes of the ampulla of Vater are:

Superior: Lymph nodes superior to the head and body of the pancreas

Inferior: Lymph nodes inferior to the head and body of the pancreas

Anterior: Anterior pancreaticoduodenal, pyloric and proximal mesenteric lymph nodes

Posterior: Posterior pancreaticoduodenal, common bile duct, and proximal mesenteric

Note: The splenic lymph nodes and those at the tail of the pancreas are not regional lymph nodes; metastases to these lymph nodes are coded as M1.

Metastatic Sites. Tumors of the ampulla can spread to almost every site. However, they usually infiltrate adjacent structures at an early stage, such as the wall of the duodenum, the head of the pancreas, and the extrahepatic bile ducts. Spread to distant sites usually occurs late in the course of the disease.

RULES FOR CLASSIFICATION

Most patients are staged pathologically after examination of the surgically resected specimen. Classification is based primarily on size and local extension.

Clinical Staging. See Pathologic Staging.

Pathologic Staging. Staging depends on surgical resection and pathologic examination of the specimen and associated lymph nodes.

DEFINITION OF TNM

Primary Tumor (T)

TX Primary tumor cannot be assessed
T0 No evidence of primary tumor
Tis Carcinoma *in situ*
T1 Tumor limited to the ampulla of Vater
T2 Tumor invades duodenal wall
T3 Tumor invades 2 cm or less into the pancreas
T4 Tumor invades more than 2 cm into the pancreas and/or into other adjacent organs

Regional Lymph Nodes (N)

NX Regional lymph nodes cannot be assessed
N0 No regional lymph node metastasis
N1 Regional lymph node metastasis

Distant Metastasis (M)

MX Presence of distant metastasis cannot be assessed
M0 No distant metastasis
M1 Distant metastasis

STAGE GROUPING

Stage 0	Tis	N0	M0
Stage I	T1	N0	M0
Stage II	T2	N0	M0
	T3	N0	M0
Stage III	T1	N1	M0
	T2	N1	M0
	T3	N1	M0
Stage IV	T4	Any N	M0
	Any T	Any N	M1

DIFFERENCES BETWEEN THE 2ND AND 3RD EDITIONS

This is a new TNM classification for the ampulla of Vater.

HISTOPATHOLOGIC TYPE

The staging system applies to all primary carcinomas that arise in the ampulla or on the papilla. Adenocarcinomas are the most common type.

HISTOPATHOLOGIC GRADE (G)

GX Grade cannot be assessed
G1 Well differentiated
G2 Moderately well differentiated
G3 Poorly differentiated
G4 Undifferentiated

BIBLIOGRAPHY

1. Braasch JW, Camer SJ: Periampullary carcinoma. Med Clin North Am, 59:309–314, 1975
2. Edmondson HA: Tumors of the gallbladder and extrahepatic bile ducts. Atlas of Tumor Pathology, Fascicle 26, Section 7. Armed Forces Institute of Pathology, Washington, DC, 1967
3. Knox RA, Kingston RD. Carcinoma of the ampulla of Vater. Br J Surg 73:72–73, 1986
4. Makipour H, Cooperman A, Danzi JT et al: Carcinoma of the ampulla of Vater. Ann Surg 183:341–344, 1976
5. Wise L, Pizzimbono C, Dehner IP: Periampullary cancer. Am J Surg 131:141–148, 1976

AMPULLA OF VATER

Data Form for Cancer Staging

Patient identification
Name _____
Address _____
Hospital or clinic number _____
Age _____ Sex _____ Race _____

Institution identification
Hospital or clinic _____
Address _____

Oncology Record

Anatomic site of cancer _____
Histologic type _____
Grade (G) _____
Date of classification _____

Chronology of classification
  (use separate form for each time staged)
[ ] Clinical (use all data prior to first treatment)
[ ] Pathologic (if definitively resected specimen available)

Definitions

Primary Tumor (T)

[ ] TX   Primary tumor cannot be assessed
[ ] T0   No evidence of primary tumor
[ ] Tis Carcinoma *in situ*
[ ] T1   Tumor limited to ampulla of Vater
[ ] T2   Tumor invades duodenal wall
[ ] T3   Tumor invades 2 cm or less into pancreas
[ ] T4   Tumor invades more than 2.0 cm into pancreas and/or into other adjacent organs

Lymph Node (N)

[ ] NX   Regional lymph nodes cannot be assessed
[ ] N0   No regional lymph node metastasis
[ ] N1   Regional lymph node metastasis

Distant Metastasis (M)

[ ] MX   Presence of distant metastasis cannot be assessed
[ ] M0   No distant metastasis
[ ] M1   Distant metastasis

Stage Grouping

[ ]	0	Tis	N0	M0
[ ]	I	T1	N0	M0
[ ]	II	T2	N0	M0
		T3	N0	M0
[ ]	III	T1	N1	M0
		T2	N1	M0
		T3	N1	M0
[ ]	IV	T4	Any N	M0
		Any T	Any N	M1

Histopathologic Grade (G)

[ ] GX   Grade cannot be assessed
[ ] G1   Well differentiated
[ ] G2   Moderately well differentiated
[ ] G3   Poorly differentiated
[ ] G4   Undifferentiated

Location in Pancreas

[ ] Head
[ ] Body
[ ] Tail
[ ] Diffuse
Size (largest diameter) _____ cm

Illustration

Indicate on diagram primary tumor and regional nodes involved.

Histopathologic Type

The staging system applies to all primary carcinomas that arise in the ampulla or on the papilla. Adenocarcinomas are the most common type.

Sites of Distant Metastasis

Pulmonary   PUL
Osseous   OSS
Hepatic   HEP
Brain   BRA
Lymph nodes   LYM
Bone marrow   MAR
Pleura   PLE
Peritoneum   PER
Skin   SKI
Other   OTH

Staged by _____ M.D.
_____ Registrar
Date _____

17

Exocrine Pancreas

In the United States, pancreatic cancer is the third most common malignancy of the gastrointestinal tract. The disease is often difficult to diagnose, especially in the early stages. Cancers of the exocrine pancreas are almost always fatal. Nearly all patients die within 2 years following diagnosis. Most cancers arise in the head of the pancreas, eventually causing extrahepatic bile duct obstruction and clinical jaundice. Cancers arising in either the body or the tail of the pancreas are insidious in their development and often far advanced when first detected. Most cancers are adenocarcinomas that can arise from either the pancreatic ducts or from the acini. There are no known predisposing or etiological factors. Tumors of the islets of Langerhans are relatively rare and are not covered by this staging classification. Staging depends on the size and extension of the primary tumor.

ANATOMY

Primary Site. The exocrine pancreas (head, ICD-O 157.0; body, 157.1; tail, 157.2; duct, 157.3; and pancreas, 157.9) is a long, coarsely lobulated gland that lies transversely in the posterior abdomen. It is located retroperitoneally in the concavity of the duodenum on its right end and touching the spleen with its left end or tail. The shape of the pancreas can be compared to the letter "J" placed sideways. The organ is divided into a head with a small uncinate process, a neck, a body, and a tail that is usually in contact with the spleen. The body is in direct relation anteriorly with the stomach and posteriorly with the aorta, splenic veins, and left kidney.

Regional Lymph Nodes. There is a rich lymphatic network surrounding the pancreas, with left splenic and superior and inferior right side truncal drainage. The regional lymph nodes are the peripancreatic nodes, which may be subdivided as follows:

Superior: Lymph nodes superior to the head and body of the pancreas

Inferior: Lymph nodes inferior to the head and body of the pancreas

Anterior: Anterior pancreaticoduodenal, pyloric, and proximal mesenteric lymph nodes

Posterior: Posterior pancreaticoduodenal, common bile duct or pericholedochal, and proximal mesenteric nodes

Splenic: Hilum of the spleen and tail of the pancreas

The following nodes are also considered regional:

Peripancreatic
Hepatic artery
Infrapyloric (for tumors in the head only)
Subpyloric (for tumors in the head only)
Celiac (for tumors in the head only)
Superior mesenteric
Pancreaticolienal (for tumors in the body and tail only)
Splenic (for tumors in the body and tail only)
Retroperitoneal
Lateral aortic

All other nodes are considered distant and should be coded as M1. The peripancreatic lymph nodes are often referred to as the superior pancreatic, anterior pancreatic, and inferior pancreatic.

Metastatic Sites. Distant spread occurs mainly to the liver and lungs. Other sites can also be involved including the bones.

RULES FOR CLASSIFICATION

Clinical Staging. The pancreas is inaccessible to physical examination. Laboratory and radiographic procedures are available but are largely diagnostic and investigative. These include imaging procedures such as ultrasonic scanning and computed tomography, along with cytology and laparoscopy. Laparotomy and surgical exploration of the pancreas with biopsy is a more accurate means of assessing the extent of the tumor and staging the patient.

Pathologic Staging. Complete or subtotal resection of the pancreas along with the tumor and associated regional lymph nodes provides the information necessary for staging. A single TNM classification serves both clinical and pathologic staging. The anatomic subdivisions are as follows:

Tumors of the head of the pancreas are those arising to the right of the left border of the superior mesenteric vein. The uncinate process is considered as part of the head.

Tumors of the body of the pancreas are those arising between the left border of the superior mesenteric vein and the left border of the aorta.

Tumors of the tail of the pancreas are those arising between the left border of the aorta and the hilum of the spleen.

DEFINITION OF TNM

Primary Tumor (T)

TX Primary tumor cannot be assessed
T0 No evidence of primary tumor
T1 Tumor limited to the pancreas
    T1a Tumor 2 cm or less in greatest dimension
    T1b Tumor more than 2 cm in greatest dimension
T2 Tumor extends directly to the duodenum, bile duct, or peripancreatic tissues
T3 Tumor extends directly to the stomach, spleen, colon, or adjacent large vessels

Regional Lymph Nodes (N)

NX Regional lymph nodes cannot be assessed
N0 No regional lymph node metastasis
N1 Regional lymph node metastasis

Distant Metastasis (M)

MX Presence of distant metastasis cannot be assessed
M0 No distant metastasis
M1 Distant metastasis

STAGE GROUPING

Stage	T	N	M
Stage I	T1	N0	M0
	T2	N0	M0
Stage II	T3	N0	M0
Stage III	Any T	N1	M0
Stage IV	Any T	Any N	M1

DIFFERENCES BETWEEN THE 2ND AND 3RD EDITIONS

In the new classification, T1 is subdivided into T1a and T1b based on the size of the primary tumor. For T2 and T3, the anatomic sites are specified and the term "surgical resection" is no longer used. The staging categories also have been redefined.

HISTOPATHOLOGIC TYPE

The staging system applies to all carcinomas. Endocrine tumors and carcinoids are excluded. The following carcinomas are included:

Duct cell carcinoma
Pleomorphic giant cell carcinoma
Giant cell carcinoma, osteoclastoid type
Adenocarcinoma
Adenosquamous carcinoma
Mucinous (colloid) carcinoma
Cystadenocarcinoma
Acinar cell adenocarcinoma
Papillary carcinoma
Small cell (oat cell) carcinoma
Pancreaticoblastoma
Mixed cell type
Carcinoma, NOS

HISTOPATHOLOGIC GRADE (G)

GX Grade cannot be assessed
G1 Well differentiated
G2 Moderately well differentiated
G3 Poorly differentiated
G4 Undifferentiated

BIBLIOGRAPHY

1. Compagno J, Oertel JE: Mucinous cystic neoplasms of the pancreas with overt and latent malignancy (cystadenocarcinoma and cystadenoma). Am J Clin Pathol 69:573–580, 1978
2. Cubilla AL, Fitzgerald PJ: Tumors of the exocrine pancreas. Atlas of Tumor Pathology, Second Series, Fascicle 19, Armed Forces Institute of Pathology, Washington, DC, 1984
3. Cubilla AL, Fortner J, Fitzgerald PJ: Lymph node involvement in carcinoma of the head of the pancreas area. Cancer 41:880–887, 1978
4. Gullick HD: Carcinoma of the pancreas: A review and critical study of 100 cases. Medicine 38:47–84, 1959
5. Levison DA: Carcinoma of the pancreas. J Pathol 129:203–223, 1979
6. Moossa AR, Levin B: The diagnosis of "early" pancreatic cancer. Cancer 47:1688–1697, 1981
7. Pollard HM et al: Staging of cancer of the pancreas. Cancer 47:1631–1637, 1981
8. Sugarbaker EV: Patterns of metastasis in human malignancies. In Fidler IJ (ed): Cancer Metastases. New York, Marcel Dekker, 1977

EXOCRINE PANCREAS

Data Form for Cancer Staging

Patient identification
Name _____
Address _____
Hospital or clinic number _____
Age _____ Sex _____ Race _____

Institution identification
Hospital or clinic _____
Address _____

Oncology Record

Anatomic site of cancer _____
Histologic type _____
Grade (G) _____
Date of classification _____

Chronology of classification
(use separate form for each time staged)
[ ] Clinical (use all data prior to first treatment)
[ ] Pathologic (if definitively resected specimen available)

Definitions

Primary Tumor (T)

[ ] TX Primary tumor cannot be assessed
[ ] T0 No evidence of primary tumor
[ ] T1 Tumor limited to the pancreas
  [ ] T1a Tumor 2 cm or less in greatest dimension
  [ ] T1b Tumor more than 2 cm in greatest dimension
[ ] T2 Tumor extends directly to the duodenum, bile duct, or peripancreatic tissues
[ ] T3 Tumor extends directly to the stomach, spleen, colon, or adjacent large vessels

Lymph Node (N)

[ ] NX Regional lymph nodes cannot be assessed
[ ] N0 No regional lymph node metastasis
[ ] N1 Regional lymph node metastasis

Distant Metastasis (M)

[ ] MX Presence of distant metastasis cannot be assessed
[ ] M0 No distant metastasis
[ ] M1 Distant metastasis

Illustration

Indicate on diagram primary tumor and regional nodes involved.

Histopathologic Type

The staging system applies to all primary carcinomas that arise in the ampulla or on the papilla. Adenocarcinomas are the most common type.

Stage Grouping

Stage	T	N	M
Stage I	T1	N0	M0
	T2	N0	M0
Stage II	T3	N0	M0
Stage III	Any T	N1	M0
Stage IV	Any T	Any N	M1

Sites of Distant Metastasis

Pulmonary PUL
Osseous OSS
Hepatic HEP
Brain BRA
Lymph nodes LYM
Bone marrow MAR
Pleura PLE
Peritoneum PER
Skin SKI
Other OTH

Histopathologic Grade (G)

[ ] GX Grade cannot be assessed
[ ] G1 Well differentiated
[ ] G2 Moderately well differentiated
[ ] G3 Poorly differentiated
[ ] G4 Undifferentiated

Location in Pancreas

[ ] Head
[ ] Body
[ ] Tail
[ ] Diffuse
Size (largest diameter) _____ cm

Staged by _____ M.D.
_____ Registrar
Date _____

American Joint Committee on Cancer—1988

LUNG

18

Lung cancers are one of the few cancers that have a known etiology. If present trends continue, lung cancer will become the leading cause of cancer deaths in women, surpassing breast cancer. The disease is difficult to treat and the 5-year survival is less than 15%. For these reasons, control of this disease is directed at its prevention. Though somewhat complex, the staging of lung cancer is based on the extent of disease, location of the primary tumor, and the associated clinical complications. Important for staging and patient evaluation is the assessment of both extrapulmonic and extrathoracic metastasis.*

ANATOMY

Primary Site. The mucosa lining the bronchus is the usual site of origin for carcinoma of the lung (ICD-O 162.2–162.9). The trachea, which lies in the anterior mediastinum, divides into the right and left main bronchi, which extend into the right and left lungs, respectively, and then further subdivide into the lobar bronchi for the upper, middle, and lower lobes on the right and the upper and lower lobes on the left. The lungs are encased in membranes called the visceral pleura and the inside of the chest cavity is lined by a similar membrane called the parietal pleura. The potential space between these two membranes is the pleural space. The lungs are separated in the midline by the mediastinum, which contains the heart, thymus, great vessels, and other structures.

Regional Lymph Nodes. The regional lymph nodes are the intrathoracic, scalene, and supraclavicular nodes. The intrathoracic nodes include:

---

*Permission was given by the AJCC for presentation of the lung classification at a national meeting and for publication while this manual was in preparation (bibliography entry 13).

115

Peribronchial
Intrapulmonic
Hilar
Paratracheal
Anterior mediastinal
Posterior mediastinal
Paraesophageal
Aortic
Carinal
Subcarinal
Pretracheal

Metastatic Sites. The most common metastatic sites are the cervical lymph nodes, liver, brain, bones, adrenal glands, kidneys, and the contralateral lung. No organ is safe.

RULES FOR CLASSIFICATION

Clinical Staging. The clinical staging is based on the anatomic extent of disease that can be demonstrated before instituting definitive therapy. This includes a medical history, physical examination, various imaging procedures, endoscopic studies (including bronchoscopy, esophagoscopy, mediastinoscopy, mediastinotomy, thoracentesis or thoracoscopy), and other tests designed to demonstrate extrathoracic metastasis and regional extension.

To aid in the classification of pleural effusion, a footnote has been added to the T categories regarding the implications of pleural fluid as a staging variable. Patients with a malignant pleural effusion are coded as T4.

Lung cancer detected by sputum cytology but not seen radiographically or during bronchoscopy is known as occult carcinoma and is coded as TX. Occult cancers without evidence of regional lymph node involvement or distant metastasis are coded as TX, N0, M0.

Vocal cord paralysis, superior vena caval obstruction, and compression of the trachea or the esophagus are usually related to metastases in the mediastinal lymph nodes and should be classified as N2 or N3, depending on whether the nodes are ipsilateral or contralateral.

T2 is used when there is direct extension into the visceral pleura, but T3 is used if the lesion invades directly the parietal pleura covering the mediastinum and pericardium as well as that lining the chest wall and covering the diaphragm. A discontinuous lesion outside the parietal pleura in the chest wall or in the diaphragm should be designated as M1.

Many cases of lung cancer will be staged clinically and treated by radiation.

Pathologic Staging. Pathologic staging is based on the information obtained from clinical staging, from thoracotomy, and from the pathologic examination of the resected specimen, including lymph nodes. The histologic type of cancer should be recorded because it has a bearing on prognosis. The same classification is used for both clinical and pathologic staging.

Multiple synchronous tumors of different histologic cell types should be considered separate primary lung cancers and each one should be staged separately.

DEFINITION OF TNM
Primary Tumor (T)

TX Primary tumor cannot be assessed, or tumor proven by the presence of malignant cells in sputum or bronchial washings but not visualized by imaging or bronchoscopy

T0 No evidence of primary tumor

Tis Carcinoma *in situ*

T1 Tumor 3 cm or less in greatest dimension, surrounded by lung or visceral pleura, without bronchoscopic evidence of invasion more proximal than the lobar bronchus,* (*i.e.*, not in the main bronchus)

T2 Tumor with *any* of the following features of size or extent:
- More than 3 cm in greatest dimension
- Involves main bronchus, 2 cm or more distal to the carina
- Invades the visceral pleura
- Associated with atelectasis or obstructive pneumonitis that extends to the hilar region but does not involve the entire lung

T3 Tumor of any size that directly invades any of the following: chest wall (including superior sulcus tumors), diaphragm, mediastinal pleura, parietal pericardium; or tumor in the main bronchus less than 2 cm distal to the carina* but without involvement of the carina; or associated atelectasis or obstructive pneumonitis of the entire lung

T4 Tumor of any size that invades any of the following: mediastinum, heart, great vessels, trachea, esophagus, vertebral body, carina; or tumor with a malignant pleural effusion.†

Note: The uncommon superficial tumor of any size with its invasive component limited to the bronchial wall, which may extend proximal to the main bronchus, is also classified T1.

Lung

†*Note: Most pleural effusions associated with lung cancer are due to tumor. However, there are a few patients in whom multiple cytopathologic examinations of pleural fluid are negative for tumor. In these cases, fluid is non-bloody and is not an exudate. When these elements and clinical judgment dictate that the effusion is not related to the tumor, the effusion should be excluded as a staging element and the patient should be staged T1, T2, or T3.*

Regional Lymph Nodes (N)

NX Regional lymph nodes cannot be assessed
N0 No regional lymph node metastasis
N1 Metastasis in ipsilateral peribronchial and/or ipsilateral hilar lymph nodes, including direct extension
N2 Metastasis in ipsilateral mediastinal and/or subcarinal lymph node(s)
N3 Metastasis in contralateral mediastinal, contralateral hilar, ipsilateral or contralateral scalene, or supraclavicular lymph node(s)

Distant Metastasis (M)

MX Presence of distant metastasis cannot be assessed
M0 No distant metastasis
M1 Distant metastasis

STAGE GROUPING

Occult carcinoma	TX	N0	M0
Stage 0	Tis	N0	M0
Stage I	T1	N0	M0
	T2	N0	M0
Stage II	T1	N1	M0
	T2	N1	M0
Stage IIIA	T1	N2	M0
	T2	N2	M0
	T3	N0, N1, N2	M0
Stage IIIB	Any T	N3	M0
	T4	Any N	M0
Stage IV	Any T	Any N	M1

DIFFERENCES BETWEEN THE 2ND AND 3RD EDITIONS

A T4 category has been added in order to classify tumors that have invaded the mediastinum or extrapulmonic structures in the thorax. The lymph node categories were increased from three to four to provide more detail in coding contralateral as opposed to ipsilateral spread. The stage groupings have been redefined according to specific T, N, and M categories. Seven stages are now listed instead of the previous five. The new grouping excludes tumors with lymph node metastasis from Stage I disease.

HISTOPATHOLOGIC TYPE

There are four common types of lung cancer, or bronchogenic carcinoma:

Squamous cell or epidermoid carcinoma
Adenocarcinoma
Large cell carcinoma
Small cell or oat cell carcinoma

Less common types include:

Bronchial-alveolar carcinoma
Giant cell carcinoma
Adenoid-cystic carcinoma
Clear cell carcinoma
Basal cell carcinoma
Scar cancer (a type of adenocarcinoma)

This staging system applies only to the carcinomas. Sarcomas and other rare tumors are excluded.

HISTOPATHOLOGIC GRADE (G)

GX Grade cannot be assessed
G1 Well differentiated
G2 Moderately well differentiated
G3 Poorly differentiated
G4 Undifferentiated

BIBLIOGRAPHY

1. Byhardt RW, Hartz A, Libnoch JA, et al: Prognostic influence of TNM staging and LDH levels in small cell carcinoma of the lung (SCCL). Int J Radiat Oncol Biol Phys 12:771–777, 1986
2. Carr DT, Mountain CF: The staging of lung cancer. Semin Oncol 1:229–234, 1974
3. Carter D, Eggleston JC: Tumors of the lower respiratory tract, Atlas of Tumor Pathology, Armed Forces Institute of Pathology, Washington, DC, 1980
4. Cooksey JA, Bitran JD, Desser RK et al: Small-cell carcinoma of the lung: The prognostic significance of stage on survival. European Journal of Cancer and Clinical Oncology 15:859–865, 1979
5. Gail MH, Eagan RT, Feld R et al: Prognostic factors in patients with resected stage I non-small cell lung cancer. Cancer 54:1802–1813, 1984

6. Feinstein AR, Wells CK: Lung cancer staging: A critical evaluation. Clin Chest Med 3:291–305, 1982
7. Harper PG, Souhami RL, Spiro SG et al: Tumor size, response rate, and prognosis in small cell carcinoma of the bronchus treated by combination chemotherapy. Cancer Treat Rep 66:463–470, 1982
8. Ishikawa S: Staging system on TNM classification for lung cancer. Jpn J Clin Oncol 6:19–30, 1973
9. Little AG, DeMeester TR, MacMahon H: The staging of lung cancer. Semin Oncol 10:56–70, 1983
10. Martini N: Improved methods of recording data in lung cancer. Clin Bull 6:93–98, 1976
11. Matthews MJ, Kanhouwa S, Pickren J et al: Frequency of residual and metastatic tumor in patients undergoing curative surgical resection for lung cancer. Cancer Treatment Reports 4(2):63–67, 1973
12. Mountain CF: A method for the assessment of operation in the control of lung cancer. Ann Thorac Surg 24:365–373, 1977
13. Mountain CF: A new international staging system for lung cancer. Chest (Suppl) 225S–233S, 1986
14. Naruke T, Suemasu K, Ishikawa S: Lymph node mapping and curability at various levels of metastasis in resected lung cancer. J Thorac Cardiovasc Surg 76:832–839, 1978
15. Pater JL, Loeb M: Nonanatomic prognostic factors in carcinoma of the lung. Cancer 50:326–331, 1982
16. Shields TW, Keehn RJ: Postresection stage groupings in carcinoma of the lung. Surg Gynecol Obstet 145:725–728, 1977
17. Spiro SG: The diagnosis and staging of lung cancer. Manage Malignant Dis Ser 6:36–52, 1984
18. Stanley KD: Prognostic factors for survival in patients with inoperable lung cancer. J Natl Cancer Inst 65:25–32, 1980
19. Williams DE, Pairolero PC, Davis CS et al: Survival of patients surgically treated for stage I lung cancer. J Thorac Cardiovasc Surg 82:70–76, 1981

LUNG

Data Form for Cancer Staging

Patient identification
Name _____
Address _____
Hospital or clinic number _____
Age _____ Sex _____ Race _____

Institution identification
Hospital or clinic _____
Address _____

Oncology Record

Anatomic site of cancer _____
Histologic type _____
Grade (G) _____
Date of classification _____

Chronology of classification
 (use separate form for each time staged)
[ ] Clinical (use all data prior to first treatment)
[ ] Pathologic (if definitively resected specimen available)

Definitions

Primary Tumor (T)

[ ] TX Primary tumor cannot be assessed, or tumor proven by presence of malignant cells in sputum or bronchial washings but not visualized by imaging or bronchoscopy
[ ] T0 No evidence of primary tumor
[ ] Tis Carcinoma *in situ*
[ ] T1 Tumor 3 cm or less in greatest dimension, surrounded by lung or visceral pleura, without bronchoscopic evidence of invasion more proximal than the lobar bronchus
[ ] T2 Tumor with *any* of the following features of size or extent:
  More than 3 cm in greatest dimension
  Involves main bronchus, 2 cm or more distal to the carina
  Invades the visceral pleura
  Associated with atelectasis or obstructive pneumonitis which extends to the hilar region but does not involve the entire lung
[ ] T3 Tumor of any size that directly invades any of the following: chest wall (including superior sulcus tumors), diaphragm, mediastinal pleura, parietal pericardium; or tumor in the main bronchus less than 2 cm distal to the carina but without involvement of the carina; or associated atelectasis or obstructive pneumonitis of the entire lung
[ ] T4 Tumor of any size that invades any of the following: mediastinum, heart, great vessels, trachea, esophagus, vertebral body, carina; or tumor with a malignant pleural effusion

Lymph Node (N)

[ ] NX Regional lymph nodes cannot be assessed
[ ] N0 No regional lymph node metastasis
[ ] N1 Metastasis in ipsilateral peribronchial and/or ipsilateral hilar lymph nodes, including direct extension
[ ] N2 Metastasis in ipsilateral mediastinal and/or subcarinal lymph node(s)
[ ] N3 Metastasis in contralateral mediastinal, contralateral hilar, ipsilateral or contralateral scalene or supraclavicular lymph node(s)

Distant Metastases (M)

[ ] MX Presence of distant metastasis cannot be assessed
[ ] M0 No distant metastasis
[ ] M1 Distant metastasis

Stage Grouping

[ ] Occult Carcinoma
       TX   N0   M0
[ ] 0 Tis   N0   M0
[ ] I T1   N0   M0
       T2   N0   M0
[ ] II T1   N1   M0
       T2   N1   M0
[ ] IIIA T1   N2   M0
       T2   N2   M0
       T3   N0   M0
       T3   N1   M0
       T3   N2   M0
[ ] IIIB Any T N3   M0
       T4   Any N   M0
[ ] IV Any T   Any N   M1

Histopathologic Grade (G)

[ ] GX Grade cannot be assessed
[ ] G1 Well differentiated
[ ] G2 Moderately well differentiated
[ ] G3 Poorly differentiated
[ ] G4 Undifferentiated

Sites of Distant Metastasis

Pulmonary PUL
Osseous OSS
Hepatic HEP
Brain BRA
Lymph nodes LYM
Bone marrow MAR
Pleura PLE
Peritoneum PER
Skin SKI
Other OTH

Staged by _____ M.D.
_____ Registrar
Date _____

American Joint Committee on Cancer—1988

Illustrations

N–Regional nodes

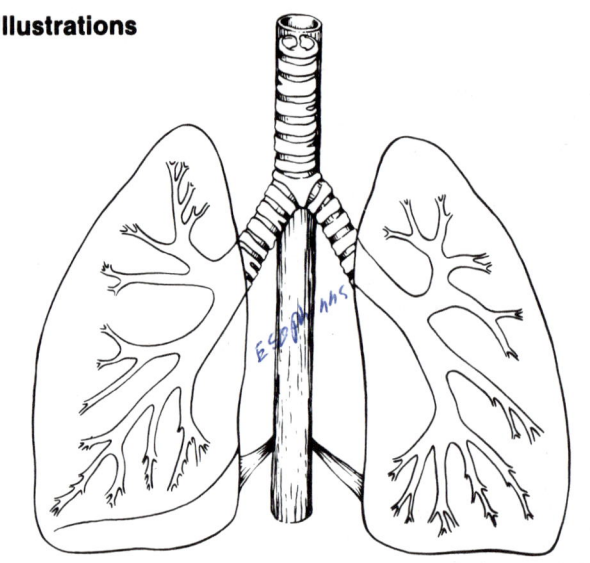

Show primary tumor, indicating size in cm (greatest diameter) and measurability:

EV = evaluable
ME = measurable
NE = nonevaluable

Show lymph node metastasis.

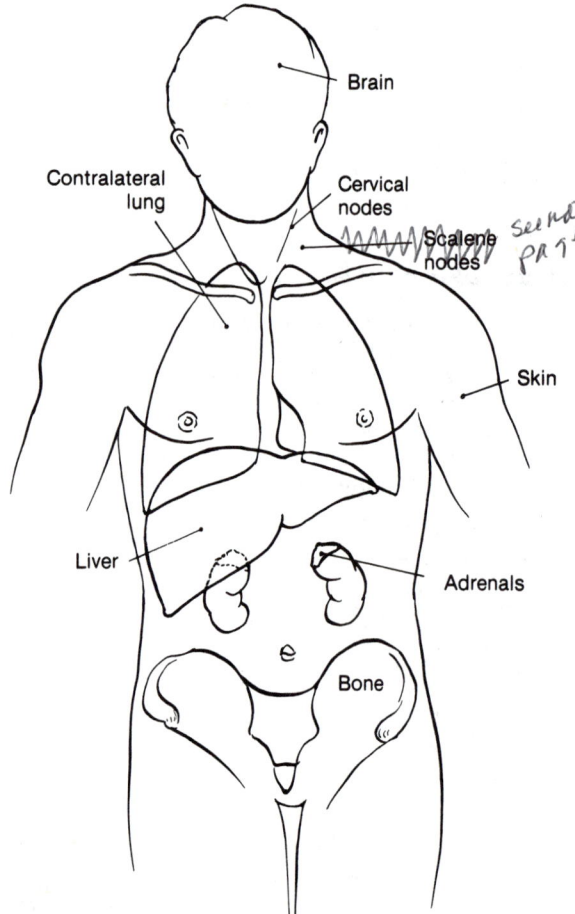

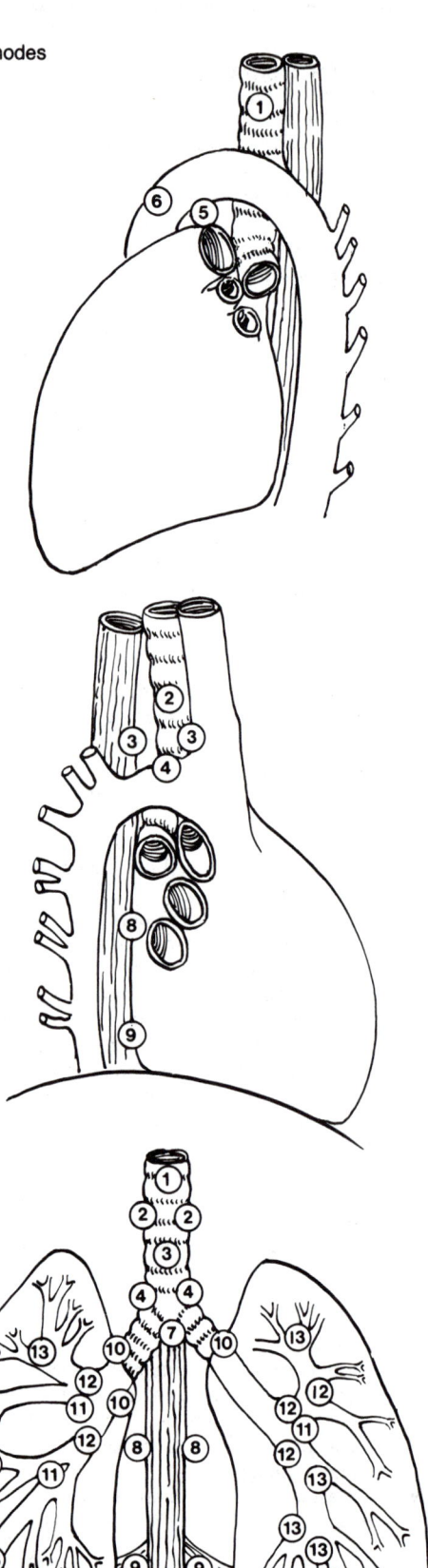

Distant metastases beyond hemithorax

Indicate all known metastases.

Indicate on diagrams primary tumor and regional nodes involved.

N2 Nodes

Superior mediastinal nodes
1. Highest mediastinal
2. Upper paratracheal
3. Pre- and retrotracheal
4. Lower paratracheal (including azygos nodes)

Aortic nodes
5. Subaortic (aortic window)
6. Para-aortic (ascending aorta or phrenic)

Inferior mediastinal nodes
7. Subcarinal
8. Paraesophageal (below carina)
9. Pulmonary ligament

N1 Nodes
10. Hilar
11. Interlobar
12. Lobar
13. Segmental

Histopathologic Type

There are four common types of lung cancer, or bronchogenic carcinoma:

Squamous cell or epidermoid carcinoma
Adenocarcinoma
Large cell carcinoma
Small cell or oat cell carcinoma

Less common types include:

Bronchial-alveolar carcinoma
Giant cell carcinoma
Adenoid-cystic carcinoma
Clear cell carcinoma
Basal cell carcinoma
Scar cancer (a type of adenocarcinoma)

This staging system applies only to the carcinomas. Sarcomas and other rare tumors are excluded.

Sites of Distant Metastasis

Pulmonary	PUL
Osseous	OSS
Hepatic	HEP
Brain	BRA
Lymph nodes	LYM
Bone marrow	MAR
Pleura	PLE
Peritoneum	PER
Skin	SKI
Other	OTH

Lung, Chapter 18, page 120

Scalene nodes are no longer considered distant. Please remove Scalene Nodes from the diagram depicting *distant metastasis beyond hemithorax* at the bottom left of the page.

MUSCULOSKELETAL SITES

Bone

This classification is used for all primary malignant tumors of bone except multiple myeloma, juxtacortical osteosarcoma, and juxtacortical chondrosarcoma. There should be histologic confirmation of the disease to permit division of cases by histologic type.

ANATOMY

Primary Site. All bones (ICD-O 170) of the skeleton.

Regional Lymph Nodes. The regional lymph nodes are those appropriate to the location of the primary tumor.

Metastatic Sites. A metastatic site includes any site beyond the regional lymph nodes of the primary site. Spread to the lungs is frequent.

RULES FOR CLASSIFICATION

Clinical Staging. All data available prior to definitive treatment are to be used for staging.

Pathologic Staging. All clinical and pathologic data obtained on examination of the resected tissue are to be used for staging.

HISTOPATHOLOGIC GRADE (G)

GX Grade cannot be assessed
G1 Well differentiated
G2 Moderately differentiated
G3 Poorly differentiated
G4 Undifferentiated

Note: Ewing's sarcoma and malignant lymphoma are defined as G4.

DEFINITION OF TNM

Primary Tumor (T)

TX Primary tumor cannot be assessed
T0 No evidence of primary tumor
T1 Tumor confined within the cortex
T2 Tumor invades beyond the cortex

Regional Lymph Nodes (N)

NX Regional lymph nodes cannot be assessed
N0 No regional lymph node metastasis
N1 Regional lymph node metastasis

Distant Metastasis (M)

MX Presence of distant metastasis cannot be assessed
M0 No distant metastasis
M1 Distant metastasis

STAGE GROUPING

Stage IA	G1, 2	T1	N0	M0
Stage IB	G1, 2	T2	N0	M0
Stage IIA	G3, 4	T1	N0	M0
Stage IIB	G3, 4	T2	N0	M0
Stage III	Not defined			
Stage IVA	Any G	Any T	N1	M0
Stave IVB	Any G	Any T	Any N	M1

DIFFERENCES BETWEEN THE 2ND AND 3RD EDITIONS

This classification is the same as that published in the second edition of the *Manual.*

HISTOPATHOLOGIC TYPE

See bibliography for reference material.

A. Bone-forming
  1. Osteosarcoma (osteogenic sarcoma)
  2. Juxtacortical osteosarcoma (parosteal osteosarcoma)
B. Cartilage-forming
  1. Chondrosarcoma
  2. Juxtacortical chondrosarcoma
  3. Mesenchymal chondrosarcoma
C. Giant cell tumor, malignant
D. Marrow tumors
  1. Ewing's sarcoma
  2. Malignant lymphoma of bone
  3. Myeloma
E. Vascular tumors
  1. Hemangioendothelioma
  2. Hemangiopericytoma
  3. Angiosarcoma
F. Connective tissue tumors
  1. Fibrosarcoma
  2. Liposarcoma
  3. Malignant mesenchymoma
  4. Undifferentiated sarcoma
G. Other tumors
  1. Chordoma
  2. Adamantinoma of long bones

BIBLIOGRAPHY

1. World Health Organization: Histological Typing of Bone Tumours: International Histological Classification of Tumours, No. 6. Geneva, World Health Organization, 1972
2. American Joint Committee on Cancer: Manual for Staging of Cancer, second edition. New York, JB Lippincott, 1983

BONE

Data Form for Cancer Staging

Patient identification
Name _____
Address _____
Hospital or clinic number _____
Age _____ Sex _____ Race _____

Institution identification
Hospital or clinic _____
Address _____

Oncology Record

Anatomic site of cancer _____
Histologic type _____
Grade (G) _____
Date of classification _____

Chronology of classification
  (use separate form for each time staged)
[ ] Clinical (use all data prior to first treatment)
[ ] Pathologic (if definitively resected specimen available)

Definitions

Primary Tumor (T)

[ ] TX   Primary tumor cannot be assessed
[ ] T0   No evidence of primary tumor
[ ] T1   Tumor confined within the cortex
[ ] T2   Tumor invades beyond the cortex

Lymph Node (N)

[ ] NX   Regional lymph nodes cannot be assessed
[ ] N0   No regional lymph node metastasis
[ ] N1   Regional lymph node metastasis

Distant Metastasis (M)

[ ] MX   Presence of distant metastasis cannot be assessed
[ ] M0   No distant metastasis
[ ] M1   Distant metastasis

Stage Grouping

[ ]	IA	G1	T1	N0	M0
		G2	T1	N0	M0
[ ]	IB	G1	T2	N0	M0
		G2	T2	N0	M0
[ ]	IIA	G3	T1	N0	M0
		G4	T1	N0	M0
[ ]	IIB	G3	T2	N0	M0
		G4	T2	N0	M0
[ ]	III	Not defined			
[ ]	IVA	Any G	Any T	N1	M0
[ ]	IVB	Any G	Any T	Any N	M1

Histopathologic Grade (G)

[ ] GX   Grade cannot be assessed
[ ] G1   Well differentiated
[ ] G2   Moderately well differentiated
[ ] G3   Poorly differentiated
[ ] G4   Undifferentiated

Histopathologic Type

A. Bone-forming
   1. Osteosarcoma (osteogenic sarcoma)
   2. Juxtacortical osteosarcoma (parosteal osteosarcoma)
B. Cartilage-forming
   1. Chondrosarcoma
   2. Juxtacortical chondrosarcoma
   3. Mesenchymal chondrosarcoma
C. Giant cell tumor, malignant
D. Marrow tumors
   1. Ewing's sarcoma
   2. Malignant lymphoma of bone
   3. Myeloma
E. Vascular tumors
   1. Hemangioendothelioma
   2. Hemangiopericytoma
   3. Angiosarcoma
F. Connective tissue tumors
   1. Fibrosarcoma
   2. Liposarcoma
   3. Malignant mesenchymoma
   4. Undifferentiated sarcoma
G. Other tumors
   1. Chordoma
   2. "Adamantinoma" of long bones

Sites of Distant Metastasis

Pulmonary	PUL
Osseous	OSS
Hepatic	HEP
Brain	BRA
Lymph nodes	LYM
Bone marrow	MAR
Pleura	PLE
Peritoneum	PER
Skin	SKI
Other	OTH

Staged by _____ M.D.
_____ Registrar
Date _____

American Joint Committee on Cancer—1988

20 Soft Tissues

The staging system applies to all soft-tissue sarcomas except Kaposi's sarcoma, dermatofibrosarcoma, and desmoid type of fibrosarcoma grade 1. Excluded from the staging system are those sarcomas arising within the confines of the dura mater, including the brain, and sarcomas arising in parenchymatous organs and from hollow viscera. The system is based on an analysis of 1215 cases obtained from 13 institutions. Cases were collected on the basis of histology, diagnosis, and type of soft tissue and include all age groups. For the most part, recommendations regarding staging of soft-tissue sarcomas in children are the same as the AJCC staging system for adults. Grading of soft-tissue sarcomas has not been utilized, however, in the stage grouping for pediatric tumors.

In the analysis, it was determined that, in addition to clinical information, the histologic type, grade, and tumor size are essential for a meaningful staging system. The histologic diagnosis identifying the type of tumor and the pathologist's assessment of the inherent extent of malignancy (differentiation of the tumor) are fundamentals on which the staging is based.

Determination of the histologic grade and type of tumor is required for staging soft-tissue sarcomas and must be established by a qualified pathologist working with an adequate sample of the tumor.

ANATOMY

Primary Site. A variety of soft tissues can give rise to these sarcomas. The tissues include fibrous connective tissue, fat, smooth or striated muscle, vascular tissue, and peripheral neural tissue, as well as undifferentiated mesenchyme.

Connective, subcutaneous and other soft tissues (ICD-O 171)
Retroperitoneum (ICD-O 158.0)
Mediastinum (ICD-O 164.2,3)

Regional Lymph Nodes. The regional lymph nodes are related to the site of origin of the sarcoma.

Metastatic Sites. The lung is the most common site, but any body site may be involved.

RULES FOR CLASSIFICATION

Clinical Staging. Clinical staging includes physical examination, imaging, clinical laboratory tests, and biopsy of the sarcoma for microscopic diagnosis and grading.

Pathologic Staging. Pathologic (pGTNM) staging consists of the removal and pathologic evaluation of the primary tumor and, if indicated, extensions of the tumor, nodes, or suspected metastases.

HISTOPATHOLOGIC GRADE (G)

After the histologic type has been determined, the tumor should be graded according to the accepted criteria of malignancy, including cellularity, cellular pleomorphism, mitotic activity, and necrosis. The amount of intercellular substance, such as collagen or mucoid material, should be considered as favorable in assessing grade.

GX	Grade cannot be assessed
G1	Well differentiated
G2	Moderately well differentiated
G3-4	Poorly differentiated; undifferentiated

DEFINITION OF TNM

Primary Tumor (T)

TX	Primary tumor cannot be assessed
T0	No evidence of primary tumor
T1	Tumor 5 cm or less in greatest dimension
T2	Tumor more than 5 cm in greatest dimension

Regional Lymph Nodes (N)

NX	Regional lymph nodes cannot be assessed
N0	No regional lymph node metastasis
N1	Regional lymph node metastasis

Distant Metastasis (M)

MX	Presence of distant metastasis cannot be assessed
M0	No distant metastasis
M1	Distant metastasis

STAGE GROUPING

Stage IA	G1	T1	N0	M0
Stage IB	G1	T2	N0	M0
Stage IIA	G2	T1	N0	M0
Stage IIB	G2	T2	N0	M0
Stage IIIA	G3-4	T1	N0	M0
Stage IIIB	G3-4	T2	N0	M0
Stage IVA	Any G	Any T	N1	M0
Stage IVB	Any G	Any T	Any N	M1

DIFFERENCES BETWEEN THE 2ND AND 3RD EDITIONS

1. T3 of the second edition has been eliminated. T3 was formerly defined as: clear radiographic evidence of destruction of cortical bone, with invasion; histopathologic confirmation of invasion of major artery or nerve.
2. N1 in the second edition categorized a case as Stage IIIC. In the third edition Stage IIIC has been eliminated and N1 now categorizes a case as Stage IVA.
3. Stage IVA has been redefined:
   IVA second edition: Any G T3 Any N M0
   IVA third edition: Any G Any T N1 M0

HISTOPATHOLOGIC TYPE

Tumors included in the analysis are listed below:

Alveolar soft-part sarcoma
Angiosarcoma
Epithelioid sarcoma
Extraskeletal chondrosarcoma
Extraskeletal osteosarcoma
Fibrosarcoma
Leiomyosarcoma
Liposarcoma
Malignant fibrous histiocytoma
Malignant hemangiopericytoma
Malignant mesenchymoma
Malignant schwannoma
Rhabdomyosarcoma
Synovial sarcoma
Sarcoma, NOS (not otherwise specified)

BIBLIOGRAPHY

1. Castro EB, Hajdu SI, Fortner JG: Surgical therapy of fibrosarcoma of extremities. Arch Surg 107:284–286, 1973
2. Enzinger FM, Lattes R, Torloni H: Histological Typing of Soft Tissue Tumours. International Histological Classification of Tumours, No. 3. Geneva, World Health Organization, 1969
3. Enzinger FM, Shiraki M: Alveolar rhabdomyosarcoma: An analysis of 110 cases. Cancer 24:18–31, 1969
4. Hajdu SI: Pathology of Soft Tissue Tumours. Philadelphia, Lea & Febiger, 1979

5. Heise HW, Myers MH, Russell WO et al: Recurrence-free survival time for surgically-treated soft tissue sarcoma patients. Cancer 57:172–177, 1986
6. Pritchard J, Soule EH, Taylor WF et al: Fibrosarcoma: A clinicopathologic and statistical study of 1969 tumors of the soft tissues of the extremities and trunk. Cancer 33:888–897, 1974
7. Russell WO, Cohen J, Enzinger F et al: A clinical and pathological staging system for soft tissue sarcomas. Cancer 40:1562–1570, 1977
8. Soule EH, Geitz M, Henderson ED: Embryonal rhabdomyosarcoma of the limbs and the limb-girdles. Cancer 23:1336–1346, 1969
9. Suit HD, Russell WO, Martin RG: Sarcoma of soft tissue: Clinical and histopathologic parameters and response to treatment. Cancer 35:1478–1483, 1975
10. Sutow WW, Sullivan MP, Ried HL et al: Prognosis in childhood rhabdomyosarcoma. Cancer 35:1384–1390, 1970
11. Van der Werf-Messing B, van Unnik JAM: Fibrosarcoma of the soft tissues: A clinicopathologic study. Cancer 18:1113–1123, 1965

SOFT TISSUES

Data Form for Cancer Staging

Patient identification
Name _____
Address _____
Hospital or clinic number _____
Age _____ Sex _____ Race _____

Institution identification
Hospital or clinic _____
Address _____

Oncology Record

Anatomic site of cancer _____
Histologic type _____
Grade (G) _____
Date of classification _____

Chronology of classification
(use separate form for each time staged)
[ ] Clinical (use all data prior to first treatment)
[ ] Pathologic (if definitively resected specimen available)

Definitions

Primary Tumor (T)
[ ] TX Primary tumor cannot be assessed
[ ] T0 No evidence of primary tumor
[ ] T1 Tumor 5 cm or less in greatest dimension
[ ] T2 Tumor more than 5 cm in greatest dimension

Lymph Node (N)
[ ] NX Regional lymph nodes cannot be assessed
[ ] N0 No regional lymph node metastasis
[ ] N1 Regional lymph node metastasis

Distant Metastasis (M)
[ ] MX Presence of distant metastasis cannot be assessed
[ ] M0 No distant metastasis
[ ] M1 Distant metastasis

Stage Grouping

[ ] IA	G1	T1	N0	M0
[ ] IB	G1	T2	N0	M0
[ ] IIA	G2	T1	N0	M0
[ ] IIB	G2	T2	N0	M0
[ ] IIIA	G3	T1	N0	M0
	G4	T1	N0	M0
[ ] IIIB	G3	T2	N0	M0
	G4	T2	N0	M0
[ ] IVA	Any G	Any T	N1	M0
[ ] IVB	Any G	Any T	Any N	M1

Histopathologic Grade (G)

[ ] GX Grade cannot be assessed
[ ] G1 Well differentiated
[ ] G2 Moderately well differentiated
[ ] G3 Poorly differentiated
[ ] G4 Undifferentiated

Histopathologic Type

Tumors included in the analysis are listed below:

Alveolar soft-part sarcoma
Angiosarcoma
Epithelioid sarcoma
Extraskeletal chondrosarcoma
Extraskeletal osteosarcoma
Fibrosarcoma
Leiomyosarcoma
Liposarcoma
Malignant fibrous histiocytoma
Malignant hemangiopericytoma
Malignant mesenchymoma
Malignant schwannoma
Rhabdomyosarcoma
Synovial sarcoma
Sarcoma, NOS (not otherwise specified)

Sites of Distant Metastasis

Pulmonary   PUL
Osseous   OSS
Hepatic   HEP
Brain   BRA
Lymph nodes   LYM
Bone marrow   MAR
Pleura   PLE
Peritoneum   PER
Skin   SKI
Other   OTH

Staged by _____ M.D.
_____ Registrar
Date _____

21

Carcinoma of the Skin (excluding eyelid, vulva, and penis)

The skin is the covering for the body. Though a variety of tumor types are found in the skin, this chapter is concerned with only two: squamous cell carcinomas and basal cell carcinomas. Skin cancers are relatively common and for the most part have a good prognosis. Basal cell carcinomas are the most common cancer in humans and easily treated with surgery. Staging of skin cancer depends on the size of the primary tumor. Refer to Chapter 36 for lesions on the eyelid.

ANATOMY

Primary Site. The skin (ICD-O 173.0, 173.2–173.9, 187.7 [scrotum]) has two layers, an outer epidermis and the inner dermis. The epidermis consists predominantly of stratified squamous epithelium, the external layer of which is keratinized. The dermis contains dense connective tissue and elastic fibers. Immediately below the dermis is the subcutaneous tissue. The sebaceous and other glands of the skin are found in the dermis and adjacent subcutaneous tissue. All of the components of the skin—epidermis, dermis and adnexal structures—can give rise to malignant neoplasms.

Cancers can arise from any area of the skin. They are most common on those surfaces exposed to sunlight, which include the face, ears, hands, and scalp. Cancers can also arise on the truncal regions and on the extremities. Basal cell carcinomas often occur on the face.

This classification also includes tumors arising in the anal margin.

Regional Lymph Nodes. The regional lymph nodes are those appropriate to the situation of the primary tumor.

Unilateral Tumors

Head, neck	Ipsilateral preauricular, cervical, and supraclavicular lymph nodes
Thorax	Ipsilateral axillary lymph nodes
Arm	Ipsilateral epitrochlear and axillary lymph nodes
Abdomen, loins and buttocks	Ipsilateral inguinal lymph nodes
Leg	Ipsilateral popliteal and inguinal lymph nodes
Anal margin and perianal skin	Ipsilateral inguinal lymph nodes

With tumors in the boundary zones between the above: the lymph nodes pertaining to the regions on both sides of the boundary zone are considered to be regional lymph nodes. The following 4-cm-wide bands are considered as boundary zones:

Between (Right/left)	*Along (Mid line)*
Head and neck/thorax	Claviculo-acromion-upper shoulder blade edge
Thorax/arm	Shoulder-axilla-shoulder
Thorax/abdomen, loins, and buttocks	Front: Middle between navel and costal arch
	Back: Lower border of thoracic vertebrae (midtransverse-axis)
Abdomen, loins, and buttock/leg	Groin-trochanter-gluteal sulcus

For tumors arising on the leg, the iliac nodes are considered sites of distant metastasis and should be coded as M1.

Metastatic Sites. The most common metastatic site is the lung, especially for the squamous cell carcinomas. Other sites of distant spread are unusual. Basal cell carcinomas tend to erode locally, although rarely these tumors may metastasize.

RULES FOR CLASSIFICATION

The clinical and pathologic classifications are identical. However, pathologic staging uses the symbol *p* as a prefix.

The classification applies only to carcinomas. There should be microscopic verification of the disease to permit division of cases by histologic type. The following are suggested procedures for assessment of the T, N, and M categories.

Clinical Staging. The assessment of skin cancer is based upon inspection and palpation of the involved area and the regional lymph nodes. Imaging studies of the underlying bony structures is important, especially in the scalp, if the lesion is fixed.

T categories: Clinical Examination
N categories: Clinical Examination
M categories: Examination and Imaging

Pathologic Staging. Complete resection of the entire site is indicated. Confirmation of lymph node involvement is also required.

DEFINITION OF TNM

Definitions for clinical (cTNM) and pathologic (pTNM) classifications are the same.

Primary Tumor (T)

TX Primary tumor cannot be assessed
T0 No evidence of primary tumor
Tis Carcinoma *in situ*
T1 Tumor 2 cm or less in greatest dimension
T2 Tumor more than 2 cm but not more than 5 cm in greatest dimension
T3 Tumor more than 5 cm in greatest dimension
T4 Tumor invades deep extradermal structures (*i.e.*, cartilage, skeletal muscle or bone)

Note: In the case of multiple simultaneous tumors, the tumor with the highest T category will be classified and the number of separate tumors will be indicated in parentheses (e.g., T2 (5)).

Regional Lymph Nodes (N)

NX Regional lymph nodes cannot be assessed
N0 No regional lymph node metastasis
N1 Regional lymph node metastasis

Distant Metastasis (M)

MX Presence of distant metastasis cannot be assessed
M0 No distant metastasis
M1 Distant metastasis

STAGE GROUPING

Stage 0	Tis	N0	M0
Stage I	T1	N0	M0
Stage II	T2	N0	M0
	T3	N0	M0
Stage III	T4	N0	M0
	Any T	N1	M0
Stage IV	Any T	Any N	M1

DIFFERENCES BETWEEN THE 2ND AND 3RD EDITIONS

The T categories have been redefined and simplified. Dermal infiltration as a criterion for T assignment has been deleted. The N categories have been reduced from five to three, removing the concept of "fixed" versus "movable" lymph nodes. For better discrimination, five stage groupings are listed, as opposed to three in the previous edition.

HISTOPATHOLOGIC TYPE

The staging system is utilized primarily for squamous cell and basal cell carcinomas of the skin. It does not apply to the adenocarcinomas that develop from sweat or sebaceous glands.

A spindle cell variant of squamous cell carcinoma exists, which is included under the classification. Squamous cell tumors may also be described as verrucous.

A form of *in situ* carcinoma or intraepidermal carcinoma is often referred to as Bowen's disease. This lesion should be coded as Tis.

HISTOPATHOLOGIC GRADE (G)

GX Grade cannot be assessed
G1 Well differentiated
G2 Moderately well differentiated
G3 Poorly differentiated
G4 Undifferentiated

BIBLIOGRAPHY

1. Edmundson WF: Microscopic grading of cancer and its practical implications. Arch Dermatol & Syph 57:141, 1948
2. Katz AD: The frequency and risk of metastases in squamous cell carcinoma of the skin. Cancer 10: 1162–1166, 1957
3. Lund HZ: How often does squamous cell carcinoma of the skin metastasize? Arch Dermatol 92:635–637, 1965
4. Pollack SV, Goslen JB, Sherertz EF et al: The biology of basal cell carcinoma: A review. J Am Acad Dermatol 7:569–577, 1982
5. Safai B, Good RA: Basal cell carcinoma with metastasis: Review of literature. Arch Pathol Lab Med 101:327–331, 1977
6. Strayer DS, Santa Crus DJ: Carcinoma in-situ of the skin: A review of histopathology. J Cutan Pathol 7:244–259, 1980

CARCINOMA OF THE SKIN (EXCLUDING EYELID, VULVA, AND PENIS)

Data Form for Cancer Staging

Patient identification
Name _____
Address _____
Hospital or clinic number _____
Age _____ Sex _____ Race _____

Institution identification
Hospital or clinic _____
Address _____

Oncology Record

Anatomic site of cancer _____
Histologic type _____
Grade (G) _____
Date of classification _____

Chronology of classification
(use separate form for each time staged)
[ ] Clinical (use all data prior to first treatment)
[ ] Pathologic (if definitively resected specimen available)

Definitions

Primary Tumor (T)
[ ] TX Primary tumor cannot be assessed
[ ] T0 No evidence of primary tumor
[ ] Tis Carcinoma *in situ*
[ ] T1 Tumor 2 cm or less in greatest dimension
[ ] T2 Tumor more than 2 cm but not more than 5 cm in greatest dimension
[ ] T3 Tumor more than 5 cm in greatest dimension
[ ] T4 Tumor invades deep extradermal structures, *i.e.*, cartilage, skeletal muscle or bone

Lymph Node (N)
[ ] NX Regional lymph nodes cannot be assessed
[ ] N0 No regional lymph node metastasis
[ ] N1 Regional lymph node metastasis

Distant Metastasis (M)
[ ] MX Presence of distant metastasis cannot be assessed
[ ] M0 No distant metastasis
[ ] M1 Distant metastasis

Stage Grouping
[ ] 0   Tis   N0   M0
[ ] I   T1   N0   M0
[ ] II   T2   N0   M0
         T3   N0   M0
[ ] III T4   N0   M0
         Any T   N1   M0
[ ] IV   Any T   Any N   M1

Histopathologic Grade (G)
[ ] GX Grade cannot be assessed
[ ] G1 Well differentiated
[ ] G2 Moderately well differentiated
[ ] G3 Poorly differentiated
[ ] G4 Undifferentiated

Illustrations

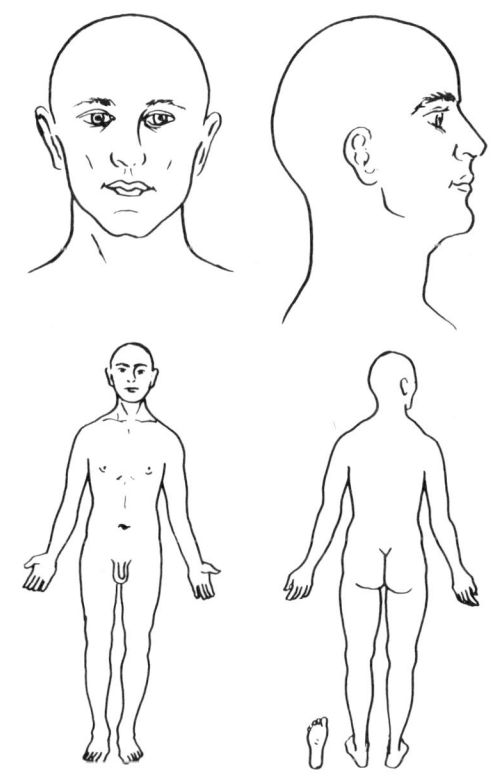

Indicate on diagrams primary tumor and regional nodes involved.

Histopathologic Type

The staging system applies only to squamous cell and to basal cell carcinomas of the skin. It does not apply to the adenocarcinomas that develop from sweat or sebaceous glands. These adnexal tumors rarely metastasize.

A spindle cell variant of squamous cell carcinoma exists, which is included under the classification. Squamous cell tumors may also be described as verrucous.

A form of *in situ* carcinoma or intraepidermal carcinoma is often referred to as Bowen's disease. This lesion should be coded as T1.

Staged by _____ M.D.
          _____ Registrar
Date _____

Sites of Distant Metastasis

Pulmonary	PUL
Osseous	OSS
Hepatic	HEP
Brain	BRA
Lymph nodes	LYM
Bone marrow	MAR
Pleura	PLE
Peritoneum	PER
Skin	SKI
Other	OTH

Melanoma of the Skin (excluding eyelid)

Malignant melanomas are most common in fair-skinned individuals who often have a history of chronic sun exposure. They can occur in any area of the skin, including the palms of the hands and soles of the feet and in the nail beds. Rarely, melanomas may arise in other sites, for example, from the mucous membranes of the oral cavity, nasopharynx, vagina, urethra, and anal canal. Melanomas may also arise from the pigmented tissues of the eye and from giant hairy nevi. In some cases of disseminated disease, a primary lesion may not be found. Melanomas can be transmitted from mother to infant during pregnancy. Early detection and treatment of incipient melanomas have resulted in a significant decrease in the mortality from this disease. The staging classification outlined in this chapter applies only to melanomas arising in the skin. These tumors are staged histologically by measuring the thickness of the lesion or its depth of penetration into the underlying dermis. The depth of penetration is usually expressed as the level of invasion with the cutaneous anatomic structures used as reference.

ANATOMY

Primary Site. The great majority of melanomas (skin ICD-O 173, vulva 184.4, penis 187.4, scrotum 187.7) arise from the pigmented melanocytes located in the basal layer of the epidermis. The tumor often develops from a pre-existing pigmented lesion, although some arise from apparently normal skin. Melanomas are found on all skin surfaces of the body. The tumor may grow into the dermis (nodular type) or spread horizontally along the skin (superficial spreading type). Multiple primary tumors may occur.

Regional Lymph Nodes. The regional lymph nodes depend on the location of the primary tumor. Regional nodes are as follows:

Unilateral Tumors

Head, neck	Ipsilateral preauricular, cervical, and supraclavicular lymph nodes
Thorax	Ipsilateral axillary lymph nodes
Arm	Ipsilateral epitrochlear and axillary lymph nodes
Abdomen, loins, and buttocks	Ipsilateral inguinal lymph nodes
Leg	Ipsilateral popliteal and inguinal lymph nodes
Anal margin and perianal skin	Ipsilateral inguinal lymph nodes

With tumors in the boundary zones between the above, the lymph nodes pertaining to the regions on both sides of the boundary zone are considered to be regional lymph nodes. The following 4-cm-wide bands are considered as boundary zones:

Between (Right/left)	*Along* (Mid line)
Head and neck/thorax	Claviculo-acromion-upper shoulder blade edge
Thorax/arm	Shoulder-axilla-shoulder
Thorax/abdomen, loins, and buttocks	Front: Middle between navel and costal arch
	Back: Lower border of thoracic vertebrae (midtransverse-axis)
Abdomen, loins, and buttock/leg	Groin-trochanter-gluteal sulcus

Iliac nodes are considered sites of distant metastasis and should be coded as M1.

Lesions arising in the midtransverse axis of the trunk at a level between the umbilicus and the lower costal margin anteriorly and extending laterally to the posterior level between the tenth thoracic spine (T10) and the first lumbar spine (L1) may spread with equal propensity to either contralateral or to ipsilateral, or to both, axillary or inguinal nodes.

Metastatic Sites. Melanomas can metastasize widely. No organ or tissue is exempt. In some cases, metastatic deposits may not become apparent for years. Melanomas commonly involve skin, subcutaneous tissues, lymph nodes, liver, bone, lung, brain, and visceral organs.

For staging purposes, two sub–M categories, identified as *a* and *b*, are included. Metastasis to the skin or to subcutaneous tissue beyond the site of the primary lymph node drainage is considered M1a whereas metastasis to other distant sites—often referred to as visceral metastasis—is considered M1b. This distinction is based on the more favorable response to therapy of patients with only skin or subcutaneous metastases.

RULES FOR CLASSIFICATION

Clinical Staging. Clinical T classification is ordinarily not possible. Biopsy and pathologic interpretation of the primary lesion are necessary for proper staging. Ulceration of the primary lesion may indicate a bad prognosis.

Pathologic Staging. The pathologic staging of the primary melanoma is based on the microscopic assessment of the depth of invasion and thickness of the primary tumor. Therefore, evaluation of the entire primary tumor is always advised, rather than a wedge or punch biopsy. The entire thickness of the skin is needed for accurate classification. Regional nodes should be carefully evaluated, if available, and the number of positive nodes should be identified with the total number of lymph nodes removed.

Both the thickness and the level of invasion have prognostic significance, and both parameters should be reported by the pathologist.

Maximal thickness of the tumor is measured with an ocular micrometer at right angle to the adjacent normal skin. The upper reference point is the top of the granular cell layer of the epidermis of the overlying skin or the base of the lesion if the tumor is ulcerated. The lower reference point is usually the deepest point of invasion. It may be the invading edge of a single tumor mass or an isolated cell or group of cells deep to the main mass. Actual measurement should be recorded.

If no primary lesion is found, the tumor is coded TX.

DEFINITION OF TNM

Both the level of invasion and the maximum thickness determine the T classification and should be recorded. If the depth of invasion and the thickness do not match, the lesion is assigned to the higher T classification, that is, the least favorable finding. Satellite lesions or nodules within 2 cm of the primary tumor are considered in the T category and the primary tumor is assigned T4, regardless of the thickness or depth of invasion. Satellite lesions or subcutaneous nodules more than 2 cm from the primary tumor but not beyond the site of the primary lymph node drainage are considered *in-transit metastases* and are listed under the N categories.

The extent of tumor is classified after excision.

Melanoma of the Skin (excluding eyelid)

Primary Tumor (pT)

pTX Primary tumor cannot be assessed
pT0 No evidence of primary tumor
pTis Melanoma *in situ* (atypical melanocytic hyperplasia, severe melanocytic dysplasia), not an invasive lesion (Clark's Level I)
pT1 Tumor 0.75 mm or less in thickness and invades the papillary dermis (Clark's Level II)
pT2 Tumor more than 0.75 mm but not more than 1.5 mm in thickness and/or invades to papillary-reticular dermal interface (Clark's Level III)
pT3 Tumor more than 1.5 mm but not more than 4 mm in thickness and/or invades the reticular dermis (Clark's Level IV)
    pT3a Tumor more than 1.5 mm but not more than 3 mm in thickness
    pT3b Tumor more than 3 mm but not more than 4 mm in thickness
pT4 Tumor more than 4 mm in thickness and/or invades the subcutaneous tissue (Clark's Level V) and/or satellite(s) within 2 cm of the primary tumor
    pT4a Tumor more than 4 mm in thickness and/or invades the subcutaneous tissue
    pT4b Satellite(s) within 2 cm of the primary tumor

Regional Lymph Nodes (N)

NX Regional lymph nodes cannot be assessed
N0 No regional lymph node metastasis
N1 Metastasis 3 cm or less in greatest dimension in any regional lymph node(s)
N2 Metastasis more than 3 cm in greatest dimension in any regional lymph node(s) and/or in-transit metastasis
    N2a Metastasis more than 3 cm in greatest dimension in any regional lymph node(s)
    N2b In-transit metastasis
    N2c Both (N2a and N2b)

Distant Metastasis (M)

MX Presence of distant metastasis cannot be assessed
M0 No distant metastasis
M1 Distant metastasis
    M1a Metastasis in skin or subcutaneous tissue or lymph node(s) beyond the regional lymph nodes
    M1b Visceral metastasis

Note: In-transit metastasis involves skin or subcutaneous tissue more than 2 cm from the primary tumor not beyond the regional lymph nodes.

STAGE GROUPING

Stage	pT	N	M
Stage I	pT1	N0	M0
	pT2	N0	M0
Stage II	pT3	N0	M0
Stage III	pT4	N0	M0
	Any pT	N1, N2	M0
Stage IV	Any pT	Any N	M1

DIFFERENCES BETWEEN THE 2ND AND 3RD EDITIONS

In this edition the T3 category has been subdivided into T3a and T3b in order to provide more detail in recording the thickness of the tumor. Also, the T4 category has been split into T4a and T4b in order to record separately satellite lesions that are within 2 cm of the primary tumor. A new T category—Tis—has been introduced in order to stage the atypical melanocytic hyperplasias or *in situ* lesions. In the new system, T0 refers to "no evidence of tumor." In the 1983 edition, T0 referred to the atypical hyperplastic melanocytic lesions.

The N categories have been complctcly redefined. The diameter of the involved nodes has been reduced from 5 to 3 cm. Also, the N2 category has been split into three groups for more specificity. In this edition, the M1 category is subdivided into M1a and M1b, depending on the location of the metastatic lesions. The symbol M2 is no longer used.

HISTOPATHOLOGIC TYPE

The types of malignant melanoma are as follows:

Lentigo maligna (Hutchinson's freckle)
Radial spreading (superficial spreading)
Nodular
Acral lentiginous
Unclassified

A rare desmoplastic variant also exists.

Melanomas are identified according to site (mucosal, ocular, vaginal, anal, urethral, etc.). The staging classification described in this chapter applies only to those arising in the skin.

HISTOPATHOLOGIC GRADE (G) (RARELY USED WITH MELANOMAS)

GX Grade cannot be assessed
G1 Well differentiated
G2 Moderately well differentiated
G3 Poorly differentiated
G4 Undifferentiated

BIBLIOGRAPHY

1. Balch CM, Murad TM, Soong SJ et al: A multifactorial analysis of melanoma: Prognostic histopathological features comparing Clark's and Breslow's staging lesions. Ann Surg 188:732–742, 1978
2. Breslow A: Thickness, cross-sectional areas and depth of invasion in the prognosis of cutaneous melanoma. Ann Surg 172:902–908, 1970
3. Breslow A: Prognosis in cutaneous melanoma: Tumor thickness as a guide to treatment. Pathol Annu Part 1:1–20, 1980
4. Clark WH Jr: The histogenesis and biological behavior of primary malignant melanoma of the skin. Cancer Res 29:705–717, 1969
5. Kopf AW, Rodriquez-Sains RS, Rigel DS et al: "Small" melanomas: Relation of prognostic variables to diameter of superficial spreading melanomas. J Dermatol Surg Oncol 8:765–770, 1982

MELANOMA OF THE SKIN (EXCLUDING EYELID)

Data Form for Cancer Staging

Patient identification
Name _____
Address _____
Hospital or clinic number _____
Age _____ Sex _____ Race _____

Institution identification
Hospital or clinic _____
Address _____

Oncology Record

Anatomic site of cancer _____
Histologic type _____
Grade (G) _____
Date of classification _____

Chronology of classification
(use separate form for each time staged)
[ ] Clinical (use all data prior to first treatment)
[ ] Pathologic (if definitively resected specimen available)

Definitions

Primary Tumor (pT)

[ ] pTX Primary tumor cannot be assessed
[ ] pT0 No evidence of primary tumor
[ ] pTis Melanoma in situ (atypical melanotic hyperplasia, severe melanotic dysplasia), not an invasive lesion (Clark's Level I)
[ ] pT1 Tumor 0.75 mm or less in thickness and invades the papillary dermis (Clark's Level II)
[ ] pT2 Tumor more than 0.75 mm but not more than 1.5 mm in thickness and/or invades to papillary-reticular dermal interface (Clark's Level III)
[ ] pT3 Tumor more than 1.5 mm but not more than 4 mm in thickness and/or invades the reticular dermis (Clark's Level IV)
  [ ] pT3a Tumor more than 1.5 mm but not more than 3 mm in thickness
  [ ] pT3b Tumor more than 3 mm but not more than 4 mm in thickness
[ ] pT4 Tumor more than 4 mm in thickness and/or invades the subcutaneous tissue (Clark's Level V) and/or satellite(s) within 2 cm of the primary tumor
  [ ] pT4a Tumor more than 4 mm in thickness and/or invades the subcutaneous tissue
  [ ] pT4b Satellite(s) with 2 cm of primary tumor

Lymph Node (N)

[ ] NX Regional lymph nodes cannot be assessed
[ ] N0 No regional lymph node metastasis
[ ] N1 Metastasis 3 cm or less in greatest dimension in any regional lymph node(s)
[ ] N2 Metastasis more than 3 cm in greatest dimension in any regional lymph node(s) and/or in-transit metastasis
  [ ] N2a Metastasis more than 3 cm in greatest dimension in any regional lymph node(s)
  [ ] N2b In-transit metastasis
  [ ] N2c Both (N2a and N2b)

Distant Metastasis (M)

[ ] MX Presence of distant metastasis cannot be assessed
[ ] M0 No distant metastasis
[ ] M1 Distant metastasis
  [ ] M1a Metastasis in skin or subcutaneous tissue or lymph node(s) beyond the regional lymph nodes
  [ ] M1b Visceral metastasis

Stage Grouping

See Bottom page 144
See attached

[ ]	I	pT1	N0	M0
[ ]	II	pT2	N0	M0
[ ]	III	pT3	N0	M0
		Any pT	N1	M0
		Any pT	N2	M0
[ ]	IV	Any pT	Any N	M1

Histopathologic Grade (G)

[ ] GX Grade cannot be assessed
[ ] G1 Well differentiated
[ ] G2 Moderately well differentiated
[ ] G3 Poorly differentiated
[ ] G4 Undifferentiated

Histopathologic Type

The types of malignant melanoma are as follows:

Lentigo maligna (Hutchinson's freckle)
Radial spreading (superficial spreading)
Nodular
Acral lentiginous
Unclassified

A rare desmoplastic variant also exists.
Melanomas are identified according to site (mucosal, ocular, vaginal, anal, urethral, and so forth). The staging classification described in this chapter applies only to those arising in the skin.

Sites of Distant Metastasis

Pulmonary	PUL
Osseous	OSS
Hepatic	HEP
Brain	BRA
Lymph nodes	LYM
Bone marrow	MAR
Pleura	PLE
Peritoneum	PER
Skin	SKI
Other	OTH

Staged by _____ M.D.
_____ Referral
Date _____

American Joint Committee on Cancer—1988

Illustrations

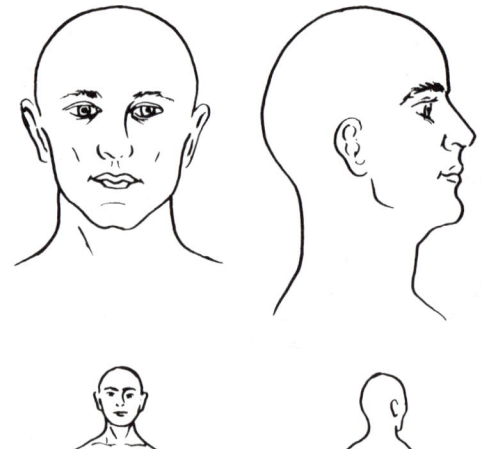

Depth of Invasion
[ ] Level I (not a melanoma and further characterization is not necessary)
[ ] Level II   [ ] Level IV
[ ] Level III   [ ] Level V
Other description _____
Maximal thickness (mm) _____
Site of primary lesion (check diagram)

Extent of primary lesion (include all pigmentation)
_____

Size in greatest diameter _____ cm

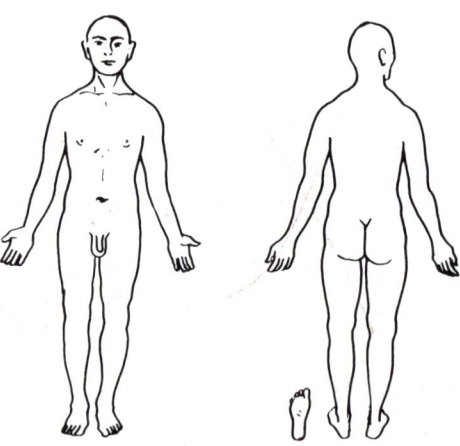

Indicate on diagrams primary tumor and regional nodes involved.

The correct stage grouping is as follows:

Stage I	pT1	N0	M0
	pT2	N0	M0
Stage II	pT3	N0	M0
	pT4	N0	M0
Stage III	Any pT	N1	M0
	Any pT	N2	M0
Stage IV	Includes all patients with a M1 disease irrespective of pTN classification.		

12-90

BREAST

23

The following TNM definitions and stage groupings for carcinoma of the breast are the same for the AJCC and the UICC/TNM projects. This staging system for carcinoma of the breast applies to infiltrating and *in situ* carcinomas. Microscopic confirmation of the diagnosis is mandatory and the histologic type of carcinoma should be recorded.

ANATOMY

Primary Site. The mammary gland (ICD-O 174, 175), situated on the anterior chest wall, is composed of glandular tissue within a dense fibroareolar stroma. The glandular tissue consists of approximately 20 lobes, each of which terminates in a separate excretory duct in the nipple.

Regional Lymph Nodes. The breast lymphatics drain by way of three major routes: axillary, transpectoral, and internal mammary. Intramammary lymph nodes are considered axillary for staging purposes. Metastases to any other lymph nodes are considered distant (M1), including supraclavicular, cervical, or contralateral internal mammary.

Metastatic Sites. All distant visceral sites are potential sites of metastases. The four major sites of involvement are bone, lung, brain, and liver, but this widely metastasizing disease has been found in almost any remote site.

RULES FOR CLASSIFICATION

Clinical Staging. Clinical staging includes physical examination, with careful inspection and palpation of the skin, mammary gland, and lymph nodes (axillary, supraclavicular, and cervical) and pathologic examination of the breast *or* other tissues to establish the diagnosis of breast carcinoma. The extent of tissues examined pathologically for clinical staging is less than that required for pathologic staging (see pathologic staging). Appropriate operative findings are elements of clinical staging, including the size of the primary tumor and chest wall invasion and the presence or absence of regional or distant metastasis.

IIIA. Based on survival data gleaned from the Surveillance Epidemiology and End Results (SEER) program of the National Cancer Institute (NCI), the 5-year survival of T3 N0 M0 (76%) is more closely aligned with Stage II (75%) than with Stage IIIA (56%). Therefore, T3 N0 M0 is now classified Stage IIB.

HISTOPATHOLOGIC TYPE

The histologic types are the following:

Cancer, NOS (not otherwise specified)
Ductal
    Intraductal (*in situ*)
    Invasive with predominant intraductal component
    Invasive, NOS (not otherwise specified)
    Comedo
    Inflammatory
    Medullary with lymphocytic infiltrate
    Mucinous (colloid)
    Papillary
    Scirrhous
    Tubular
    Other
Lobular
    In situ
    Invasive with predominant *in situ* component
    Invasive
Nipple
    Paget's disease, NOS (not otherwise specified)
    Paget's disease with intraductal carcinoma
    Paget's disease with invasive ductal carcinoma
Other

HISTOPATHOLOGIC GRADE (G)

GX Grade cannot be assessed
G1 Well differentiated
G2 Moderately well differentiated
G3 Poorly differentiated
G4 Undifferentiated

BREAST

Data Form for Cancer Staging

Patient identification
Name _____
Address _____
Hospital or clinic number _____
Age _____ Sex _____ Race _____

Institution identification
Hospital or clinic _____
Address _____

Oncology Record

Anatomic site of cancer _____
Histologic type _____
Grade (G) _____
Date of classification _____

Chronology of classification
  (use separate form for each time staged)
[ ] Clinical (use all data prior to first treatment)
[ ] Pathologic (if definitively resected specimen available)

Definitions

Primary Tumor (T)

[ ] TX   Primary tumor cannot be assessed
[ ] T0   No evidence of primary tumor
[ ] Tis   Carcinoma *in situ*: Intraductal carcinoma, lobular carcinoma *in situ*, or Paget's disease of the nipple with no tumor.
[ ] T1   Tumor 2 cm or less in greatest dimension
  [ ] T1a   0.5 cm or less in greatest dimension
  [ ] T1b   More than 0.5 cm but not more than 1 cm in greatest dimension
  [ ] T1c   More than 1 cm but not more than 2 cm in greatest dimension
[ ] T2   Tumor more than 2 cm but not more than 5 cm in greatest dimension
[ ] T3   Tumor more than 5 cm in greatest dimension
[ ] T4   Tumor of any size with direct extension to chest wall or skin.
  [ ] T4a   Extension to chest wall
  [ ] T4b   Edema (including peau d'orange) or ulceration of the skin of breast or satellite skin nodules confined to same breast
  [ ] T4c   Both T4a and T4b
  [ ] T4d   Inflammatory carcinoma

Lymph Node (N)

[ ] NX   Regional lymph nodes cannot be assessed
[ ] N0   No regional lymph node metastasis
[ ] N1   Metastasis to movable ipsilateral axillary lymph node(s)
[ ] N2   Metastasis to ipsilateral axillary lymph node(s) fixed to one another or to other structures
[ ] N3   Metastasis to ipsilateral internal mammary lymph node(s)

Pathologic Classification (pN)

[ ] pNX   Regional lymph nodes cannot be assessed
[ ] pN0   No regional lymph node metastasis
[ ] pN1   Metastasis to movable ipsilateral axillary lymph node(s)
  [ ] pN1a   Only micrometastasis (none larger than 0.2 cm)
  [ ] pN1b   Metastasis to lymph nodes, any larger than 0.2 cm
    [ ] pN1bi   Metastasis in 1 to 3 lymph nodes, any more than 0.2 cm and all less than 2 cm in greatest dimension
    [ ] pN1bii   Metastasis to 4 or more lymph nodes, any more than 0.2 cm and all less than 2 cm in greatest dimension
    [ ] pN1biii   Extension of tumor beyond the capsule of a lymph node metastasis less than 2 cm in greatest dimension
    [ ] pN1biv   Metastasis to a lymph node 2 cm or more in greatest dimension
[ ] pN2   Metastasis to ipsilateral axillary lymph nodes that are fixed to one another or to other structures
[ ] pN3   Metastasis to ipsilateral internal mammary lymph node(s)

Distant Metastasis (M)

[ ] MX   Presence of distant metastasis cannot be assessed
[ ] M0   No distant metastasis
[ ] M1   Distant metastasis (includes metastasis to ipsilateral supraclavicular lymph nodes

Stage Grouping

[ ] 0	Tis	N0	M0
[ ] I	T1	N0	M0
[ ] IIA	T0	N1	M0
	T1	N1*	M0
	T2	N0	M0
[ ] IIB	T2	N1	M0
	T3	N0	M0
[ ] IIIA	T0	N2	M0
	T1	N2	M0
	T2	N2	M0
	T3	N1	M0
	T3	N2	M0
[ ] IIIB	T4	Any N	M0
	Any T	N3	M0
[ ] IV	Any T	Any N	M1

Note: The prognosis of patients with pN1a is similar to that of patients with pN0.

Histopathologic Grade (G)

[ ] GX   Grade cannot be assessed
[ ] G1   Well differentiated
[ ] G2   Moderately well differentiated
[ ] G3   Poorly differentiated
[ ] G4   Undifferentiated

Staged by _____ M.D.
_____ Registrar
Date _____

American Joint Committee on Cancer—1988

Illustration

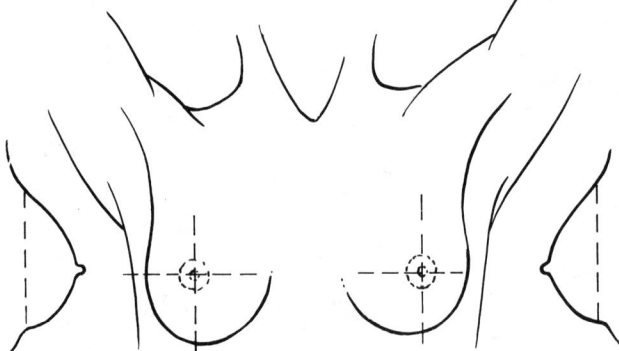

Indicate on diagram primary tumor and regional nodes involved.

Histopathologic Type

The histologic types are the following:

Cancer, NOS (not otherwise specified)
Ductal
    Intraductal (*in situ*)
    Invasive with predominant intraductal component
    Invasive, NOS (not otherwise specified)
    Comedo
    Inflammatory
    Medullary with lymphocytic infiltrate
    Mucinous (colloid)
    Papillary
    Scirrhous
    Tubular
    Other
Lobular
    In situ
    Invasive with predominant *in situ* component
    Invasive
Nipple
    Paget's disease, NOS (not otherwise specified)
    Paget's disease with intraductal carcinoma
    Paget's disease with invasive ductal carcinoma
Other

Sites of Distant Metastasis

Pulmonary	PUL
Osseous	OSS
Hepatic	HEP
Brain	BRA
Lymph nodes	LYM
Bone marrow	MAR
Pleura	PLE
Peritoneum	PER
Skin	SKI
Other	OTH

GYNECOLOGIC SITES

24

Cervix Uteri

Cervix uteri, corpus uteri, ovary, vagina, and vulva are the sites included in this section. Cervix uteri and corpus uteri were among the first sites to be classified by the TNM system. The League of Nations stages for carcinoma of the cervix have been used with minor modifications for nearly 50 years, and, because these are accepted by the Federation Internationale de Gynecologie et d'Obstetrique (FIGO), the TNM categories have been defined to correspond to the FIGO stages. Some amendments have been made in collaboration with FIGO, and the classifications now published have the approval of FIGO, AJCC, and all other national TNM committees of the Union Internationale Contre le Cancer (UICC).

The AJCC has worked closely with the International Federation of Gynecology and Obstetrics (FIGO) in classification of cancer at gynecologic sites. Staging of malignant tumors is essentially the same and stages are comparable by the two systems.

ANATOMY

Primary Site. The cervix (ICD-O 180) is the lower third of the uterus. It is roughly cylindrical in shape, projects through the upper anterior vaginal wall, and communicates with the vagina through an orifice called the external os. Cancer of the cervix may originate on the vaginal surface or in the canal.

Regional Lymph Nodes. The cervix is drained by preureteral, postureteral, and uterosacral routes into the following first station nodes: parametrial, hypogastric (obturator), external iliac, internal iliac, sacral, pericervical, presacral, and common iliac. Para-aortic node involvement is considered distant metastasis and is coded M1.

Metastatic Sites. The most common sites of distant spread are the lungs and skeleton.

RULES FOR CLASSIFICATION

The classification applies only to carcinoma. There should be histologic confirmation of the disease.

Clinical Staging. Careful clinical examination should be performed in all cases, preferably by an experienced examiner and with anesthesia. The clinical staging must not be changed because of subsequent findings. When there is doubt as to which stage a particular cancer should be allocated, the earlier stage is mandatory. The following examinations are permitted: palpation, inspection, colposcopy, endocervical curettage, hysteroscopy, cystoscopy, proctoscopy, intravenous urography, and x-ray examination of the lungs and skeleton. Suspected bladder or rectal involvement should be confirmed by biopsy and histologic evidence. Optional examinations include lymphangiography, arteriography, venography, laparoscopy, and other imaging methods. Because these are not yet generally available and because the interpretation of results is variable, the findings of optional studies should not be the basis for changing the clinical staging.

Pathologic Staging. In cases treated by surgical procedures, the pathologist's findings in the removed tissues can be the basis for extremely accurate statements on the extent of disease. These findings should not be allowed to change the clinical staging but should be recorded in the manner described for the pathologic staging of disease. The pTNM nomenclature is appropriate for this purpose. Infrequently hysterectomy is carried out in the presence of unsuspected extensive invasive cervical carcinoma. Such cases cannot be clinically staged or included in therapeutic statistics, but it is desirable that they be reported separately. Only if the rules for clinical staging are strictly observed will it be possible to compare results among clinics and by differing modes of therapy.

Anatomic Subsites

Endocervix (ICD-O 180.0)
Exocervix (ICD-O 180.1)

DEFINITION OF TNM

The definitions of the T categories correspond to the several stages accepted by FIGO. Both systems are included for comparison.

Primary Tumor (T)

TNM	FIGO	DEFINITION
TX		Primary tumor cannot be assessed
T0		No evidence of primary tumor
Tis	0	Carcinoma *in situ*
T1	I	Cervical carcinoma confined to uterus (extension to corpus should be disregarded)
T1a	Ia	Preclinical invasive carcinoma, diagnosed by microscopy only
T1a1	Iaa1	Minimal microscopic stromal invasion
T1a2	Ia2	Tumor with invasive component 5 mm or less in depth taken from the base of the epithelium and 7 mm or less in horizontal spread
T1b	Ib	Tumor larger than T1a2
T2	II	Cervical carcinoma invades beyond uterus but not to pelvic wall or to the lower third of vagina
T2a	IIa	Without parametrial invasion
T2b	IIb	With parametrial invasion
T3	III	Cervical carcinoma extends to the pelvic wall and/or involves lower third of vagina and/or causes hydronephrosis or nonfunctioning kidney
T3a	IIIa	Tumor involves lower third of the vagina, no extension to pelvic wall
T3b	IIIb	Tumor extends to pelvic wall and/or causes hydronephrosis or nonfunctioning kidney
T4*	IVa	Tumor invades mucosa of bladder or rectum and/or extends beyond true pelvis.
M1	IVb	Distant metastasis

Regional Lymph Nodes (N)

Regional lymph nodes include paracervical, parametrial, hypogastric (obturator), common, internal and external iliac, presacral and sacral.

NX Regional lymph nodes cannot be assessed
N0 No regional lymph node metastasis
N1 Regional lymph node metastasis

Note: Presence of bullous edema is not sufficient evidence to classify a tumor T4

Cervix Uteri

Distant Metastasis (M)

MX	Presence of distant metastasis cannot be assessed
M0	No distant metastasis
M1 IVb	Distant metastasis

pTNM Pathologic Classification

The pT, pN, and pM categories correspond to the T, N, and M categories.

STAGE GROUPING

Stage 0	Tis	N0	M0
Stage IA	T1a	N0	M0
Stage IB	T1b	N0	M0
Stage IIA	T2a	N0	M0
Stage IIB	T2b	N0	M0
Stage IIIA	T3a	N0	M0
Stage IIIB	T1	N1	M0
	T2	N1	M0
	T3a	N1	M0
	T3b	Any N	M0
Stage IVA	T4	Any N	M0
Stage IVB	Any T	Any N	M1

DIFFERENCES BETWEEN THE 2ND AND 3RD EDITIONS

The extent of micro-invasion in Stage Ia is defined with greater precision in this edition of the *Manual.*

HISTOPATHOLOGIC TYPE

Cases should be classified as carcinoma of the cervix if the primary growth is in the cervix. All histologic types must be included. Grading is encouraged but is not a basis for modifying the stage groupings. When surgery is the primary treatment, the histologic findings permit the case to have pathologic staging. In this, the pTNM nomenclature is to be used.

HISTOPATHOLOGIC GRADE (G)

GX	Grade cannot be assessed
G1	Well differentiated
G2	Moderately well differentiated
G3	Poorly differentiated
G4	Undifferentiated

CERVIX UTERI

Data Form for Cancer Staging

Patient identification
Name _____
Address _____
Hospital or clinic number _____
Age _____ Sex _____ Race _____

Institution identification
Hospital or clinic _____
Address _____

Oncology Record

Anatomic site of cancer _____
Histologic type _____
Grade (G) _____
Date of classification _____

Chronology of classification
  (use separate form for each time staged)
[ ] Clinical (use all data prior to first treatment)
[ ] Pathologic (if definitively resected specimen available)

Definitions

Primary Tumor (T)

[ ] TX Primary tumor cannot be assessed
[ ] T0 No evidence of primary tumor
[ ] Tis Carcinoma *in situ*
[ ] T1 Cervical carcinoma confined to uterus
  [ ] T1a Preclinical invasive carcinoma, diagnosed by microscopy only
    [ ] T1a1 Minimal microscopic stromal invasion
    [ ] T1a2 Tumor with invasive component 5 mm or less in depth taken from the base of the epithelium and 7 mm or less in horizontal spread
  [ ] T1b Tumor larger than T1a2
[ ] T2 Cervical carcinoma invades beyond uterus but not to pelvic wall or to the lower third of vagina
  [ ] T2a Tumor without parametrial invasion
  [ ] T2b Tumor with parametrial invasion
[ ] T3 Cervical carcinoma extends to pelvic wall and/or involves lower third of vagina and/or causes hydronephrosis or nonfunctioning kidney
  [ ] T3a Tumor involves lower third of the vagina, no extension to pelvic wall
  [ ] T3b Tumor extends to pelvic wall and/or causes hydronephrosis or nonfunctioning kidney
[ ] T4 Tumor invades mucosa of bladder or rectum and/or extends beyond the true pelvis

Lymph Node (N)

[ ] NX Regional lymph nodes cannot be assessed
[ ] N0 No regional lymph node metastasis
[ ] N1 Regional lymph node metastasis

Distant Metastasis (M)

[ ] MX Presence of distant metastasis cannot be assessed
[ ] M0 No distant metastasis
[ ] M1 Distant metastasis

Stage Grouping

[ ] 0	Tis	N0	M0
[ ] IA	T1a	N0	M0
[ ] IB	T1b	N0	M0
[ ] IIA	T2a	N0	M0
[ ] IIB	T2b	N0	M0
[ ] IIIA	T3a	N0	M0
[ ] IIIB	T1	N1	M0
	T2	N1	M0
	T3a	N1	M0
	T3b	Any N	M0
[ ] IVA	T4	Any N	M0
[ ] IVB	Any T	Any N	M1

Histopathologic Grade (G)

[ ] GX Grade cannot be assessed
[ ] G1 Well differentiated
[ ] G2 Moderately well differentiated
[ ] G3 Poorly differentiated
[ ] G4 Undifferentiated

Histopathologic Type

Cases should be classified as carcinoma of the cervix if the primary growth is in the cervix. All histologic types must be included. Grading is encouraged but is not a basis for modifying the stage groupings. When surgery is the primary treatment, the histologic findings permit the case to have pathologic staging. In this, the pTNM nomenclature is to be used.

Staged by _____ M.D.
          _____ Registrar
Date _____

Sites of Distant Metastasis

Pulmonary	PUL
Osseous	OSS
Hepatic	HEP
Brain	BRA
Lymph nodes	LYM
Bone marrow	MAR
Pleura	PLE
Peritoneum	PER
Skin	SKI
Other	OTH

Illustrations

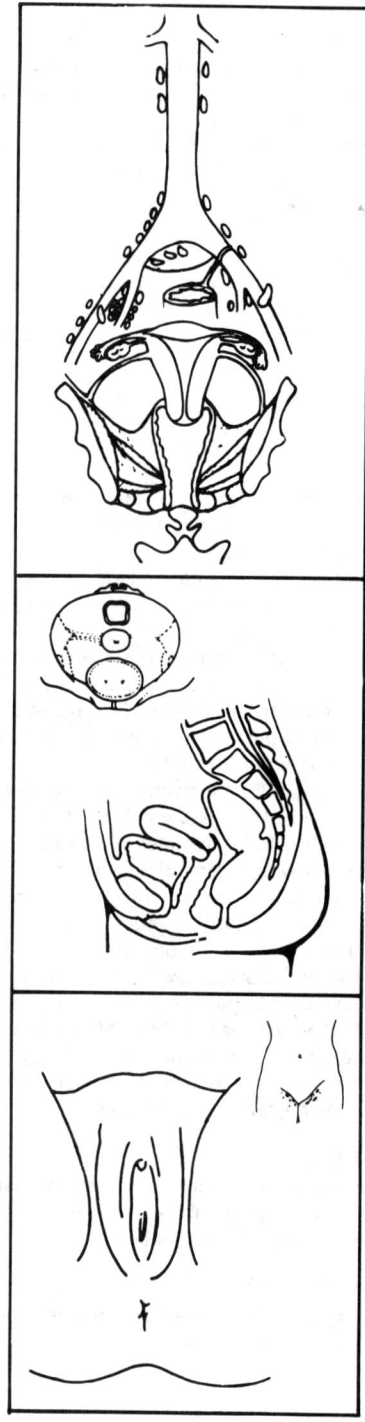

Indicate on diagrams primary tumor and regional nodes involved.

25

Corpus Uteri

ANATOMY

Primary Site. The upper two thirds of the uterus above the level of the internal cervical os is called the corpus (ICD-O 182). The fallopian tubes enter at the upper lateral corners of a pear-shaped body. The portion of the muscular organ that is above a line joining the tubo uterine orifices is often referred to as the *fundus*.

Regional Lymph Nodes. The major lymphatic trunks are the utero-ovarian (infundibulopelvic), parametrial, and presacral, which drain into the internal iliac, pericervical, obturator, hypogastric, external iliac, common iliac, and presacral nodes.

Metastatic Sites. The vagina and lung are the common metastatic sites.

RULES FOR CLASSIFICATION

The classification applies only to carcinoma. There should be histologic verification and grading of the tumor.

Clinical Staging. Careful clinical examination should be performed, preferably by an experienced examiner and with anesthesia, before any definitive therapy. The clinical staging must not be changed because of subsequent findings. When there is doubt as to which stage a particular cancer should be allocated, the earlier stage is mandatory. The following examinations are permitted: palpation, inspection, colposcopy, endocervical curettage, hysteroscopy, cystoscopy, proctoscopy, intravenous urography, and imaging examination of lungs and skeleton. Optional examinations include lymphangiography, arteriography, venography, and laparoscopy. Sounding and determination of the depth of the uterine cavity is an important step. Fractional curettage is essential with separation of endometrial and endocervical curettings. Careful inspection and palpation of the vagina should be carried out to assess the entire length of the vaginal tube from the apex to the urethra.

Pathologic Staging. Hysterectomy with or without pelvic node dissection provides the basis for surgical-pathologic staging and should not be substituted for clinical staging.

Anatomic Subsites

Corpus uteri (ICD-O 182.0)
Isthmus uteri (ICD-O 182.1)

DEFINITION OF TNM

The definitions of the T categories correspond to the several stages accepted by FIGO. (FIGO stages are further subdivided by histologic grade of tumor.) Both systems are included for comparison.

Primary Tumor (T)

TNM	FIGO	DEFINITION
TX		Primary tumor cannot be assessed
T0		No evidence of primary tumor
Tis	0	Carcinoma *in situ*
T1	I	Tumor confined to corpus
T1a	Ia	Uterine cavity 8 cm or less in length
T1b	Ib	Uterine cavity more than 8 cm in length
T2	II	Tumor invades cervix but does not extend beyond uterus
T3	III	Tumor extends beyond uterus but not outside true pelvis
T4*	IVa	Tumor invades mucosa of bladder or rectum and/or extends beyond the true pelvis
M1	IVb	Distant metastasis

Regional Lymph Nodes (N)

Regional lymph nodes include hypogastric (obturator); common, internal, and external iliac; parametrial and sacral nodes.

NX	Regional lymph nodes cannot be assessed
N0	No regional lymph node metastasis
N1	Regional lymph node metastasis

Distant Metastasis (M)

TNM	FIGO	DEFINITION
MX		Presence of distant metastasis cannot be assessed
M0		No distant metastasis
M1	IVb	Distant metastasis

*Note: The presence of bullous edema is not sufficient evidence to classify a tumor T4.

pTNM Pathologic Classification

The pT, pN, and pM categories correspond to the T, N, and M categories.

STAGE GROUPING

Stage 0	Tis	N0	M0
Stage IA	T1a	N0	M0
Stage IB	T1b	N0	M0
Stage II	T2	N0	M0
Stage III	T1	N1	M0
	T2	N1	M0
	T3	Any N	M0
Stage IVA	T4	Any N	M0
Stage IVB	Any T	Any N	M1

DIFFERENCES BETWEEN THE 2ND AND 3RD EDITIONS

This classification is the same as that published in the second edition of the *Manual*.

NOTES ABOUT STAGING

Studies of large series of cases of endometrial carcinoma limited to the corpus have shown that the prognosis is related to some extent to the size of the uterus. However, an enlargement of the uterus may be caused by fibroids, adenomyosis, and other disorders. Therefore, the size of the uterus cannot serve as a basis for subgrouping Stage I cases. The length and the width of the uterine cavity are related to the prognosis. The great majority of cases of corpus cancer belong to Stage I. A subdivision of these cases is desirable. Therefore, the Cancer Committee recommends a subdivision of Stage I cases with regard to the length of the sound used and to the histologic examination of the curettings.

Extension of the carcinoma to the endocervix is confirmed by fractional curettage, hysterography, or hysteroscopy. Scraping the cervix should be the first step of the curettage and the specimens from the cervix should be examined separately. Occasionally, it may be difficult to decide whether the endocervix is involved by the cancer. In such cases, the simultaneous presence of normal cervical glands and cancer in the same section will give the final diagnosis.

Extension of the carcinoma outside the uterus should refer a case to Stage III or Stage IV. The presence of metastases in the vagina or in the ovary permits allotment of a case to Stage III.

Corpus Uteri

HISTOPATHOLOGIC TYPE

It is desirable that Stage I cases be subgrouped according to the degree of differentiation described on microscopic examination. The predominant lesion is adenocarcinoma, but all histologic types should be reported. However, choriocarcinomas, sarcomas, mixed mesodermal tumors, and carcinosarcomas should be presented separately.

HISTOPATHOLOGIC GRADE (G)

- GX Grade cannot be assessed
- G1 Well differentiated
- G2 Moderately well differentiated
- G3–4 Poorly differentiated or undifferentiated

CORPUS UTERI

Data Form for Cancer Staging

Patient identification
Name _____
Address _____
Hospital or clinic number _____
Age _____ Sex _____ Race _____

Institution identification
Hospital or clinic _____
Address _____

Oncology Record

Anatomic site of cancer _____
Histologic type _____
Grade (G) _____
Date of classification _____

Chronology of classification
 (use separate form for each time staged)
[ ] Clinical (use all data prior to first treatment)
[ ] Pathologic (if definitively resected specimen available)

Definitions

Primary Tumor (T)

TNM	FIGO	DEFINITION
TX		Primary tumor cannot be assessed
T0		No evidence of primary tumor
Tis	0	Carcinoma *in situ*
T1	I	Tumor confined to corpus
T1a	Ia	Uterine cavity 8 cm or less in length
T1b	Ib	Uterine cavity more than 8 cm in length
T2	II	Tumor invades cervix but does not extend beyond uterus
T3	III	Tumor extends beyond uterus but not outside true pelvis
T4*	IVa	Tumor invades mucosa of bladder or rectum and/or extends beyond the true pelvis
M1	IVb	Distant metastasis

*Note: The presence of bullous edema is not sufficient evidence to classify a tumor T4.

Lymph Node (N)

[ ] NX Regional lymph nodes cannot be assessed
[ ] N0 No regional lymph node metastasis
[ ] N1 Regional lymph node metastasis

Distant Metastasis (M)

TNM	FIGO	DEFINITION
MX		Presence of distant metastasis cannot be assessed
M0		No distant metastasis
M1	IVb	Distant metastasis

Stage Grouping

[ ]	0	Tis	N0	M0
[ ]	IA	T1a	N0	M0
[ ]	IB	T1b	N0	M0
[ ]	II	T2	N0	M0
[ ]	III	T1	N1	M0
		T2	N1	M0
		T3	Any N	M0
[ ]	IVA	T4	Any N	M0
[ ]	IVB	Any T	Any N	M1

Histopathologic Type

It is desirable that Stage I cases be subgrouped according to the degree of differentiation described on microscopic examination. The predominant lesion is adenocarcinoma, but all histologic types should be reported. However, choriocarcinomas, sarcomas, mixed mesodermal tumors, and carcinosarcomas should be presented separately.

Histopathologic Grade (G)

[ ] GX Grade cannot be assessed
[ ] G1 Well differentiated
[ ] G2 Moderately well differentiated
[ ] G3-4 Poorly differentiated or undifferentiated

Sites of Distant Metastasis

Pulmonary	PUL
Osseous	OSS
Hepatic	HEP
Brain	BRA
Lymph nodes	LYM
Bone marrow	MAR
Pleura	PLE
Peritoneum	PER
Skin	SKI
Other	OTH

Staged by _____ M.D.
_____ Registrar
Date _____

Illustrations

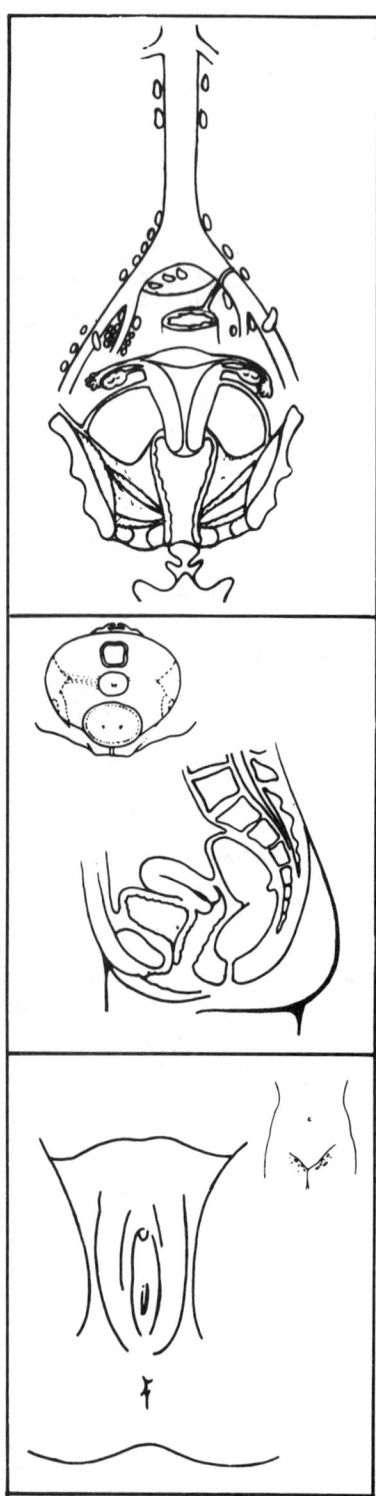

Indicate on diagrams primary tumor and regional nodes involved.

26

Ovary

ANATOMY

Primary Site. Ovaries (ICD-O 183.0) are a pair of solid bodies, flattened ovoids 2 to 4 cm in diameter, that are connected by a peritoneal fold to the broad ligament and by the infundibulopelvic ligament to the lateral wall of the pelvis.

Regional Lymph Nodes. The lymphatic drainage occurs by the utero-ovarian and round ligament trunks and an external iliac accessory route into the following regional nodes: external iliac, common iliac, hypogastric, internal iliac, obturator, lateral sacral, and paraaortic nodes and, rarely, to inguinal nodes.

Metastatic Sites. The peritoneum, including the omentum and pelvic and abdominal viscera, are common sites for seeding. Diaphragmatic involvement and liver metastases are common. Pulmonary and pleural involvement also occur.

RULES FOR CLASSIFICATION

There should be histologic confirmation of the disease to permit division of cases by histopathologic type. In accordance with FIGO, a simplified version of the WHO histologic typing (1973 publication No. 9) is recommended. The degree of differentiation (grade) should be recorded.

It is desirable to have a clinical stage grouping of ovarian tumors similar to those already existing for other malignant tumors in the female pelvis. Rarely is it possible to come to a final diagnosis by inspection or palpation or by any of the other methods recommended for clinical staging of carcinoma of the uterus and vagina. Therefore, the Cancer Committee of FIGO has recommended that the clinical staging of primary carcinoma of the ovary should be based on findings by laparoscopy or laparotomy, as well as on the usual clinical examination and roentgen studies.

Clinical Staging. Although clinical studies similar to those for other sites may be used, the establishment of a diagnosis most often requires a laparotomy, which is most widely accepted in surgical-pathologic staging. Clinical studies, if carcinoma of the ovary is diagnosed, include routine radiography of the chest. CT or other imaging studies may be helpful in both initial staging and follow-up of the tumors.

Pathologic Staging. This should include laparotomy and resection of ovarian masses, as well as hysterectomy. Biopsies of all suspicious sites, such as the omentum, mesentery, liver, diaphragm, and pelvic and para-aortic nodes, are required.

DEFINITION OF TNM

The definitions of the T categories correspond to the several stages accepted by FIGO. Both systems are included for comparison.

Primary Tumor (T)

TNM	FIGO	DEFINITION
TX		Primary tumor cannot be assessed
T0		No evidence of primary tumor
T1	I	Tumor limited to ovaries
T1a	Ia	Tumor limited to one ovary; capsule intact, no tumor on ovarian surface
T1b	Ib	Tumor limited to both ovaries; capsules intact, no tumor on ovarian surface
T1c	Ic	Tumor limited to one or both ovaries with any of the following: capsule ruptured, tumor on ovarian surface, malignant cells in ascites, or peritoneal washing
T2	II	Tumor involves one or both ovaries with pelvic extension
T2a	IIa	Extension and/or implants on uterus and/or tube(s)
T2b	IIb	Extension to other pelvic tissues
T2c	IIc	Pelvic extension (2a or 2b) with malignant cells in ascites or peritoneal washing
T3 and/or N1	III	Tumor involves one or both ovaries with microscopically confirmed peritoneal metastasis outside the pelvis and/or regional lymph node metastasis
T3a	IIIa	Microscopic peritoneal metastasis beyond pelvis
T3b	IIIb	Macroscopic peritoneal metastasis beyond pelvis 2 cm or less in greatest dimension
T3c and/or N1	IIIc	Peritoneal metastasis beyond pelvis more than 2 cm in greatest dimension and/or regional lymph node metastasis
M1	IV	Distant metastasis (excludes peritoneal metastasis)

Note: Liver capsule metastasis is T3/Stage III, liver parenchymal metastasis M1/Stage IV. Pleural effusion must have positive cytology for M1/Stage IV.

Regional Lymph Nodes (N)

Regional lymph nodes include hypogastric (obturator), common iliac, external iliac, internal iliac, lateral sacral, para-aortic, and inguinal.

NX Regional lymph nodes cannot be assessed
N0 No regional lymph node metastasis
N1 Regional lymph node metastasis

Distant Metastasis (M)

TNM	FIGO	DEFINITION
MX		Presence of distant metastasis cannot be assessed
M0		No distant metastasis
M1	IV	Distant metastasis (excludes peritoneal metastasis)

Note: The presence of nonmalignant ascites is not classified. The presence of ascites does not affect staging unless malignant cells are present.

pTNM Pathologic Classification

The pT, pN, and pM categories correspond to the T, N, and M categories.

STAGE GROUPING

Stage IA	T1a	N0	M0
Stage IB	T1b	N0	M0
Stage IC	T1c	N0	M0
Stage IIA	T2a	N0	M0
Stage IIB	T2b	N0	M0
Stage IIC	T2c	N0	M0
Stage IIIA	T3a	N0	M0
Stage IIIB	T3b	N0	M0
Stage IIIC	T3c	N0	M0
	Any T	N1	M0
Stage IV	Any T	Any N	M1

Ovary

DIFFERENCES BETWEEN THE 2ND AND 3RD EDITIONS

Recommendations in the two editions of the *Manual* are essentially the same.

HISTOPATHOLOGIC TYPE

The task force of the AJCC endorses the histologic typing of ovarian tumors as presented in the WHO publication no. 9, 1973, and recommends that all ovarian epithelial tumors be subdivided according to a simplified version of this. The types recommended at the present time are as follows: serous tumors, mucinous tumors, endometrioid tumors, clear cell (mesonephroid) tumors, undifferentiated tumors, and unclassified tumors.

A. Serous cystomas
   1. Serous benign cystadenomas
   2. Serous cystadenomas with proliferating activity of the epithelial cells and nuclear abnormalities, but with no infiltrative destructive growth (low potential malignancy)
   3. Serous cystadenocarcinomas
B. Mucinous cystomas
   1. Mucinous benign cystadenomas
   2. Mucinous cystadenomas with proliferating activity of the epithelial cells and nuclear abnormalities, but with no infiltrative destructive growth (low potential malignancy)
   3. Mucinous cystadenocarcinomas
C. Endometrioid tumors (similar to adenocarcinomas in the endometrium)
   1. Endometrioid benign cysts
   2. Endometrioid tumors with proliferating activity of the epithelial cells and nuclear abnormalities, but with no infiltrative destructive growth (low potential malignancy)
   3. Endometrioid adenocarcinomas
D. Clear cell (mesonephroid) tumors
   1. Benign clear cell tumors
   2. Clear cell tumors with proliferating activity of the epithelial cells and nuclear abnormalities, but with no infiltrative destructive growth (low potential malignancy)
   3. Clear cell cystadenocarcinomas
E. Unclassified tumors that cannot be allotted to one of the groups A–D
F. No histology
G. Other malignant tumors: Malignant tumors other than those of the common epithelial types are not to be included with the categories listed above. However, the more common ones such as granulosa cell tumor, immature teratoma, dysgerminoma, and endodermal sinus tumor may be collected and reported separately by institutions so desiring, particularly those with a pediatric population among their patients.

In some cases of inoperable widespread malignant tumor, it may be impossible for the gynecologist and the pathologist to decide the origin of the growth. In order to evaluate the results obtained in the treatment of carcinoma of the ovary, however, it is necessary that all patients are reported on, including those who are thought to have a malignant ovarian tumor. If clinical examination cannot exclude the possibility that the lesion is a primary ovarian carcinoma, a case should be reported in the group "special category" and will belong to either histologic group E or F. Cases in which exploratory surgery has shown that obvious ovarian malignant tumor is present but in which no biopsy has been taken should be classified as ovarian carcinoma, "no histology."

HISTOPATHOLOGIC GRADE (G)

GX	Grade cannot be assessed
GB	Borderline malignancy
G1	Well differentiated
G2	Moderately well differentiated
G3–4	Poorly differentiated or undifferentiated

OVARY

Data Form for Cancer Staging

Patient identification
Name ___
Address ___
Hospital or clinic number ___
Age ___ Sex ___ Race ___

Institution identification
Hospital or clinic ___
Address ___

Oncology Record

Anatomic site of cancer ___
Histologic type ___
Grade (G) ___
Date of classification ___

Chronology of classification
(use separate form for each time staged)
[ ] Clinical (use all data prior to first treatment)
[ ] Pathologic (if definitively resected specimen available)

Definitions

Primary Tumor (T)

TNM	FIGO	DEFINITION
[ ] TX		Primary tumor cannot be assessed
[ ] T0		No evidence of primary tumor
[ ] T1	I	Tumor limited to ovaries
[ ] T1a	Ia	Tumor limited to one ovary; capsule intact, no tumor on ovarian surface
[ ] T1b	Ib	Tumor limited to both ovaries; capsules intact, no tumor on ovarian surface
[ ] T1c	Ic	Tumor limited to one or both ovaries with any of the following: capsule ruptured, tumor on ovarian surface, malignant cells in ascites, or peritoneal washings
[ ] T2	II	Tumor involves one or both ovaries with pelvic extension
[ ] T2a	IIa	Extension or implants on uterus or tubes
[ ] T2b	IIb	Extension to other pelvic tissues
[ ] T2c	IIc	Pelvic extension (2a or 2b) with malignant cells in ascites or peritoneal washing
[ ] T3 and/or N1	III	Tumor involves one or both ovaries with microscopically confirmed peritoneal metastasis outside the pelvis or regional lymph node metastasis
[ ] T3a	IIIa	Microscope peritoneal metastasis beyond pelvis
[ ] T3b	IIIb	Macroscopic peritoneal metastasis beyond pelvis 2 cm or less in greatest dimension
[ ] T3c and/or N1	IIIc	Peritoneal metastasis beyond pelvis more than 2 cm in greatest dimension or regional lymph node metastasis
M1	IV	Distant metastasis (excludes peritoneal metastasis)

*Note: Liver capsule metastasis is T3/Stage III, liver parenchymal metastasis M1/Stage IV. Pleural effusion must have positive cytology for M1/Stage IV.

Lymph Node (N)

[ ] NX Regional lymph nodes cannot be assessed
[ ] N0 No regional lymph node metastasis
[ ] N1 Regional lymph node metastasis

Distant Metastasis (M)

TNM	FIGO	DEFINITION
[ ] MX		Presence of distant metastasis cannot be assessed
[ ] M0		No distant metastasis
[ ] M1	IV	Distant metastasis (excludes peritoneal metastasis)

Stage Grouping

[ ] IA	T1a	N0	M0
[ ] IB	T1b	N0	M0
[ ] IC	T1c	N0	M0
[ ] IIA	T2a	N0	M0
[ ] IIB	T2b	N0	M0
[ ] IIC	T2c	N0	M0
[ ] IIIA	T3a	N0	M0
[ ] IIIB	T3b	N0	M0
[ ] IIIC	T3c	N0	M0
	Any T	N1	M0
[ ] IV	Any T	Any N	M1

Histopathologic Grade (G)

[ ] GX Grade cannot be assessed
[ ] GB Borderline malignancy
[ ] G1 Well differentiated
[ ] G2 Moderately well differentiated
[ ] G3-G4 Poorly differentiated or undifferentiated

Histopathologic Type

The task force of the AJCC endorses the histologic typing of ovarian tumors as presented in the WHO publication no. 9, 1973, and recommends that all ovarian epithelial tumors be subdivided according to a simplified version of this. The types recommended at the present time are as follows: serous tumors, mucinous tumors, endometrioid tumors, clear cell (mesonephroid) tumors, undifferentiated tumors, and unclassified tumors.

Staged by ___ M.D.
___ Registrar
Date ___

A. Serous cystomas
   1. Serous benign cystadenomas
   2. Serous cystadenomas with proliferating activity of the epithelial cells and nuclear abnormalities, but with no infiltrative destructive growth (low potential malignancy)
   3. Serous cystadenocarcinomas
B. Mucinous cystomas
   1. Mucinous benign cystadenomas
   2. Mucinous cystadenomas with proliferating activity of the epithelial cells and nuclear abnormalities, but with no infiltrative destructive growth (low potential malignancy)
   3. Mucinous cystadenocarcinomas
C. Endometrioid tumors (similar to adenocarcinomas in the endometrium)
   1. Endometrioid benign cysts
   2. Endometrioid tumors with proliferating activity of the epithelial cells and nuclear abnormalities, but with no infiltrative destructive growth (low potential malignancy)
   3. Endometrioid adenocarcinomas
D. Clear cell (mesonephroid) tumors
   1. Benign clear cell tumors
   2. Clear cell tumors with proliferating activity of the epithelial cells and nuclear abnormalities, but with no infiltrative destructive growth (low potential malignancy)
   3. Clear cell cystadenocarcinomas
E. Unclassified tumors that cannot be allotted to one of the groups A–D
F. No histology
G. Other malignant tumors: Malignant tumors other than those of the common epithelial types are not to be included with the categories listed above. However, the more common ones such as granulosa cell tumor, immature teratoma, dysgerminoma, and endodermal sinus tumor may be collected and reported separately by institutions so desiring, particularly those with a pediatric population among their patients.

In some cases of inoperable widespread malignant tumor, it may be impossible for the gynecologist and the pathologist to decide the origin of the growth. In order to evaluate the results obtained in the treatment of carcinoma of the ovary, however, it is necessary that all patients are reported on, as well as those who are thought to have a malignant ovarian tumor. If clinical examination cannot exclude the possibility that the lesion is a primary ovarian carcinoma, a case should be reported in the group "special category" and will belong to either histologic group E or F. Cases in which exploratory surgery has shown that obvious ovarian malignant tumor is present, but in which no biopsy has been taken, should be classified as ovarian carcinoma, "no histology."

Sites of Distant Metastasis

Pulmonary	PUL
Osseous	OSS
Hepatic	HEP
Brain	BRA
Lymph nodes	LYM
Bone marrow	MAR
Pleura	PLE
Peritoneum	PER
Skin	SKI
Other	OTH

Illustrations

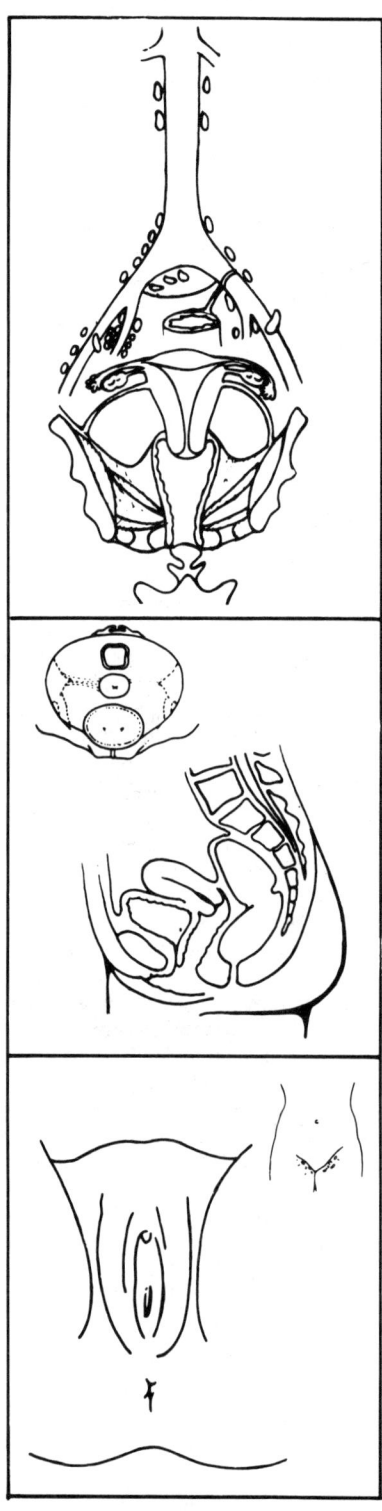

Indicate on diagrams primary tumor and regional nodes involved.

Vagina

ANATOMY

Primary Site. The vagina (ICD-O 184.0) extends from the vulva upward to the uterine cervix.

Regional Lymph Nodes. The femoral, inguinal, common iliac, internal iliac, external iliac and hypogastric nodes are the sites of regional spread.

Metastatic Sites. The most common sites of distant spread include the lungs and skeleton.

RULES FOR CLASSIFICATION

The classification applies to primary carcinoma only.

A tumor that has extended to the portio and reached the external os should be classified as carcinoma of the cervix.

A tumor involving the vulva should be classified as carcinoma of the vulva.

There should be histologic confirmation of the disease. Any unconfirmed cases must be reported separately.

Clinical Staging. All data available prior to first definitive treatment should be used.

Pathologic Staging. In addition to data used for clinical staging, additional information available from examination of the resected specimen is to be used.

DEFINITION OF TNM

The definitions of the T categories correspond to the several stages accepted by FIGO. Both systems are included for comparison.

Primary Tumor (T)

TNM	FIGO	DEFINITION
TX		Primary tumor cannot be assessed
T0		No evidence of primary tumor
Tis	0	Carcinoma *in situ*
T1	I	Tumor confined to vagina
T2	II	Tumor invades paravaginal tissues but not to pelvic wall
T3	III	Tumor extends to pelvic wall
T4*	IVa	Tumor invades *mucosa* of bladder or rectum and/or extends beyond the true pelvis
M1	IVb	Distant metastasis

*Note: The presence of bullous edema is not sufficient evidence to classify a tumor T4. If the mucosa is not involved the tumor is Stage III.

Regional Lymph Nodes (N)

NX Regional lymph nodes cannot be assessed
N0 No regional lymph node metastasis

Upper two-thirds of vagina:
N1 Pelvic lymph node metastasis

Lower one-third of vagina:
N1 Unilateral inguinal lymph node metastasis
N2 Bilateral inguinal lymph node metastasis

Distant Metastasis (M)

TNM	FIGO	DEFINITION
MX		Presence of distant metastasis cannot be assessed
M0		No distant metastasis
M1	IVb	Distant metastasis

pTNM Pathological Classification

The pT, pN, and pM categories correspond to the T, N, and M categories.

STAGE GROUPING

Stage 0	Tis	N0	M0
Stage I	T1	N0	M0
Stage II	T2	N0	M0
Stage III	T1	N1	M0
	T2	N1	M0
	T3	N0, N1	M0
Stage IVA	T1	N2	M0
	T2	N2	M0
	T3	N2	M0
	T4	Any N	M0
Stage IVB	Any T	Any N	M1

DIFFERENCES BETWEEN THE 2ND AND 3RD EDITIONS

Stage grouping recommendations were not made in the second edition but are made in this edition of the *Manual.*

HISTOPATHOLOGIC TYPE

Cases are classified as carcinoma if they have their origin in the vagina.

HISTOPATHOLOGIC GRADE (G)

GX Grade cannot be assessed
G1 Well differentiated
G2 Moderately well differentiated
G3 Poorly differentiated
G4 Undifferentiated

VAGINA

Data Form for Cancer Staging

Patient identification
Name _____
Address _____
Hospital or clinic number _____
Age _____ Sex _____ Race _____

Institution identification
Hospital or clinic _____
Address _____

Oncology Record

Anatomic site of cancer _____
Histologic type _____
Grade (G) _____
Date of classification _____

Chronology of classification
(use separate form for each time staged)
[ ] Clinical (use all data prior to first treatment)
[ ] Pathologic (if definitively resected specimen available)

Definitions

Primary Tumor (T)

TNM	FIGO	DEFINITION
[ ] TX		Primary tumor cannot be assessed
[ ] T0		No evidence of primary tumor
[ ] Tis	0	Carcinoma *in situ*
[ ] T1	I	Tumor confined to vagina
[ ] T2	II	Tumor invades paravaginal tissues but not to pelvic wall
[ ] T3	III	Tumor extends to pelvic wall
[ ] T4*	IVa	Tumor invades *mucosa* of bladder or rectum or extends beyond the true pelvis
[ ] M1	IVb	Distant metastasis

Note: The presence of bullous edema is not sufficient evidence to classify a tumor T4. If the mucosa is not involved the tumor is stage III.

Lymph Node (N)

[ ] NX   Regional lymph nodes cannot be assessed
[ ] N0   No regional lymph node metastasis

Upper two-thirds of vagina:
[ ] N1   Pelvic lymph node metastasis

Lower one-third of vagina:
[ ] N1   Unilateral inguinal lymph node metastasis
[ ] N2   Bilateral inguinal lymph node metastasis

Distant Metastasis (M)

TNM	FIGO	DEFINITION
[ ] MX		Presence of distant metastasis cannot be assessed
[ ] M0		No distant metastasis
[ ] M1	IVb	Distant metastasis

Stage Grouping

[ ]	0	Tis	N0	M0
[ ]	I	T1	N0	M0
[ ]	II	T2	N0	M0
[ ]	III	T1	N1	M0
		T2	N1	M0
		T3	N0	M0
		T3	N1	M0
[ ]	IVA	T1	N2	M0
		T2	N2	M0
		T3	N2	M0
		T4	Any N	M0
[ ]	IVB	Any T	Any N	M1

Histopathologic Type

Cases are classified as carcinoma if they have their origin in the vagina.

Histopathologic Grade (G)

[ ] GX   Grade cannot be assessed
[ ] G1   Well differentiated
[ ] G2   Moderately well differentiated
[ ] G3   Poorly differentiated
[ ] G4   Undifferentiated

Sites of Distant Metastasis

Pulmonary	PUL
Osseous	OSS
Hepatic	HEP
Brain	BRA
Lymph nodes	LYM
Bone marrow	MAR
Pleura	PLE
Peritoneum	PER
Skin	SKI
Other	OTH

Staged by _____ M.D.
_____ Registrar
Date _____

Illustrations

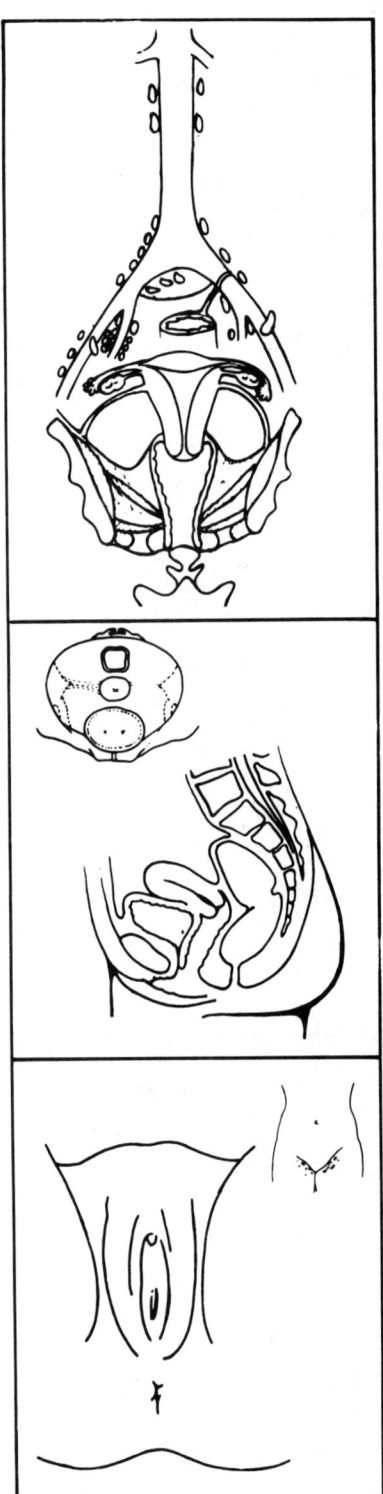

Indicate on diagrams primary tumor and regional nodes involved.

28

Vulva

The staging classification for carcinomas of the vulva is taken directly from the FIGO.

While it is not consistent with the principles of TNM classification used for other anatomic sites, it is accepted in the spirit of unanimity so that data accumulated throughout the world will be comparable.

Cases should be classified as carcinoma of the vulva when the primary site of the growth is in the vulva. Tumors present in the vulva as secondary growths from either a genital or extra-genital site should be excluded. Malignant melanoma should be reported separately.

A carcinoma of the vulva that has extended to the vagina should be considered a carcinoma of the vulva.

ANATOMY

Primary Site. The vulva (ICD-O 184.4) is the anatomic area immediately external to the vagina.

Regional Lymph Nodes. The femoral, inguinal, internal iliac, external iliac, and hypogastric nodes are the sites of regional spread.

Metastatic Sites. Any site beyond the area of the regional lymph nodes.

RULES FOR CLASSIFICATION

The classification applies only to primary carcinoma of the vulva. There should be histologic confirmation of the cancer. A carcinoma of the vulva that has extended to the vagina should be classified as carcinoma of the vulva. Malignant melanoma should be reported separately.

Clinical Staging. The rules for staging are similar to those for carcinoma of the cervix.

Pathologic Staging. The rules for staging are similar to those for carcinoma of the cervix.

DEFINITION OF TNM

TNM classification of carcinoma of the vulva is based on the FIGO classification.

Primary Tumor (T)

TX Primary tumor cannot be assessed
T0 No evidence of primary tumor
Tis Pre-invasive carcinoma (carcinoma *in situ*)
T1 Tumor confined to the vulva, 2 cm or less in greatest dimension
T2 Tumor confined to the vulva, more than 2 cm in greatest dimension
T3 Tumor invades any of the following: urethra, vagina, perineum, or anus
T4 Tumor invades any of the following: bladder mucosa, upper part of urethral mucosa, rectal mucosa or tumor fixed to the bone

Regional Lymph Nodes (N)

NX Regional lymph nodes cannot be assessed
N0 No nodes palpable
N1 Nodes palpable in either groin, not enlarged, mobile (not clinically suspicious of neoplasm)
N2 Nodes palpable in either groin, enlarged, firm and mobile (clinically suspicious of neoplasm)
N3 Fixed or ulcerated nodes

Distant Metastasis (M)

MX Presence of distant metastasis cannot be assessed
M0 No clinical metastasis
M1a Palpable deep pelvic lymph nodes
M1b Other distant metastases

STAGE GROUPING: DEFINITIONS OF THE CLINICAL STAGES IN CARCINOMA OF THE VULVA

(Correlation of the FIGO, UICC, and AJCC nomenclatures)

Stage 0
Tis Carcinoma *in situ*, intraepithelial carcinoma

Stage I
T1 N0 M0   Tumor confined to the vulva; 2 cm or
T1 N1 M0   less in greatest dimension. Nodes are not palpable, or are palpable in either groin, not enlarged, mobile (not clinically suspicious of neoplasm)

Stage II
T2 N0 M0   Tumor confined to the vulva; more
T2 N1 M0   than 2 cm in greatest dimension. Nodes are not palpable, or are palpable in either groin, not enlarged, mobile (not clinically suspicious of neoplasm)

Stage III
T3 N0 M0   Tumor of any size with
T3 N1 M0   (1) Adjacent spread to the lower ure-
T3 N2 M0   thra and/or the vagina, the peri-
T1 N2 M0   neum, or the anus, and/or
T2 N2 M0   (2) nodes palpable in either one or both groins (enlarged, firm, and mobile, not fixed but clinically suspicious of neoplasm)

Stage IV
T4 N0 M0   Tumor of any size
T4 N1 M0   (1) infiltrating the bladder mu-
T4 N2 M0   cosa and/or the upper part of the urethral mucosa and/or the rectal mucosa, and/or
Any T Any N M1a (2) fixed to the bone or other
Any T Any N M1b   distant metastases, and/or
Any T N3 M0   (3) Fixed or ulcerated nodes in either one or both groins

DIFFERENCES BETWEEN THE 2ND AND 3RD EDITIONS

The 1983 edition of the *Manual* did not include N2 but did include N4, which was defined as "juxtaregional node involvement." In this edition, juxtaregional metastatic nodes are considered distant metastasis and are labeled either M1a or M1b.

HISTOPATHOLOGIC TYPE

Squamous cell carcinoma is the most frequent form of cancer of the vulva. Malignant melanoma should be reported separately.

HISTOPATHOLOGIC GRADE (G)

GX Grade cannot be assessed
G1 Well differentiated
G2 Moderately well differentiated
G3 Poorly differentiated
G4 Undifferentiated

VULVA

Data Form for Cancer Staging

Patient identification
Name _____
Address _____
Hospital or clinic number _____
Age _____ Sex _____ Race _____

Institution identification
Hospital or clinic _____
Address _____

Oncology Record

Anatomic site of cancer _____
Histologic type _____
Grade (G) _____
Date of classification _____

Chronology of classification
(use separate form for each time staged)
[ ] Clinical (use all data prior to first treatment)
[ ] Pathologic (if definitively resected specimen available)

Definitions

Primary Tumor (T)

[ ] TX   Primary tumor cannot be assessed
[ ] T0   No evidence of primary tumor
[ ] Tis   Pre-invasive carcinoma (carcinoma *in situ*)
[ ] T1   Tumor confined to the vulva, 2 cm or less in greatest dimension
[ ] T2   Tumor confined to the vulva, more than 2 cm in greatest dimension
[ ] T3   Tumor invades any of the following: urethra, vagina, perineum, or anus
[ ] T4   Tumor invades any of the following: bladder mucosa, upper part of urethral mucosa, rectal mucosa or tumor fixed to the bone

Lymph Node (N)

[ ] NX   Regional lymph nodes cannot be assessed
[ ] N0   No nodes palpable
[ ] N1   Nodes palpable in either groin, not enlarged, mobile (not clinically suspicious of neoplasm)
[ ] N2   Nodes palpable in either groin, enlarged, firm and mobile (clinically suspicious of neoplasm)
[ ] N3   Fixed or ulcerated nodes

Distant Metastasis (M)

[ ] MX   Presence of distant metastasis cannot be assessed
[ ] M0   No clinical metastases
[ ] M1a   Palpable deep pelvic lymph nodes
[ ] M1b   Other distant metastases

Stage Grouping: Definitions of the Clinical Stages in Carcinoma of the Vulva

(Correlation of the FIGO, UICC, and AJCC nomenclatures)

Stage 0
[ ] Tis   Carcinoma *in situ*, intraepithelial carcinoma

Stage I
[ ] T1 N0 M0   Tumor confined to the vulva; 2 cm or
[ ] T1 N1 M0   less in greater dimension. Nodes are not palpable, or are palpable in either groin, not enlarged, mobile (not clinically suspicious of neoplasm)

Stage II
[ ] T2 N0 M0   Tumor confined to the vulva; more
[ ] T2 N1 M0   than 2 cm in greatest dimension. Nodes are not palpable, or are palpable in either groin,* not enlarged, mobile (not clinically suspicious of neoplasm)

Stage III
[ ] T3 N0 M0   Tumor of any size with
[ ] T3 N1 M0   (1) Adjacent spread to the lower
[ ] T3 N2 M0   urethra and/or the vagina, the
[ ] T1 N2 M0   perineum, or the anus, and/or
[ ] T2 N2 M0   (2) nodes palpable in either one or both groins (enlarged, firm and mobile, not fixed but clinically suspicious of neoplasm)

Stage IV
[ ] T4 N0 M0   Tumor of any size
[ ] T4 N1 M0   (1) infiltrating the bladder mucosa
[ ] T4 N2 M0   and/or the upper part of the
[ ] All conditions   urethral mucosa and/or the rectal
    containing N3   mucosa, and/or
    or M1a   (2) fixed to the bone or other distant
    or M1b   metastases or
[ ] Any T Any N   (3) Fixed or ulcerated nodes in either
    M1a   one or both groins
[ ] Any T Any N M1b
[ ] Any T N3 M0

Staged by _____ M.D.
_____ Registrar
Date _____

Histopathologic Grade (G)

[ ] GX   Grade cannot be assessed
[ ] G1   Well differentiated
[ ] G2   Moderately well differentiated
[ ] G3   Poorly differentiated
[ ] G4   Undifferentiated

Histopathologic Type

Squamous cell carcinoma is the most frequent form of cancer of the vulva. Malignant melanoma should be reported separately.

Sites of Distant Metastasis

Pulmonary	PUL
Osseous	OSS
Hepatic	HEP
Brain	BRA
Lymph nodes	LYM
Bone marrow	MAR
Pleura	PLE
Peritoneum	PER
Skin	SKI
Other	OTH

Illustrations

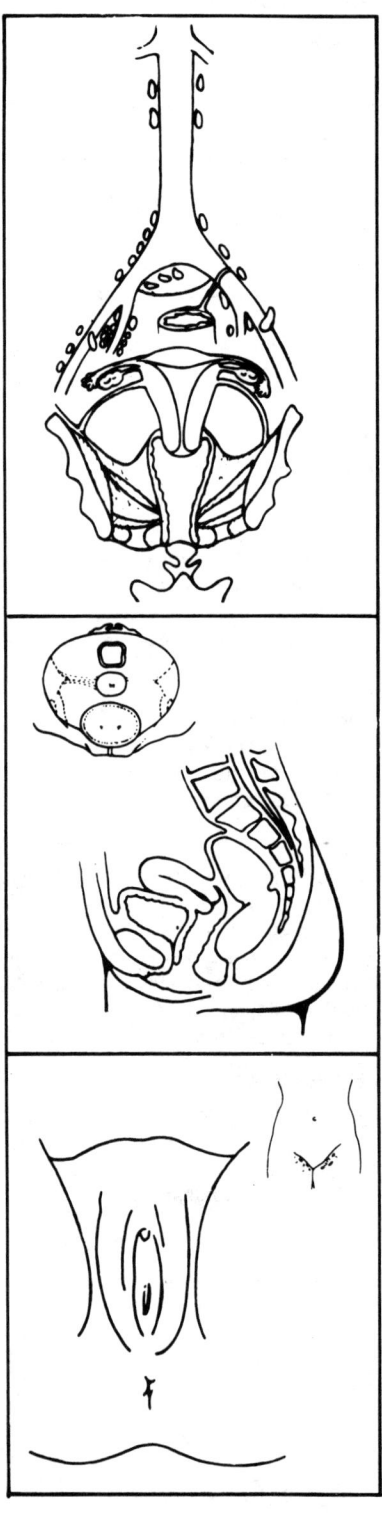

Indicate on diagrams primary tumor and regional nodes involved.

GENITOURINARY SITES

29

Prostate

Prostatic cancer has a sinister reputation. It is the second most commonly occurring cancer in men, seen predominantly in older individuals. The disease is often difficult to diagnose in its early stages. In many patients, the symptoms do not appear until the cancer has metastasized. Carcinomas of the prostate are responsive to sex hormones and presumably, therefore, have many analogies with breast cancer. They are stimulated by androgens and inhibited by estrogens. Prostatic cancer has a tendency to metastasize to bone.

ANATOMY

Primary Site. Adenocarcinoma of the prostate (ICD-O 185) usually arises within the true gland and rarely seems to begin in the benign hyperplastic enlargement that occurs around the prostatic urethra in older men. Pathologically, this cancer tends to be multifocal in origin. It is more commonly found in the peripheral posterior portion of the gland and therefore is highly amenable to early detection by rectal examination.

There is general agreement that the incidence of both clinical and latent carcinoma increases with age, but this cancer is rarely clinically diagnosed in men under age 40 years. The size or extent of the localized prostatic tumor may be estimated by digital examination or may be amplified by various imaging techniques. Diagnosis of clinically suspicious areas of the prostate is histologically confirmed by needle biopsy, endoscopic resection, or fine needle aspiration.

The grade of the prostatic cancer is as important for the prognosis as the extent of its growth. The histopathologic grading of these tumors can be complex because of the heterogeneity so often encountered in surgical specimens. This classification allows either an anaplasia or a pattern type of grading method to be used.

Regional Lymph Nodes. The regional lymph nodes are the nodes of the true pelvis, which essentially are the pelvic nodes below the bifurcation of the common iliac arteries and include the following groups:

Regional
Hypogastric
Obturator
Iliac (internal, external, NOS)
Periprostatic
Pelvic, NOS
Sacral (lateral, presacral, promontory (Gerota's), or NOS)
Superficial Inguinal (Femoral)

Distant Lymph Nodes. The anatomic boundaries are subtended by the arcuate line and planes involved. The fixed points of the pelvis are the pubic crest, perineal line, medial border of ilium, ala of sacrum, and sacral promontory.

Laterality does not affect the N classification. The significance of regional lymph node metastasis in staging prostate cancer lies in the number and size and not in whether unilateral or contralateral.

Aortic (para-aortic, peri-aortic, lumbar)
Common iliac
Inguinal
Supraclavicular, cervical, scalene

Metastatic Sites. Spread to bones, lung, liver, and distant lymph nodes often occurs.

RULES FOR CLASSIFICATION

Clinical Staging. Primary tumor assessment includes digital examination of the prostate and histologic or cytologic confirmation of prostatic carcinoma. Clinical examination, acid phosphatase determination, and imaging techniques are suggested. All information available prior to first definitive treatment may be used for clinical staging.

Pathologic Staging. Histologic examination of resected specimen is required. Total prostatoseminal vesiculectomy and pelvic lymph node dissection are required for this staging.

DEFINITION OF TNM

Primary Tumor (T)

TX Primary tumor cannot be assessed
T0 No evidence of primary tumor
T1 Tumor is incidental histologic finding
    T1a Three or fewer microscopic foci of carcinoma
    T1b More than 3 microscopic foci of carcinoma
T2 Tumor present clinically or grossly, limited to the gland
    T2a Tumor 1.5 cm or less in greatest dimension with normal tissue on at least three sides
    T2b Tumor more than 1.5 cm in greatest dimension or in more than one lobe
T3 Tumor invades the prostatic apex, or into or beyond the prostatic capsule, bladder neck, or seminal vesicle, but is not fixed
T4 Tumor is fixed or invades adjacent structures other than those listed in T3

Regional Lymph Nodes (N)

NX Regional lymph nodes cannot be assessed
N0 No regional lymph node metastasis
N1 Metastasis in a single lymph node, 2 cm or less in greatest dimension
N2 Metastasis in a single lymph node, more than 2 cm but not more than 5 cm in greatest dimension, or multiple lymph nodes, none more than 5 cm in greatest dimension
N3 Metastasis in a lymph node more than 5 cm in greatest dimension

Distant Metastasis (M)

MX Presence of distant metastasis cannot be assessed
M0 No distant metastasis
M1 Distant metastasis

HISTOPATHOLOGIC GRADE (G)

GX Grade cannot be assessed
G1 Well differentiated, slight anaplasia
G2 Moderately differentiated, moderate anaplasia
G3-4 Poorly differentiated or undifferentiated, marked anaplasia

STAGE GROUPING

Stage	T	N	M	G
Stage 0	T1a	N0	M0	G1
	T2a	N0	M0	G1
Stage I	T1a	N0	M0	G2, G3-4
	T2a	N0	M0	G2, G3-4
Stage II	T1b	N0	M0	Any G
	T2b	N0	M0	Any G
Stage III	T3	N0	M0	Any G
Stage IV	T4	N0	M0	Any G
	Any T	N1, N2, N3	M0	Any G
	Any T	Any N	M1	Any G

Table 1. A Comparison of Two Staging Systems for Prostate Cancer

	TNM		AMERICAN UROLOGICAL ASSOCIATION (A–D)
T0	No evidence of primary tumor	Stage A—	No palpable lesion
T1a	Three or fewer microscopic foci of carcinoma	A1	Focal
T1b	More than 3 microscopic foci of carcinoma	A2	Diffuse
T2	Tumor present clinically or grossly, limited to the gland	Stage B—	Confined to prostate
T2a	Tumor 1.5 cm or less in greatest dimension with normal tissue on at least 3 sides	B1	Small, discrete nodule
T2b	Tumor more than 1.5 cm in greatest dimension or in more than one lobe	B2	Large or multiple nodules or areas
T3	Tumor invades the prostatic apex, or into or beyond the prostatic capsule, bladder neck, or seminal vesicle but is not fixed	Stage C— C1	Localized to periprostatic area No involvement of seminal vesicles, <70g
T4	Tumor is fixed or invades adjacent structures other than those listed in T3	C2	Involvement of seminal vesicles, >70g
N1	Metastasis in a single lymph node, 2 cm or less in greatest dimension	Stage D—	Metastatic disease
N2	Metastasis in a single lymph node, more than 2 cm but not more than 5 cm in greatest dimension, or multiple lymph nodes, none more than 5 cm in greatest dimension	D1	Pelvic lymph node metastases or urethral obstruction causing hydronephrosis
N3	Metastasis in a lymph node more than 5 cm in greatest dimension	D2	Bone or distant lymph node or organ or soft tissue metastases
M1	Distant metastasis		

DIFFERENCES BETWEEN THE 2ND AND 3RD EDITIONS

The T categories have been slightly modified. In this edition, T1 has been added and subdivided into "a" and "b" categories. Also, T2, which is new, is subdivided. The N categories have been redefined with the emphasis on the size of the metastatic lesion as well as the number of nodes involved. Finally, the histologic grade has been added as part of the stage groupings because of its importance for prognosis.

HISTOPATHOLOGIC TYPE

The histopathologic type is almost always adenocarcinoma of variable grades.

BIBLIOGRAPHY

1. Barzell W, Bean MA, Hilaris BS et al: Prostatic adenocarcinoma: Relationship of grade and local extent to the pattern of metastases. J Urol 118:278–282, 1977
2. Donohue RE, Fauver HE, Whitesal JA et al: Staging prostatic cancer: A different distribution. J Urol 122:327–329, 1979
3. Flocks RH, Culp DA, Porto R: Lymphatic spread from prostatic cancer. J Urol 81:194–196, 1959
4. Fowler JE Jr, Whitmore WF Jr: The incidence and extent of pelvic lymph node metastases in apparently localized prostatic cancer. Cancer 47:2941–2945, 1981
5. Grossman IC, Carpiniello V, Greenberg SH et al: Staging pelvic lymphadenectomy for carcinoma of the prostate: Review of 91 cases. J Urol 124:632–634, 1980
6. Huben RP, Murphy GP: Prostate cancer: An update. CA—Cancer J Clin 36:274–292, 1986
7. Mostofi FK: Problems of grading carcinoma of prostate. Semin Oncol 3:161–169, 1976
8. Parfitt HE Jr, Smith JA Jr, Gliedman JB et al: Accuracy of staging in A1 carcinoma of the prostate. Cancer 51:2346–2350, 1983
9. Resnick ME: Non-invasive techniques in evaluating patients with carcinoma of the prostate. J Urol 17:25–30, 1981
10. Spirnak JP, Resnick M: Clinical staging of prostatic cancer: New modalities. Urol Clin North Am 11:221–235, 1984

PROSTATE

Data Form for Cancer Staging

Patient identification
Name _____
Address _____
Hospital or clinic number _____
Age _____ Sex _____ Race _____

Institution identification
Hospital or clinic _____
Address _____

Oncology Record

Anatomic site of cancer _____
Histologic type _____
Grade (G) _____
Date of classification _____

Chronology of classification
(use separate form for each time staged)
[ ] Clinical (use all data prior to first treatment)
[ ] Pathologic (if definitively resected specimen available)

Definitions

Primary Tumor (T)

[ ] TX   Primary tumor cannot be assessed
[ ] T0   No evidence of primary tumor
[ ] T1   Tumor is incidental histologic finding
    [ ] T1a   Three or fewer microscopic foci of carcinoma
    [ ] T1b   More than three microscopic foci of carcinoma
[ ] T2   Tumor present clinically or grossly, limited to the gland
    [ ] T2a   Tumor 1.5 cm or less in greatest dimension with normal tissue on at least three sides
    [ ] T2b   Tumor more than 1.5 cm in greatest dimension or in more than one lobe
[ ] T3   Tumor invades the prostatic apex, or into or beyond the prostatic capsule, bladder neck, or seminal vesicle, but is not fixed
[ ] T4   Tumor is fixed or invades adjacent structures other than those listed in T3

Lymph Node (N)

[ ] NX   Regional lymph nodes cannot be assessed
[ ] N0   No regional lymph node metastasis
[ ] N1   Metastasis in a single lymph node, 2 cm or less in greatest dimension
[ ] N2   Metastasis in a single lymph node, more than 2 cm but not more than 5 cm in greatest dimension, or multiple lymph nodes, none more than 5 cm in greatest dimension
[ ] N3   Metastasis in a lymph node more than 5 cm in greatest dimension

Distant Metastasis (M)

[ ] MX   Presence of distant metastasis cannot be assessed
[ ] M0   No distant metastasis
[ ] M1   Distant metastasis

Stage Grouping

[ ] 0	T1a	N0	M0	G1
	T2a	N0	M0	G1
[ ] I	T1a	N0	M0	G2
	T1a	N0	M0	G3
	T1a	N0	M0	G4
	T2a	N0	M0	G2
	T2a	N0	M0	G3
	T2a	N0	M0	G4
[ ] II	T1b	N0	M0	Any G
	T2b	N0	M0	Any G
[ ] III	T3	N0	M0	Any G
[ ] IV	T4	N0	M0	Any G
	Any T	N1	M0	Any G
	Any T	N2	M0	Any G
	Any T	N3	M0	Any G
	Any T	Any N	M1	Any G

Histopathologic Grade (G)

[ ] GX   Grade cannot be assessed
[ ] G1   Well differentiated, slight anaplasia
[ ] G2   Moderately well differentiated, moderate anaplasia
[ ] G3-4   Poorly differentiated or undifferentiated, marked anaplasia

Histopathologic Type

Almost always adenocarcinoma of variable grades.

Sites of Distant Metastasis

Pulmonary	PUL
Osseous	OSS
Hepatic	HEP
Brain	BRA
Lymph nodes	LYM
Bone marrow	MAR
Pleura	PLE
Peritoneum	PER
Skin	SKI
Other	OTH

Staged by _____ M.D.
_____ Registrar
Date _____

American Joint Committee on Cancer—1988

Illustrations

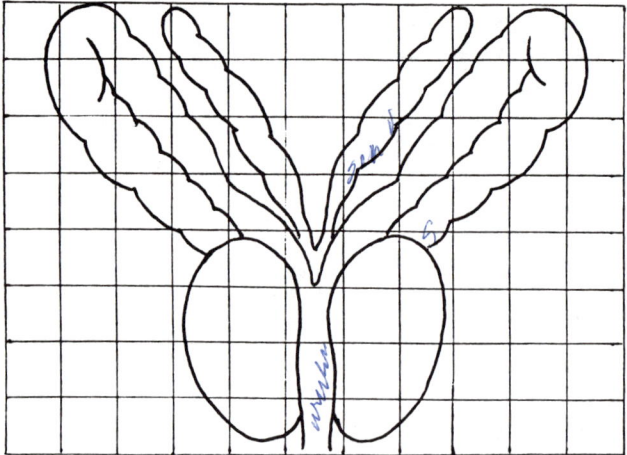

This diagram is for use with prostate diagram. Sketch in extent of tumor.

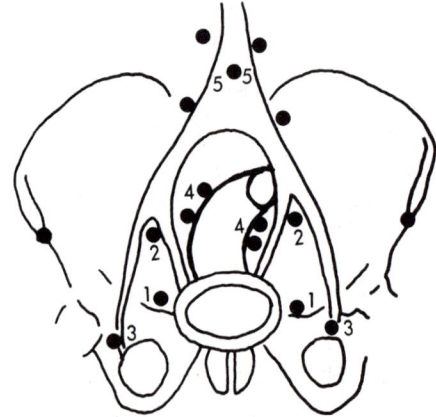

Indicate on diagram primary tumor and regional nodes involved.

182

30 Testis

Cancers of the testis are usually found in young adults. Fortunately, they are relatively rare, accounting for less than 1% of all malignancies in males. Cryptorchidism is a predisposing condition. There are two main histologic types: seminomas, which are most common, and teratomas. Most cases of testicular cancer, even when far advanced, can be successfully treated. Circulating tumor markers are found in the serum of patients with cancer of the testis, which enables the clinician to document the course of the disease. These markers are invaluable for the management of testicular malignancies. Staging is based on the extent of disease.

ANATOMY

Primary Site. The testes (ICD-O 186) are composed of convoluted seminiferous tubules with a stroma containing functional endocrine interstitial cells. Both are encased in a dense barrier capsule, the tunica albuginea, with fibrous septa extending into and separating the testes into lobules. The tubules converge and exit at the mediastinum of the testis into the rete testis and efferent ducts, which join a single duct. This duct, the epididymis, coils outside the upper and lower pole of the testicle, then joins a muscular conduit, the vas deferens, which accompanies the vessels and lymphatic channels of the spermatic cord. The major route for local extension of cancer is through the lymphatic channels. The tumor emerges from the mediastinum of the testis and courses through the spermatic cord. Occasionally, the epididymis is invaded early and then the external iliac nodes may become involved. If there has been previous scrotal or inguinal surgery with invasion of the scrotal wall (though this is rare), then the lymphatic spread may be to inguinal nodes.

Regional Lymph Nodes. The regional lymph nodes are the abdominal para-aortic nodes and the paracaval nodes, the intra-pelvic nodes, and the inguinal nodes.

Spread of the tumor into contralateral regional or first station nodes of the area occurs in 20% of cases. When there has been previous inguinal or scrotal surgery, inguinal nodes are also considered as regional or first station nodes. All nodes outside the regional nodes are distant. As defined, bulky disease has important prognostic significance.

Laterality does not affect the N classification. The significance of regional lymph node metastasis in staging testicular cancer lies in the number and size and not in whether unilateral or contralateral.

Metastatic Sites. Distant spread of testicular tumors occurs most commonly to the nodes, followed by metastases to the lung, liver, viscera, and bones. As defined, bulk of disease has important prognostic significance. Serum markers (alpha-fetoprotein [AFP]) and the β-subunit of human chorionic gonadotropin (BHCG) should be obtained prior to initial orchiectomy to establish whether the tumor marker is predictive. Markers are helpful in the management of patients with disseminated disease. Stage can be further subdivided by the presence or absence of markers.

RULES FOR CLASSIFICATION

Clinical Staging. Clinical examination and radical orchiectomy are required for clinical staging.

Pathologic Staging. Histologic evaluation of the radical orchiectomy specimen must be used for the pT stage. The specimens from a defined node-bearing area (i.e., retroperitoneal periaortic node dissection) must be used for the pN stage. Histologic verification is required.

DEFINITION OF TNM

Primary Tumor (T)

The extent of primary tumor is classified after radical orchiectomy.

- TX Primary tumor cannot be assessed (in the absence of radical orchiectomy, TX is used)
- T0 Histologic scar or no evidence of primary tumor
- Tis Intratubular tumor: preinvasive cancer
- T1 Tumor limited to testis, including rete testis
- T2 Tumor invades beyond tunica albuginea or into epididymis
- T3 Tumor invades spermatic cord
- T4 Tumor invades scrotum

Regional Lymph Nodes (N)

- NX Regional lymph nodes cannot be assessed
- N0 No regional lymph node metastasis
- N1 Metastasis in a single lymph node, 2 cm or less in greatest dimension
- N2 Metastasis in a single lymph node, more than 2 cm but not more than 5 cm in greatest dimension, or multiple lymph nodes, none more than 5 cm in greatest dimension
- N3 Metastasis in a lymph node more than 5 cm in greatest dimension

Distant Metastasis (M)

- MX Presence of distant metastasis cannot be assessed
- M0 No distant metastasis
- M1 Distant metastasis

STAGE GROUPING

Stage	T	N	M
Stage 0	Tis	N0	M0
Stage I	T1	N0	M0
	T2	N0	M0
Stage II	T3	N0	M0
	T4	N0	M0
Stage III	Any T	N1	M0
Stage IV	Any T	N2, N3	M0
	Any T	Any N	M1

DIFFERENCES BETWEEN THE 2ND AND 3RD EDITIONS

The T categories have been redefined for more precision in classification. The previous T3 is now considered T2, and T4a is now T3. T4 is no longer subdivided into "a" and "b." The N categories have also been modified. Size and the number of nodes involved are the basis for classification. Laterality is no longer a factor. The stage groupings have also been modified to correspond to the modified T and N categories.

HISTOPATHOLOGIC TYPE

Cell types can be divided into seminomatous and nonseminomatous tumors. The latter can be further divided into teratoma, embryonal carcinoma, yolk sac tumor, and choriocarcinoma. Mixtures of these types should be noted. Lymphomas are excluded. Combinations of embryonal carcinoma and teratoma can be designated as teratocarcinoma.

HISTOPATHOLOGIC GRADE (G)

Testicular tumors are not graded.

BIBLIOGRAPHY

1. Hoskin P, Dilly S, Easton D et al: Prognostic factors in stage I non-seminomatous germ-cell testicular tumors managed by orchiectomy and surveillance: Implications for adjuvant chemotherapy. J Clin Oncol 4:1031–1036, 1986
2. Javadpour N, Canning DA, O'Connell KJ et al: Predictors of recurrent clinical stage I non-seminomatous testicular cancer: A prospective clinicopathological study. Urology 276:508–511, 1986
3. Pike MC, Chilvers C, Peckham MJ: Effect of age at orchidopexy on risk of testicular cancer. Lancet 1:1246–1248, 1986
4. Rowland RG, Weisman D, Williams SD et al: Accuracy of preoperative staging in stages A and B non-seminomatous germ cell testis tumors. J Urol 127:718–720, 1982
5. Williams SD, Einhorn LH: Clinical stage I testis tumors: The medical oncologist's view. Cancer Treat Rep 66:15–18, 1981

TESTIS

Data Form for Cancer Staging

Patient identification
Name _____
Address _____
Hospital or clinic number _____
Age _____ Sex _____ Race _____

Institution identification
Hospital or clinic _____
Address _____

Oncology Record

Anatomic site of cancer _____
Histologic type _____
Grade (G) _____
Date of classification _____

Chronology of classification
  (use separate form for each time staged)
[ ] Clinical (use all data prior to first treatment)
[ ] Pathologic (if definitively resected specimen available)

Definitions

Primary Tumor (T)

[ ] TX Primary tumor cannot be assessed. (In the absence of radical orchiectomy, TX is used)
[ ] T0 Histologic scar or no evidence of primary tumor
[ ] Tis Intratubular tumor: preinvasive cancer
[ ] T1 Tumor limited to testis, including rete testis
[ ] T2 Tumor invades beyond tunica albuginea or into epididymis
[ ] T3 Tumor invades spermatic cord
[ ] T4 Tumor invades scrotum

Lymph Node (N)

[ ] NX Regional lymph nodes cannot be assessed
[ ] N0 No regional lymph node metastasis
[ ] N1 Metastasis in a single lymph node, 2 cm or less in greatest dimension
[ ] N2 Metastasis in a single lymph node, more than 2 cm but not more than 5 cm in greatest dimension, or multiple lymph nodes, none more than 5 cm in greatest dimension
[ ] N3 Metastasis in a lymph node more than 5 cm in greatest dimension

Distant Metastasis (M)

[ ] MX Presence of distant metastasis cannot be assessed
[ ] M0 No distant metastasis
[ ] M1 Distant metastasis

Stage Grouping

[ ] 0	Tis	N0	M0
[ ] I	T1	N0	M0
	T2	N0	M0
[ ] II	T3	N0	M0
	T4	N0	M0
[ ] III	Any T	N1	M0
[ ] IV	Any T	N2	M0
	Any T	N3	M0
	Any T	Any N	M1

Histopathologic Type

Cell types can be divided into seminomatous and nonseminomatous tumors. The latter can be further divided into teratoma, embryonal carcinoma, yolk sac tumor, and choriocarcinoma. Mixtures of these types should be noted. Lymphomas are excluded. Combinations of embryonal carcinoma and teratoma can be designated as teratocarcinoma.

Illustrations

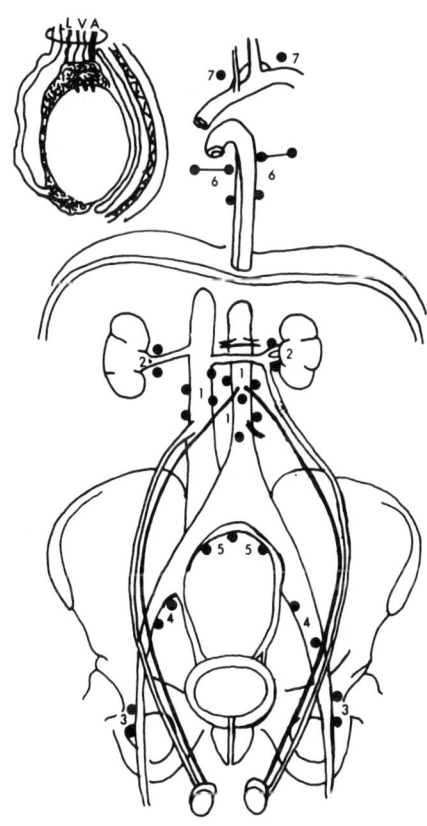

Indicate on diagram primary tumor and regional nodes involved.

Sites of Distant Metastasis

Pulmonary	PUL
Osseous	OSS
Hepatic	HEP
Brain	BRA
Lymph nodes	LYM
Bone marrow	MAR
Pleura	PLE
Peritoneum	PER
Skin	SKI
Other	OTH

Staged by _____ M.D.
_____ Registrar
Date _____

31

Penis

Cancers of the penis are rare in the United States, although the incidence varies in different countries of the world. Most are squamous cell carcinomas that arise in the skin or on the glans penis. Prognosis is favorable provided the lymph nodes are not involved. Melanomas can also occur. The staging classification, however, applies only to squamous cell tumors. (Melanomas are staged in Chapter 22.) Some cancers of the penis may be described as verrucous. These are included under this classification. An *in situ* lesion, erythroplasia of Queyrat, is also included and by definition should be coded as an *in situ* carcinoma of the penis.

ANATOMY

Primary Site. The penis (prepuce, ICD-O 187.1; glans, 187.2; skin, 187.4) is composed of three cylindrical masses of cavernous tissue bound together by fibrous tissue. Two masses are lateral and are known as the corpora cavernosa penis. The corpus spongiosum penis is a median mass and contains the greater part of the urethra. The penis is attached to the front and the sides of the pubic arch. The skin covering the penis is thin and loosely connected with the deeper parts of the organ. This skin at the root of the penis is continuous with that over the scrotum and perineum. Distally, the skin becomes folded upon itself to form the prepuce or foreskin. Circumcision has been associated with a decreased incidence of cancer of the penis.

Regional Lymph Nodes. Two divisions of lymphatics drain the penis: the superficial system and the deep system. The superficial system drains the skin of the penis to the superficial nodes immediately below the inguinal ligament. The glans and deeper penile structures drain via the deep system to the deeper subinguinal nodes. These lymphatics drain directly into the iliac nodes. Superficial and deep inguinal nodes and pelvic nodes are regional nodes.

Metastatic Sites. Lung, liver, or bone are most often involved.

RULES FOR CLASSIFICATION

Clinical Staging. Clinical examination, endoscopy where possible, and histologic confirmation are required. Imaging techniques are indicated for metastatic disease detection.

Pathologic Staging. Complete resection of the primary site with appropriate margins is required. Where regional lymph node involvement is suspected these should be included.

DEFINITION OF TNM

Primary Tumor (T)

- TX Primary tumor cannot be assessed
- T0 No evidence of primary tumor
- Tis Carcinoma *in situ*
  - Ta Noninvasive verrucous carcinoma
- T1 Tumor invades subepithelial connective tissue
- T2 Tumor invades corpus spongiosum or cavernosum
- T3 Tumor invades urethra or prostate
- T4 Tumor invades other adjacent structures

Regional Lymph Nodes (N)

- NX Regional lymph nodes cannot be assessed
- N0 No regional lymph node metastasis
- N1 Metastasis in a single superficial, inguinal lymph node
- N2 Metastasis in multiple or bilateral superficial inguinal lymph nodes
- N3 Metastasis in deep inguinal or pelvic lymph node(s) unilateral or bilateral

Distant Metastasis (M)

- MX Presence of distant metastasis cannot be assessed
- M0 No distant metastasis
- M1 Distant metastasis

STAGE GROUPING

Stage	T	N	M
Stage 0	Tis	N0	M0
	Ta	N0	M0
Stage I	T1	N0	M0
Stage II	T1	N1	M0
	T2	N0, N1	M0
Stage III	T1	N2	M0
	T2	N2	M0
	T3	N0, N1, N2	M0
Stage IV	T4	Any N	M0
	Any T	N3	M0
	Any T	Any N	M1

DIFFERENCES BETWEEN THE 2ND AND 3RD EDITIONS

The AJCC did not include the penis in its 1983 *Manual.*

HISTOPATHOLOGIC TYPE

Cell types are limited to squamous cell carcinoma.

HISTOPATHOLOGIC GRADE (G)

- GX   Grade cannot be assessed
- G1   Well differentiated
- G2   Moderately well differentiated
- G3–4 Poorly differentiated or undifferentiated

BIBLIOGRAPHY

1. Bassett JW: Carcinoma of the penis. Cancer 5:530–538, 1952
2. Colon JE: Carcinoma of the penis. J Urol 67:702–708, 1952
3. Hanash KA, Furlow WL, Utz DC et al: Carcinoma of the penis: A clinicopathologic study. J Urol 104:291–297, 1970
4. McDougal WS, Kirchner FK Jr, Edwards RH et al: Treatment of carcinoma of the penis: The case for primary lymphadenectomy. J Urol 136:38–41, 1986

PENIS

Data Form for Cancer Staging

Patient identification
Name _____
Address _____
Hospital or clinic number _____
Age _____ Sex _____ Race _____

Institution identification
Hospital or clinic _____
Address _____

Oncology Record

Anatomic site of cancer _____
Histologic type _____
Grade (G) _____
Date of classification _____

Chronology of classification
(use separate form for each time staged)
[ ] Clinical (use all data prior to first treatment)
[ ] Pathologic (if definitively resected specimen available)

Definitions

Primary Tumor (T)
[ ] TX   Primary tumor cannot be assessed
[ ] T0   No evidence of primary tumor
[ ] Tis Carcinoma *in situ*
   [ ] Ta Noninvasive verrucous carcinoma
[ ] T1   Tumor invades subepithelial connective tissue
[ ] T2   Tumor invades corpus spongiosum or cavernosum
[ ] T3   Tumor invades urethra or prostate
[ ] T4   Tumor invades other adjacent structures

Lymph Node (N)
[ ] NX   Regional lymph nodes cannot be assessed
[ ] N0   No regional lymph node metastasis
[ ] N1   Metastasis in a single, superficial inguinal lymph node
[ ] N2   Metastasis in multiple or bilateral superficial inguinal lymph nodes
[ ] N3   Metastasis in deep inguinal or pelvic lymph node(s), unilateral or bilateral

Distant Metastasis
[ ] MX   Presence of distant metastasis cannot be assessed
[ ] M0   No distant metastasis
[ ] M1   Distant metastasis

Histopathologic Grade (G)
[ ] GX   Grade cannot be assessed
[ ] G1   Well differentiated
[ ] G2   Moderately well differentiated
[ ] G3-4 Poorly differentiated or undifferentiated

Histopathologic Type

Cell types are limited to squamous cell carcinoma.

Sites of Distant Metastasis

Pulmonary   PUL
Osseous   OSS
Hepatic   HEP
Brain   BRA
Lymph nodes LYM
Bone marrow MAR
Pleura   PLE
Peritoneum   PER
Skin   SKI
Other   OTH

Stage Grouping

[ ]	0	Tis	N0	M0
		Ta	N0	M0
[ ]	I	T1	N0	M0
[ ]	II	T1	N1	M0
		T2	N0	M0
		T2	N1	M0
[ ]	III	T1	N2	M0
		T2	N2	M0
		T3	N0	M0
		T3	N1	M0
		T3	N2	M0
[ ]	IV	T4	Any N	M0
		Any T	N3	M0
		Any T	Any N	M1

Staged by _____ M.D.
                _____ Registrar
Date _____

32

Urinary Bladder

Bladder cancer is distressing for both the patient and the physician. The disease can take an unpredictable and protracted course. It can present as a low grade papillary lesion, as an indolent *in situ* lesion, which can occupy large areas of the mucosal surface, or as an infiltrative cancer that rapidly extends through the bladder wall. The papillary and *in situ* lesions can either follow a benign course or pursue a malignant course with sudden invasion of the bladder wall. Predisposing factors include the exposure to certain chemicals that are used in the dye industry and smoking. Bladder cancer is more common in men. Hematuria is the most frequent presenting sign. Staging depends on the tumor grade, size, type of tumor, and extent of penetration into the bladder wall. Two separate staging systems have been used for bladder cancer.

ANATOMY

Primary Site. The urinary bladder (ICD-O 188) consists of three layers: the mucosal and submucosal sub-epithelial connective tissue, the muscularis, and the serosa (peritoneum covering the superior surface and upper part of the base). In the male, it adjoins the rectum and seminal vesicle posteriorly, the prostate inferiorly, and the pubis and peritoneum anteriorly. In the female, the vagina is located posteriorly and the uterus superiorly. The bladder is extraperitoneal in location.

Regional Lymph Nodes. The regional lymph nodes are the nodes of the true pelvis, which essentially are the pelvic nodes below the bifurcation of the common iliac arteries.

Laterality does not affect the N classification. The significance of regional lymph node metastasis in staging bladder cancer lies in the number and size and not in whether unilateral or contralateral.

Regional nodes include:

Hypogastric
Obturator
Iliac, internal, external, NOS
Perivesical
Pelvis, NOS
Sacral, lateral, NOS
Presacral

The common iliac nodes are considered sites of distant metastasis and should be coded as M1.

Metastatic Sites. Distant spread to lymph nodes, lung, bone, and liver is most common.

RULES FOR CLASSIFICATION

Clinical Staging. Primary tumor assessment includes bimanual examination under anesthesia before and after endoscopic surgery (biopsy or transurethral resection) or histologic verification of the presence or absence of tumor when indicated. Add "m" for multiple tumors. Appropriate imaging techniques for lymph node evaluation should be used as indicated. When indicated, evaluation for distant metastases includes imaging of the chest, biochemical studies, and isotopic studies to detect common metastatic sites. Computed body scan or other modalities may subsequently be used to supply information concerning minimal requirements for staging. The primary tumor biopsy may be superficial or invasive and can be partially or totally resected with sufficient tissue from the tumor base for full evaluation of depth of tumor invasion. Visually adjacent cystoscopically normal mucosa should be considered for biopsy; urinary cytology and pyelography are important.

Pathologic Staging. Histologic examination and confirmation of extent is required. Total cystectomy and lymph node dissection are required for this staging.

DEFINITION OF TNM

Primary Tumor (T)

The suffix "m" should be added to the appropriate T category to indicate multiple tumors. The suffix "is" may be added to any T to indicate the presence of associated carcinoma *in situ*.

TX Primary tumor cannot be assessed
T0 No evidence of primary tumor
Tis Carcinoma *in situ:* "flat tumor"
    Ta Noninvasive papillary carcinoma
T1 Tumor invades subepithelial connective tissue
T2* Tumor invades superficial muscle (inner half)
T3* Tumor invades deep muscle or perivesical fat
    T3a* Tumor invades deep muscle (outer half)
    T3b Tumor invades perivesical fat
T4 Tumor invades any of the following: prostate, uterus, vagina, pelvic wall, abdominal wall

Note: If pathology report does not specify that tumor invades muscle, consider as invasion of subepithelial connective tissue. If depth of muscle invasion is not specified by the surgeon, code as T2. (Superficial = inner half; deep = outer half.)

Regional Lymph Nodes (N)

Regional lymph nodes are those within the true pelvis; all others are distant nodes.

NX Regional lymph nodes cannot be assessed
N0 No regional lymph node metastasis
N1 Metastasis in a single lymph node, 2 cm or less in greatest dimension
N2 Metastasis in a single lymph node, more than 2 cm but not more than 5 cm in greatest dimension, or multiple lymph nodes, none more than 5 cm in greatest dimension
N3 Metastasis in a lymph node more than 5 cm in greatest dimension

Distant Metastasis (M)

MX Presence of distant metastasis cannot be assessed
M0 No distant metastasis
M1 Distant metastasis

STAGE GROUPING

Stage	T	N	M
Stage 0	Tis	N0	M0
	Ta	N0	M0
Stage I	T1	N0	M0
Stage II	T2	N0	M0
Stage III	T3a	N0	M0
	T3b	N0	M0
Stage IV	T4	N0	M0
	Any T	N1, N2, N3	M0
	Any T	Any N	M1

DIFFERENCES BETWEEN THE 2ND AND 3RD EDITIONS

The T categories have been redefined. The criteria used for staging by physical examination have been eliminated from this edition. In the N category, the size of the metastatic tumor in the regional nodes determines the classification, not the laterality, as previously published.

HISTOPATHOLOGIC TYPE

The histologic types are:

Urothelial carcinoma
Papillary carcinoma
Transitional cell carcinoma

The predominant cancer is a transitional cell cancer. Grading of the tumor is as follows.

HISTOPATHOLOGIC GRADE (G)

GX Grade cannot be assessed
G1 Well differentiated
G2 Moderately well differentiated
G3-4 Poorly differentiated or undifferentiated

BIBLIOGRAPHY

1. deVere White RW, Olsson CA, Deitch AD: Flow cytometry: Role in monitoring transitional cell carcinoma of bladder. Urology 28:15–20, 1986
2. Jewett HJ, Strong GH: Infiltrating carcinoma of the bladder—Relation of depth of penetration of the bladder wall to incidence of local extension and metastasis. J Urol 55:366–372, 1946
3. Mostofi FK: Pathological aspects and spread of carcinoma of bladder. JAMA 206:1764–1769, 1968
4. Smith JA Jr, Whitmore WF Jr: Regional lymph node metastasis from bladder cancer. J Urol 126:591–593, 1981
5. Whitmore WF Jr: Management of bladder cancer. Curr Probl Cancer 4:3–48, 1979

URINARY BLADDER

Data Form for Cancer Staging

Patient identification
Name _____
Address _____
Hospital or clinic number _____
Age _____ Sex _____ Race _____

Institution identification
Hospital or clinic _____
Address _____

Oncology Record

Anatomic site of cancer _____
Histologic type _____
Grade (G) _____
Date of classification _____

Chronology of classification
  (use separate form for each time staged)
[ ] Clinical (use all data prior to first treatment)
[ ] Pathologic (if definitively resected specimen available)

Definitions

Primary Tumor (T)

[ ] TX   Primary tumor cannot be assessed
[ ] T0   No evidence of primary tumor
[ ] Tis Carcinoma *in situ:* "flat tumor"
  [ ] Ta Noninvasive papillary carcinoma
[ ] T1   Tumor invades subepithelial connective tissue
[ ] T2   Tumor invades superficial muscle (inner half)
[ ] T3   Tumor invades deep muscle or perivesical fat
  [ ] T3a Tumor invades deep muscle (outer half)
  [ ] T3b Tumor invades perivesical fat
[ ] T4   Tumor invades any of the following: prostate, uterus, vagina, pelvic wall, abdominal wall

Lymph Node (N)

[ ] NX   Regional lymph nodes cannot be assessed
[ ] N0   No regional lymph node metastasis
[ ] N1   Metastasis in a single lymph node, 2 cm or less in greatest dimension
[ ] N2   Metastasis in a single lymph node, more than 2 cm but not more than 5 cm in greatest dimension, or multiple lymph nodes, none more than 5 cm in greatest dimension
[ ] N3   Metastasis in a lymph node more than 5 cm in greatest dimension

Distant Metastasis (M)

[ ] MX   Presence of distant metastasis cannot be assessed
[ ] M0   No distant metastasis
[ ] M1   Distant metastasis

Histopathologic Grade (G)

[ ] GX   Grade cannot be assessed
[ ] G1   Well differentiated
[ ] G2   Moderately well differentiated
[ ] G3-4   Poorly differentiated or undifferentiated

Histopathologic Type

The histologic types are:

Urothelial carcinoma
Papillary carcinoma
Transitional cell carcinoma

  The predominant cancer is a transitional cell cancer.

Sites of Distant Metastasis

Pulmonary	PUL
Osseous	OSS
Hepatic	HEP
Brain	BRA
Lymph nodes	LYM
Bone marrow	MAR
Pleura	PLE
Peritoneum	PER
Skin	SKI
Other	OTH

Stage Grouping

[ ]	0	Tis	N0	M0
		Ta	N0	M0
[ ]	I	T1	N0	M0
[ ]	II	T2	N0	M0
[ ]	III	T3a	N0	M0
		T3b	N0	M0
[ ]	IV	T4	N0	M0
		Any T	N1	M0
		Any T	N2	M0
		Any T	N3	M0
		Any T	Any N	M1

Staged by _____ M.D.
_____ Registrar
Date _____

Illustrations

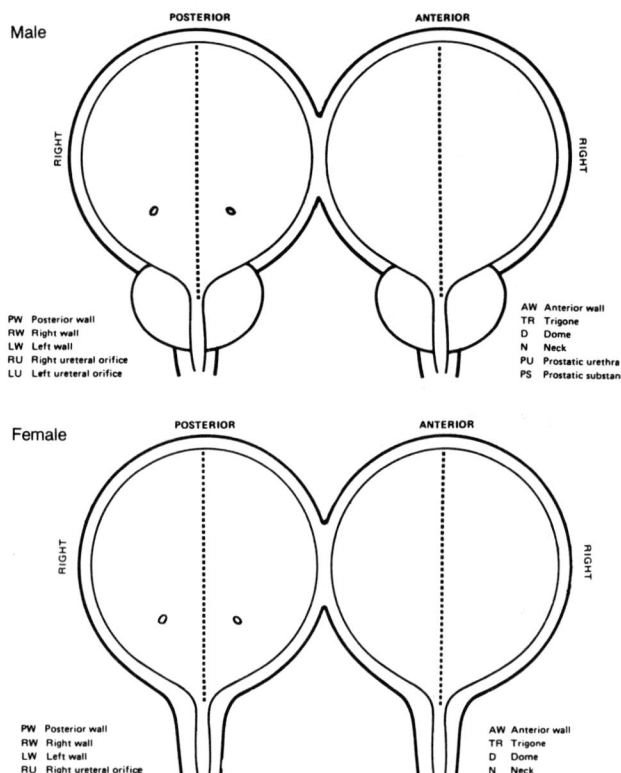

Indicate on diagrams primary tumor and regional nodes involved.

33

Kidney

Cancers of the kidney are relatively rare, accounting for less than 3% of all malignancies. Nearly all malignant tumors are carcinomas that arise from the renal tubular epithelium or less frequently from the renal pelvis. These tumors are more common in males. Pain and hematuria are usually the presenting features. Renal carcinomas may be associated with erythrocytosis, secondary to release of erythropoietin from the tumor cells. These carcinomas have a tendency to extend along the renal vein and even the inferior vena cava. They also may regress spontaneously. Staging depends upon the size of the primary tumor, invasion of the adjacent structures and vascular extension. Only a single TNM classification is used.

ANATOMY

Primary Site. The kidney (ICD-O 189.0) is encased by a fibrous capsule and is surrounded by perirenal fat. The kidney is composed of the cortex (glomeruli, convoluted tubules) and the medulla (Henle's loops, pyramids of converging tubules). Each papilla opens into the minor calices; these in turn unite in the major calices and drain into the renal pelvis. At the hilus are the pelvis, ureter, and renal artery and vein. Gerota's fascia overlies the psoas and quadrants lumborum.

Regional Lymph Nodes. The regional lymph nodes are the abdominal para-aortic, paracaval, and hilar nodes.

Laterality does not affect the N classification. The significance of regional lymph node metastasis in staging kidney cancer lies in the number and size and not in whether unilateral or contralateral.

Metastatic Sites. Common metastatic sites include bone, liver, lung, brain, and distant nodes.

RULES FOR CLASSIFICATION

The classification applies only to renal-cell carcinoma. Adenoma is excluded. There should be histologic confirmation of the disease.

Clinical Staging. Clinical examination, urography, and appropriate imaging techniques are required for assessment of the primary tumor and its extensions both local and distant. Evaluation for distant metastases should be done by laboratory biochemical studies, chest x-rays, and isotopic studies. Clinical staging may also include laparotomy and biopsy of distant sites.

Pathologic Staging. Histologic examination and confirmation of extent is required. Resection of the primary tumor, kidney, adrenal gland, Gerota's fascia, perinephric fat, renal vein, and appropriate lymph nodes is required.

DEFINITION OF TNM

Primary Tumor (T)

TX Primary tumor cannot be assessed
T0 No evidence of primary tumor
T1 Tumor 2.5 cm or less in greatest dimension limited to the kidney
T2 Tumor more than 2.5 cm in greatest dimension limited to the kidney
T3 Tumor extends into major veins or invades adrenal gland or perinephric tissues but not beyond Gerota's fascia
    T3a Tumor invades adrenal gland or perinephric tissues but not beyond Gerota's fascia
    T3b Tumor grossly extends into renal vein(s) or vena cava
T4 Tumor invades beyond Gerota's fascia

Regional Lymph Nodes (N)

NX Regional lymph nodes cannot be assessed
N0 No regional lymph node metastasis
N1 Metastasis in a single lymph node, 2 cm or less in greatest dimension
N2 Metastasis in a single lymph node, more than 2 cm but not more than 5 cm in greatest dimension, or multiple lymph nodes, none more than 5 cm in greatest dimension
N3 Metastasis in a lymph node more than 5 cm in greatest dimension

Distant Metastasis (M)

MX Presence of distant metastasis cannot be assessed
M0 No distant metastasis
M1 Distant metastasis

STAGE GROUPING

Stage	T	N	M
Stage I	T1	N0	M0
Stage II	T2	N0	M0
Stage III	T1	N1	M0
	T2	N1	M0
	T3a	N0, N1	M0
	T3b	N0, N1	M0
Stage IV	T4	Any N	M0
	Any T	N2, N3	M0
	Any T	Any N	M1

DIFFERENCES BETWEEN THE 2ND AND 3RD EDITIONS

The T categories, which have been redefined and simplified, are based on the size of the primary tumor. T1 and T2 refer to cancers that are intrarenal and have not invaded through the capsule. The T3 and T4 categories are now based on the local extension of the primary tumor.

The N classification has also been redefined and depends upon the size and number of involved lymph nodes and no longer on laterality. The T classification has been modified accordingly.

HISTOPATHOLOGIC TYPE

The histopathologic types are:

Renal cell carcinoma
  Adenocarcinoma
  Renal papillary adenocarcinoma
  Tubular carcinoma
  Granular cell carcinoma
  Clear cell carcinoma (hypernephroma)

The predominant cancer is adenocarcinoma; subtypes are clear-cell and granular-cell carcinoma. A grading system as below is recommended when feasible. The staging system does not apply to sarcomas of the kidney. A separate classification is published for nephroblastomas.

HISTOPATHOLOGIC GRADE (G)

GX Grade cannot be assessed
G1 Well differentiated
G2 Moderately well differentiated
G3–4 Poorly differentiated/undifferentiated

BIBLIOGRAPHY

1. Angervall L, Carlstrom E, Wahlquist L et al: Effects of clinical and morphological variables on spread of renal carcinoma in an operative series. Scand J Urol Nephrol 3:134–140, 1969
2. Bennington JL, Beckwith JB: *Tumors of the Kidney, Renal Pelvis, and Ureter,* Atlas of Tumor Pathology, Second Series, Fascicle 12. Washington, DC, Armed Forces Institute of Pathology, 1975
3. Holland JM: Cancer of the kidney—Natural history and staging. Cancer 32:1030–1042, 1973
4. Hulten L, Rosencrantz M, Seeman T et al: Occurrence and localization of lymph node metastases in renal carcinoma: Lymphographic and histopathologic investigation in connection with nephrectomy. Scand J Urol Nephrol 3:129–133, 1966
5. Katz SA, Davis JE: Renal adenocarcinoma: Prognostics and treatment reflected by survival. Urology 10:10–11, 1977
6. McDonald JR, Priestley JT: Malignant tumors of the kidney: Surgical and prognostic significance of tumor thrombosis of the renal vein. Surg Gynecol Obstet 77:295, 1983
7. Ramchandani P, Soulen RL, Schnall RI et al: Impact of magnetic resonance on staging of renal carcinoma. Urology 27:564–568, 1986
8. Weyman PJ, McClennan BL, Stanley RJ et al: Comparison of computer tomography and angiography in the evaluation of renal carcinoma. Radiology 137:417–424, 1980

KIDNEY

Data Form for Cancer Staging

Patient identification
Name _____
Address _____
Hospital or clinic number _____
Age _____ Sex _____ Race _____

Institution identification
Hospital or clinic _____
Address _____

Oncology Record

Anatomic site of cancer _____
Histologic type _____
Grade (G) _____
Date of classification _____

Chronology of classification
  (use separate form for each time staged)
[ ] Clinical (use all data prior to first treatment)
[ ] Pathologic (if definitively resected specimen available)

Definitions

Primary Tumor (T)

[ ] TX   Primary tumor cannot be assessed
[ ] T0   No evidence of primary tumor
[ ] T1   Tumor 2.5 cm or less in greatest dimension limited to the kidney
[ ] T2   Tumor more than 2.5 cm in greatest dimension limited to the kidney
[ ] T3   Tumor extends into major veins or invades adrenal gland or perinephric tissues but not beyond Gerota's fascia
  [ ] T3a   Tumor invades adrenal gland or perinephric tissues but not beyond Gerota's fascia
  [ ] T3b   Tumor grossly extends into renal vein(s) or vena cava
[ ] T4   Tumor invades beyond Gerota's fascia

Lymph Node (N)

[ ] NX   Regional lymph nodes cannot be assessed
[ ] N0   No regional lymph node metastasis
[ ] N1   Metastasis in a single lymph node, 2 cm or less in greatest dimension
[ ] N2   Metastasis in a single lymph node, more than 2 cm but not more than 5 cm in greatest dimension, or multiple lymph nodes, none more than 5 cm in greatest dimension
[ ] N3   Metastasis in a lymph node more than 5 cm in greatest dimension

Distant Metastasis (M)

[ ] MX   Presence of distant metastasis cannot be assessed
[ ] M0   No distant metastasis
[ ] M1   Distant metastasis

Stage Grouping

[ ]	I	T1	N0	M0
[ ]	II	T2	N0	M0
[ ]	III	T1	N1	M0
		T2	N1	M0
		T3a	N0	M0
		T3a	N1	M0
		T3b	N0	M0
		T3b	N1	M0
[ ]	IV	T4	Any N	M0
		Any T	N2	M0
		Any T	N3	M0
		Any T	Any N	M1

Histopathologic Grade (G)

[ ] GX   Grade cannot be assessed
[ ] G1   Well differentiated
[ ] G2   Moderately well differentiated
[ ] G3-4   Poorly differentiated or undifferentiated

Histopathologic Type

The histopathologic types are:

Renal cell carcinoma
  Adenocarcinoma
  Renal papillary adenocarcinoma
  Tubular carcinoma
  Granular cell carcinoma
  Clear cell carcinoma—Hypernephroma

The predominant cancer is adenocarcinoma; subtypes are clear-cell and granular-cell carcinoma. A grading system is recommended when feasible. The staging system does not apply to sarcomas of the kidney. A separate classification is published for nephroblastomas.

Staged by _____ M.D.
          _____ Registrar
Date _____

Sites of Distant Metastasis

Pulmonary	PUL
Osseous	OSS
Hepatic	HEP
Brain	BRA
Lymph nodes	LYM
Bone marrow	MAR
Pleura	PLE
Peritoneum	PER
Skin	SKI
Other	OTH

Illustrations

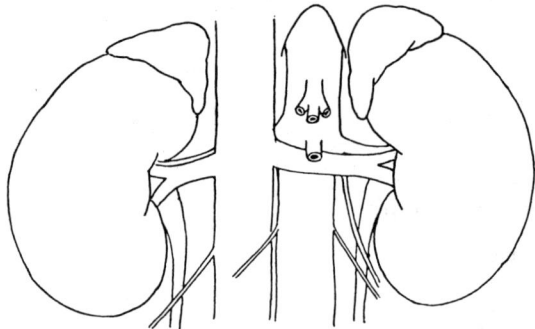

This drawing is to be used with the checklist. Sketch in the urographic, angiographic, ultrasound, or CT extent of tumor.

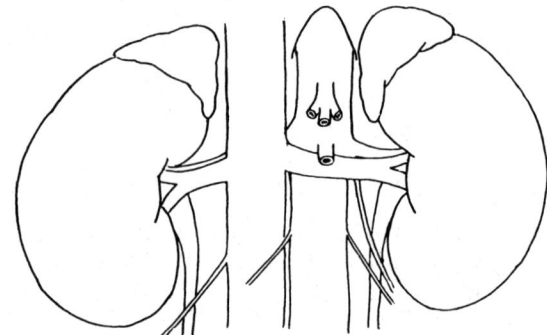

This drawing is to be used with the checklist and the upper drawing. Sketch in the pathologic extent of tumor.

Renal Pelvis and Ureter

34

Tumors of the renal pelvis and ureter are not common. Tumors of the renal pelvis comprise only 5% to 10% of all renal cancers. Most cases are found in adults. Very often, malignant tumors in the renal pelvis or ureter are multiple and associated with cancers located in other parts of the urinary tract. For instance, carcinomas of the ureter are often associated with tumors in the urinary bladder. Most tumors are transitional cell carcinomas, although other types can occur. Tumors in the renal pelvis may be associated with calculi. Staging depends on the extent of disease.

ANATOMY

Primary Site. The renal pelvis (ICD-O 189.1) and ureter (ICD-O 189.2) form a single unit, which cephalad is continuous with the collecting ducts of the renal pyramides and comprises the minor and major calyces, which are continuous with the renal pelvis. The uretero-pelvic junction is variable in position and location, but serves as a "landmark" that separates the renal pelvis and the ureter, which continues caudad and traverses the wall of the urinary bladder as the intramural ureter opening on the trigone of the bladder at the ureteral orifice. The renal pelvis and ureter are composed of the following layers: the mucosa, submucosa (lamina propria), and muscularis, which is continuous with a connective tissue adventitial layer. It is in this outer layer that the major blood supply and lymphatics are found.

The intrarenal portion of the renal pelvis is surrounded by renal parenchyma, and the extrarenal pelvis is surrounded by perihilar fat. The ureter courses through the retroperitoneum adjacent to the parietal peritoneum and rests on the retroperitoneal musculature above the pelvic vessels, and, as it crosses the vessels and enters the deep pelvis, it is surrounded by pelvic fat until it traverses the bladder wall.

Regional Lymph Nodes. The regional lymph nodes are the hilar, abdominal para-aortic, paracaval and common, internal, and external iliac nodes.

Laterality does not affect the N classification. The significance of regional lymph node metastasis in staging renal cancer lies in the number and size and not in whether unilateral or contralateral.

Metastatic Sites. Distant spread to lung, bone, and liver is most common.

RULES FOR CLASSIFICATION

Clinical Staging. Primary tumor assessment includes radiographic imaging, endoscopic evaluation, and ureteroscopy when applicable. Material in cytoscopic study should be obtained. The possible concurrent presence of bladder tumors is not a prognostic factor in this staging system. These tumors should be staged separately. Evaluation of distant metastatic sites includes radiographic, radioisotopic, and appropriate blood studies.

Pathologic Staging. Histologic confirmation of extent of disease is required. Resection of primary tumor, kidney, ureter, appropriate regional lymph nodes, and bladder cuff is usually required. Special circumstances may limit the magnitude of resection, but, at a minimum, the tumor with appropriate margins and regional lymph nodes must be available for pathologic evaluation.

DEFINITION OF TNM

Primary Tumor (T)

TX Primary tumor cannot be assessed
T0 No evidence of primary tumor
Tis Carcinoma *in situ*
 Ta Papillary noninvasive carcinoma
T1 Tumor invades subepithelial connective tissue
T2 Tumor invades muscularis
T3 Tumor invades beyond muscularis into periureteric or peripelvic fat or renal parenchyma
T4 Tumor invades adjacent organs or through the kidney into perinephric fat

Regional Lymph Nodes (N)

NX Regional lymph nodes cannot be assessed
N0 No regional lymph node metastasis
N1 Metastasis in a single lymph node, 2 cm or less in greatest dimension
N2 Metastasis in a single lymph node, more than 2 cm but not more than 5 cm in greatest dimension, or multiple lymph nodes, none more than 5 cm in greatest dimension
N3 Metastasis in a lymph node more than 5 cm in greatest dimension

Distant Metastasis (M)

MX Presence of distant metastasis cannot be assessed
M0 No distant metastasis
M1 Distant metastasis

STAGE GROUPING

Stage	T	N	M
Stage 0	Tis	N0	M0
	Ta	N0	M0
Stage I	T1	N0	M0
Stage II	T2	N0	M0
Stage III	T3	N0	M0
Stage IV	T4	N0	M0
	Any T	N1, N2, N3	M0
	Any T	Any N	M1

DIFFERENCES BETWEEN THE 2ND AND 3RD EDITIONS

Staging systems for the renal pelvis and ureter were not previously published by the AJCC.

HISTOPATHOLOGIC TYPE

The histologic types are:

Transitional cell carcinoma
Papillary carcinoma
Squamous cell carcinoma
 Epidermoid carcinoma
Adenocarcinoma
Urothelial carcinoma

HISTOPATHOLOGIC GRADE

GX   Grade cannot be assessed
G1   Well differentiated
G2   Moderately well differentiated
G3–4 Poorly differentiated/undifferentiated

BIBLIOGRAPHY

1. Batata MA, Whitmore WF, Hilaris BS et al: Primary carcinoma of the ureter: A prognostic study. Cancer 35:1626–1632, 1975
2. Bloom NA, Vidone RA, Lytton B: Primary carcinoma of the ureter. A report of 102 new cases. J Urol 103:590–598, 1970
3. Claymen RV, Williams RD, Fraley EE: The pursuit of the renal mass. N Engl J Med 300:72–74, 1979
4. Johansson S, Angervall L, Bengtsson U et al: A clinicopathologic and prognostic study of epithelial tumors of the renal pelvis. Cancer 37:1376–1383, 1976
5. Wagle DG, Moore RH, Murphy GP: Primary carcinoma of the renal pelvis. Cancer 33:1642–1648, 1974

RENAL PELVIS AND URETER

Data Form for Cancer Staging

Patient identification
Name _____
Address _____
Hospital or clinic number _____
Age _____ Sex _____ Race _____

Institution identification
Hospital or clinic _____
Address _____

Oncology Record

Anatomic site of cancer _____
Histologic type _____
Grade (G) _____
Date of classification _____

Chronology of classification
 (use separate form for each time staged)
[ ] Clinical (use all data prior to first treatment)
[ ] Pathologic (if definitively resected specimen available)

Definitions

Primary Tumor (T)
[ ] TX Primary tumor cannot be assessed
[ ] T0 No evidence of primary tumor
[ ] Tis Carcinoma *in situ*
 [ ] Ta Papillary noninvasive carcinoma
[ ] T1 Tumor invades subepithelial connective tissue
[ ] T2 Tumor invades muscularis
[ ] T3 Tumor invades beyond muscularis into periureteric or peripelvic fat or renal parenchyma
[ ] T4 Tumor invades adjacent organs or through the kidney into perinephric fat

Lymph Node (N)
[ ] NX Regional lymph nodes cannot be assessed
[ ] N0 No regional lymph node metastasis
[ ] N1 Metastasis in a single lymph node, 2 cm or less in greatest dimension
[ ] N2 Metastasis in a single lymph node, more than 2 cm but not more than 5 cm in greatest dimension, or multiple lymph nodes, none more than 5 cm in greatest dimension
[ ] N3 Metastasis in a lymph node more than 5 cm in greatest dimension

Distant Metastasis (M)
[ ] MX Presence of distant metastasis cannot be assessed
[ ] M0 No distant metastasis
[ ] M1 Distant metastasis

Stage Grouping

[ ] 0	Tis	N0	M0
	Ta	N0	M0
[ ] I	T1	N0	M0
[ ] II	T2	N0	M0
[ ] III	T3	N0	M0
[ ] IV	T4	N0	M0
	Any T	N1	M0
	Any T	N2	M0
	Any T	N3	M0
	Any T	Any N	M1

Histopathologic Grade (G)

[ ] GX Grade cannot be assessed
[ ] G1 Well differentiated
[ ] G2 Moderately well differentiated
[ ] G3-4 Poorly differentiated or undifferentiated

Histopathologic Type

The histopathologic types are:

Transitional cell carcinoma
Papillary carcinoma
Squamous cell carcinoma
 Epidermoid carcinoma
Adenocarcinoma
Urothelial carcinoma

Sites of Distant Metastasis

Pulmonary	PUL
Osseous	OSS
Hepatic	HEP
Brain	BRA
Lymph nodes	LYM
Bone marrow	MAR
Pleura	PLE
Peritoneum	PER
Skin	SKI
Other	OTH

Staged by _____ M.D.
_____ Registrar
Date _____

35

Urethra

In both sexes, cancers of the urethra are exceedingly rare. Most carcinomas of the female urethra occur at the junction of the transitional and stratified squamous epithelium at the meatus. In males, the cancer may be associated with a venereal disease, such as gonorrhea. The most common location is the bulbomembranous portion. As in the female, most tumors are squamous cell carcinomas. Transitional cell carcinomas are found in the prostatic portion. Staging depends upon the depth of penetration and local extension.

ANATOMY

Primary Site. In the *male*, the urethra (ICD-O 189.3) is divided into anterior, penile (pendulous), and posterior (bulbomembranous and prostate). The urethra consists of mucosa, submucosal stroma, and the surrounding corpus spongiosum. Histologically, the meatal and parameatal urethra are lined by squamous epithelium, the penile and bulbomembranous urethra with pseudostratified or stratified columnar epithelium, and the prostatic urethra with transitional cell epithelium. The corpora cavernosum is contiguous to the bulbous and penile urethra.

The *female* urethra (ICD-O 189.3) is divided into proximal and distal sections. The mucosa is supported on a connective tissue submucosa. The periurethral glands of Skene are concentrated near the meatus but extend along the entire urethra. The urethra is surrounded by a longitudinal layer of smooth muscle that is continuous with the bladder. The distal third of the urethra is contiguous to the vaginal wall. The mucosa of the distal two thirds of the urethra is squamous epithelium; the proximal one third is transitional; and the periurethral glands are lined by pseudostratified and stratified columnar epithelium.

Regional Lymph Nodes. The regional lymph nodes are the inguinal and common iliac, external iliac, and internal iliac nodes.

Laterality does not affect the N classification. The significance of regional lymph node metastasis in staging urethral cancer lies in the number and size and not in whether unilateral or bilateral.

Metastatic Sites. Distant spread to lung, liver, and bone is most common.

RULES FOR CLASSIFICATION

Clinical Staging. Radiographic imaging, cystourethroscopy, palpation, and biopsy or cytology of the tumor prior to definitive treatment are desirable. The site of origin should be confirmed to exclude metastatic disease.

Pathologic Staging. Histologic examination and confirmation of extent and location of disease are required. Extent of resection, including removal of regional lymph nodes, will be dependent on tumor location, depth of penetration, and sex of patient.

DEFINITION OF TNM

Primary Tumor (T) (male and female)

TX Primary tumor cannot be assessed
T0 No evidence of primary tumor
Tis Carcinoma *in situ*
  Ta Non-invasive papillary, polypoid, or verrucous carcinoma
T1 Tumor invades subepithelial connective tissue
T2 Tumor invades corpus spongiosum or prostate or periurethral muscle
T3 Tumor invades corpus cavernosum or beyond prostatic capsule or the anterior vagina or bladder neck
T4 Tumor invades other adjacent organs

Regional Lymph Nodes (N)

NX Regional lymph nodes cannot be assessed
N0 No regional lymph node metastasis
N1 Metastasis in a single lymph node, 2 cm or less in greatest dimension
N2 Metastasis in a single lymph node, more than 2 cm but not more than 5 cm in greatest dimension, or multiple lymph nodes, none more than 5 cm in greatest dimension
N3 Metastasis in a lymph node more than 5 cm in greatest dimension

Distant Metastasis (M)

MX Presence of distant metastasis cannot be assessed
M0 No distant metastasis
M1 Distant metastasis

STAGE GROUPING

Stage	T	N	M
Stage 0	Tis	N0	M0
	Ta	N0	M0
Stage I	T1	N0	M0
Stage II	T2	N0	M0
Stage III	T1	N1	M0
	T2	N1	M0
	T3	N0, N1	M0
Stage IV	T4	N0, N1	M0
	Any T	N2, N3	M0
	Any T	Any N	M1

DIFFERENCES BETWEEN THE 2ND AND 3RD EDITIONS

A staging classification for cancers of the urethra was not published in the 1983 edition of the *Manual*.

HISTOPATHOLOGIC TYPE

Cell types can be divided into transitional, squamous, and glandular.

HISTOPATHOLOGIC GRADE (G)

GX   Grade cannot be assessed
G1   Well differentiated
G2   Moderately well differentiated
G3-4 Poorly differentiated or undifferentiated

BIBLIOGRAPHY

1. Levine RL: Urethral cancer. Cancer 45:1965–1972, 1980
2. Rogers RE, Burns B: Carcinoma of the female urethra. Obstet Gynecol 33:54–57, 1969
3. Vernon HK, Wilkins RD: Primary carcinoma of the male urethra. Br J Urol 21:232–235, 1950

URETHRA

Data Form for Cancer Staging

Patient identification
Name _____
Address _____
Hospital or clinic number _____
Age _____ Sex _____ Race _____

Institution identification
Hospital or clinic _____
Address _____

Oncology Record

Anatomic site of cancer _____
Histologic type _____
Grade (G) _____
Date of classification _____

Chronology of classification
(use separate form for each time staged)
[ ] Clinical (use all data prior to first treatment)
[ ] Pathologic (if definitively resected specimen available)

Definitions

Primary Tumor (T)

[ ] TX Primary tumor cannot be assessed
[ ] T0 No evidence of primary tumor
[ ] Tis Carcinoma in situ
 [ ] Ta Noninvasive papillary, polypoid, or verrucous carcinoma
[ ] T1 Tumor invades subepithelial connective tissue
[ ] T2 Tumor invades corpus spongiosum or prostate or periurethral muscle
[ ] T3 Tumor invades corpus cavernosum or beyond prostatic capsule or the anterior vagina or bladder neck
[ ] T4 Tumor invades other adjacent organs

Lymph Node (N)

[ ] NX Regional lymph nodes cannot be assessed
[ ] N0 No regional lymph node metastasis
[ ] N1 Metastasis in a single lymph node, 2 cm or less in greatest dimension
[ ] N2 Metastasis in a single lymph node, more than 2 cm but not more than 5 cm in greatest dimension, or multiple lymph nodes, none more than 5 cm in greatest dimension
[ ] N3 Metastasis in a lymph node more than 5 cm in greatest dimension

Distant Metastasis (M)

[ ] MX Presence of distant metastasis cannot be assessed
[ ] M0 No distant metastasis
[ ] M1 Distant metastasis

Histopathologic Type

Cell types can be divided into transitional, squamous, and glandular.

Histopathologic Grade (G)

[ ] GX Grade cannot be assessed
[ ] G1 Well differentiated
[ ] G2 Moderately well differentiated
[ ] G3 4 Poorly differentiated or undifferentiated

Sites of Distant Metastasis

Pulmonary	PUL
Osseous	OSS
Hepatic	HEP
Brain	BRA
Lymph nodes	LYM
Bone marrow	MAR
Pleura	PLE
Peritoneum	PER
Skin	SKI
Other	OTH

Stage Grouping

[ ] 0	Tis	N0	M0
	Ta	N0	M0
[ ] I	T1	N0	M0
[ ] II	T2	N0	M0
[ ] III	T1	N1	M0
	T2	N1	M0
	T3	N0	M0
	T3	N1	M0
[ ] IV	T4	N0	M0
	T4	N1	M0
	Any T	N2	M0
	Any T	N3	M0
	Any T	Any N	M1

Staged by _____ M.D.
_____ Registrar
Date _____

OPHTHALMIC TUMORS

36

Carcinoma of the Eyelid

The orbit and its contents—primarily the eye—contain many types of tissues. Consequently, a wide variety of malignant tumors occur in this anatomic area. Included in this section are recommendations for staging these cancers based on data available in the literature and knowledge of the experts serving on the Task Force for Staging of Cancer of the Eye of the American Joint Committee on Cancer.

For histologic nomenclature and diagnostic criteria, reference to the WHO classification* is recommended.

The following sites are included:

Eyelid
Conjunctiva
Uvea
Retina
Orbit
Lacrimal gland

ANATOMY

Primary Site. The eyelid (ICD-O 173.1) is covered externally by epidermis and internally by conjunctiva, which becomes continuous with the conjunctiva that covers the eyeball. Basal cell carcinoma and squamous cell carcinoma arise from the epidermal surface. Sebaceous cell carcinoma arises from the meibomian glands in the tarsus, the glands of Zeis at the lid margin, and the sebaceous glands of the caruncle. Other adnexal carcinomas arise from the sweat glands of Moll and the hair follicles.

Regional Lymph Nodes. The eyelids are supplied with lymphatics that drain into the preauricular, submandibular, and cervical lymph nodes.

---

*Zimmerman LE, Sobin LH et al: Histological typing of tumors of the eye and its adnexa. In International Histological Classification of Tumours. Geneva, World Health Organization, 1980

Metastatic Sites. Tumors of the eyelids not only metastasize to distant sites by way of the regional lymphatics and bloodstream but also spread directly into the orbit, including the lacrimal gland, and into the eyeball.

RULES FOR CLASSIFICATION

The classification applies only to carcinoma.

There should be histologic verification of the cancer. This verification permits a division of cases by histologic type (*i.e.,* basal cell, squamous cell, and sebaceous carcinoma). Any unconfirmed case must be reported separately.

Clinical Staging. The assessment of the cancer is based on inspection, slit-lamp examination, palpation of the regional lymph nodes, and, when indicated, radiologic (including computed tomography [CT]) and ultrasonographic examination of the orbit, paranasal sinuses, and chest.

Pathologic Staging. Complete resection of the primary site is indicated. Histologic study of the margins and the deep aspect of resected tissues is necessary. Resection or needle biopsy of enlarged regional lymph nodes or orbital masses is desirable.

DEFINITION OF TNM

The following definitions apply to both clinical and pathologic staging.

Primary Tumor (T)

TX	Primary tumor cannot be assessed
T0	No evidence of primary tumor
Tis	Carcinoma *in situ*
T1	Tumor of any size, not invading the tarsal plate or, at the eyelid margin, 5 mm or less in greatest dimension
T2	Tumor invades tarsal plate or, at the eyelid margin, more than 5 mm but not more than 10 mm in greatest dimension
T3	Tumor involves full eyelid thickness or, at the eyelid margin, more than 10 mm in greatest dimension
T4	Tumor invades adjacent structures

Regional Lymph Nodes (N)

NX	Regional lymph nodes cannot be assessed
N0	No regional lymph node metastasis
N1	Regional lymph node metastasis

Distant Metastasis (M)

MX	Presence of distant metastasis cannot be assessed
M0	No distant metastasis
M1	Distant metastasis

STAGE GROUPING

No stage grouping is presently recommended.

DIFFERENCES BETWEEN THE 2ND AND 3RD EDITIONS

This classification is the same as that published in the second edition of the *Manual.*

HISTOPATHOLOGIC TYPE

Basal cell carcinoma
Squamous cell carcinoma
Sebaceous cell carcinoma

HISTOPATHOLOGIC GRADE (G)

GX	Grade cannot be assessed
G1	Well differentiated
G2	Moderately well differentiated
G3	Poorly differentiated
G4	Undifferentiated

CARCINOMA OF THE EYELID

Data Form for Cancer Staging

Patient identification
Name _____
Address _____
Hospital or clinic number _____
Age _____ Sex _____ Race _____

Institution identification
Hospital or clinic _____
Address _____

Oncology Record

Anatomic site of cancer _____
Histologic type _____
Grade (G) _____
Date of classification _____

Chronology of classification
(use separate form for each time staged)
[ ] Clinical (use all data prior to first treatment)
[ ] Pathologic (if definitively resected specimen available)

Definitions

Primary Tumor (T)

[ ] TX   Primary tumor cannot be assessed
[ ] T0   No evidence of primary tumor
[ ] Tis Carcinoma in situ
[ ] T1   Tumor of any size, not invading the tarsal plate or, at the eyelid margin, 5 mm or less in greatest dimension
[ ] T2   Tumor invades tarsal plate or, at the eyelid margin, more than 5 mm but not more than 10 mm in greatest dimension
[ ] T3   Tumor involves full eyelid thickness or, at the eyelid margin, more than 10 mm in greatest dimension
[ ] T4   Tumor invades adjacent structures

Lymph Node (N)

[ ] NX   Regional lymph nodes cannot be assessed
[ ] N0   No regional lymph node metastasis
[ ] N1   Regional lymph node metastasis

Distant Metastasis (M)

[ ] MX   Presence of distant metastasis cannot be assessed
[ ] M0   No distant metastasis
[ ] M1   Distant metastasis

Stage Grouping

No stage grouping is presently recommended.

Histopathologic Type

Basal cell carcinoma
Squamous cell carcinoma
Sebaceous carcinoma

Histopathologic Grade (G)

[ ] GX   Grade cannot be assessed
[ ] G1   Well differentiated
[ ] G2   Moderately well differentiated
[ ] G3   Poorly differentiated
[ ] G4   Undifferentiated

Illustration

Indicate on diagram and describe exact location and characteristics of tumor.

Sites of Distant Metastasis

Pulmonary	PUL
Osseous	OSS
Hepatic	HEP
Brain	BRA
Lymph nodes	LYM
Bone marrow	MAR
Pleura	PLE
Peritoneum	PER
Skin	SKI
Other	OTH

Staged by _____ M.D.
_____ Registrar
Date _____

37

Melanoma of the Eyelid

This chapter has been adapted from the discussion for melanoma of the skin, since that discussion is considered to be applicable to melanoma of the skin of the eyelid.

No cT categories are presently recommended.

The pT categories correspond to those in the third edition of the TNM classification and are based on Clark's "levels" and Breslow's "thickness of invasion." Thickness of invasion into the skin is recorded as an actual measurement as determined by the ocular micrometer. The measurement extends from the normal level of the basement membrane to the greatest depth of tumor penetration.

The N and M categories correspond to those of melanoma of the skin.

ANATOMY

Primary Site. The eyelid (ICD-O 173.1) is covered externally by epidermis and internally by conjunctiva, which becomes continuous with the conjunctiva that covers the eyeball.

Regional Lymph Nodes. The eyelids are supplied with lymphatics that drain into the preauricular, submandibular, and cervical lymph nodes.

Metastatic Sites. Tumors of the eyelids not only metastasize to distant sites by way of the regional lymphatics and bloodstream but also spread directly into the orbit, including the lacrimal gland, and into the eyeball.

RULES FOR CLASSIFICATION

Clinical Staging. The assessment of the cancer is based on inspection, slit-lamp examination, palpation of the regional lymph nodes, and, when indicated, radiologic (including computed tomography [CT]) and ultrasonographic examination of the orbit, paranasal sinuses, and chest.

Pathologic Staging. Complete resection of the primary site is indicated. Histologic study of the margins and the deep aspect of resected tissues is necessary. Resection or needle biopsy of enlarged regional lymph nodes or orbital masses is desirable.

DEFINITION OF TNM
Clinical Classification (cTNM)
Primary Tumor (T)
No classification is recommended at present.

Regional Lymph Nodes (N)

NX Regional lymph nodes cannot be assessed
N0 No regional lymph node metastasis
N1 Metastasis 3 cm or less in greatest dimension in any regional lymph node(s)
N2 Metastasis more than 3 cm in greatest dimension in any regional lymph node(s) and/or in-transit metastasis
    N2a Metastasis more than 3 cm in greatest dimension in any regional node(s)
    N2b In-transit metastasis
    N2c Both (N2a and N2b)

Pathologic Classification (pTNM)
Primary Tumor (pT)

pTX Primary tumor cannot be assessed
pT0 No evidence of primary tumor
pTis Melanoma *in situ* (atypical melanocytic hyperplasia, severe melanocytic dysplasia), not an invasive malignant lesion (Clark's Level I)
pT1 Tumor 0.75 mm or less in thickness and invades the papillary dermis (Clark's Level II)
pT2 Tumor more than 0.75 mm but not more than 1.5 mm in thickness and/or invades to papillary-reticular dermal interface (Clark's Level III)
pT3 Tumor more than 1.5 mm but not more than 4 mm in thickness and/or invades the reticular dermis (Clark's Level IV)
    pT3a Tumor more than 1.5 mm but not more than 3 mm in thickness
    pT3b Tumor more than 3 mm but not more than 4 mm in thickness
pT4 Tumor more than 4 mm in thickness and/or invades the subcutaneous tissue and/or satellite(s) within 2 cm of the primary tumor (Clark's Level V)
    pT4a Tumor more than 4 mm in thickness and/or invades the subcutaneous tissue
    pT4b Satellite(s) within 2 cm of the primary tumor

Regional Lymph Nodes (pN)

pNX Regional lymph nodes cannot be assessed
pN0 No regional lymph node metastasis
pN1 Metastasis 3 cm or less in greatest dimension in any regional lymph node(s)
pN2 Metastasis more than 3 cm in greatest dimension in any regional lymph node(s) and/or in-transit metastasis
    pN2a Metastasis more than 3 cm in greatest dimension
    pN2b In-transit metastasis
    pN2c Both (pN2a and pN2b)

Distant Metastasis (pM)

pMX Presence of distant metastasis cannot be assessed
pM0 No distant metastasis
pM1 Distant metastasis
    pM1a Metastasis in skin or subcutaneous tissue or lymph node(s) beyond the regional lymph nodes
    pM1b Visceral metastasis

Note: In-transit metastasis involves skin or subcutaneous tissue more than 2 cm from the primary tumor not beyond the regional lymph nodes.

STAGE GROUPING

Stage I	pT1	N0	M0
	pT2	N0	M0
Stage II	pT3	N0	M0
Stage III	pT4	N0	M0
	Any pT	N1, N2	M0
Stage IV	Any pT	Any N	M1

DIFFERENCES BETWEEN THE 2ND AND 3RD EDITIONS

The upper limit on thickness for T3 tumors is now 4 mm rather than 3 mm as in the second edition of the *Manual*. Tumors more than 4 mm in thickness are now classified as T4. The stage grouping, which is totally revised, conforms to that for melanoma of the skin.

HISTOPATHOLOGIC TYPE

This classification is only for melanoma of the eyelid.

HISTOPATHOLOGIC GRADE (G) (RARELY USED WITH MELANOMAS)

GX Grade cannot be assessed
G1 Well differentiated

G2 Moderately well differentiated
G3 Poorly differentiated
G4 Undifferentiated

BIBLIOGRAPHY

1. Breslow A: Tumor thickness, level of invasion and node dissection in Stage 1 cutaneous melanoma. Ann Surg 182:572–575, 1975
2. Breslow A: Thickness, cross-sectional areas and depth of invasion in the prognosis of cutaneous melanoma. Ann Surg 172:902–908, 1970
3. Clark WH Jr, Ainsworth AM, Bernardina EA et al: The developmental biology of primary human malignant melanomas. Semin Oncol 2:83–103, 1975
4. Elder DE, Jucovy PM, Tuthill RJ, Clark WH Jr: The classification of malignant melanoma. Am J Dermatopathol 2:315–319, 1980

MELANOMA OF THE EYELID

Data Form for Cancer Staging

Patient identification
Name _____
Address _____
Hospital or clinic number _____
Age _____ Sex _____ Race _____

Institution identification
Hospital or clinic _____
Address _____

Oncology Record

Anatomic site of cancer _____
Histologic type _____
Grade (G) _____
Date of classification _____

Chronology of classification
(use separate form for each time staged)
[ ] Clinical (use all data prior to first treatment)
[ ] Pathologic (if definitively resected specimen available)

Definitions

Primary Tumor (T)
No classification is recommended at present.

Lymph Node (N)
[ ] NX Regional lymph nodes cannot be assessed
[ ] N0 No regional lymph node metastasis
[ ] N1 Metastasis 3 cm or less in greatest dimension in any regional lymph node(s)
[ ] N2 Metastasis more than 3 cm in greatest dimension in any regional lymph node(s) and/or in-transit metastasis
   [ ] N2a Metastasis more than 3 cm in greatest dimension in any regional node(s)
   [ ] N2b In-transit metastasis
   [ ] N2c Both

Primary Tumor (pT)
[ ] pTX Primary tumor cannot be assessed
[ ] pT0 No evidence of primary tumor
[ ] pTis Melanoma *in situ* (atypical melanocytic hyperplasia, severe melanocytic dysplasia), not an invasive malignant lesion (Clark's Level I)
[ ] pT1 Tumor 0.75 mm or less in thickness and invades the papillary dermis (Clark's Level II)
[ ] pT2 Tumor more than 0.75 mm but not more than 1.5 mm in thickness and/or invades to the papillary-reticular dermal interface (Clark's Level III)
[ ] pT3 Tumor more than 1.50 mm but not more than 4 mm in thickness and/or invades the reticular dermis (Clark's Level IV)
[ ] pT4 Tumor more than 4 mm in thickness and/or invades the subcutaneous tissue (Clark's Level V)

Lymph Node (pN)
[ ] pNX Regional lymph nodes cannot be assessed
[ ] pN0 No regional lymph node metastasis
[ ] pN1 Regional lymph node metastasis

Distant Metastasis (pM)
[ ] pMX Presence of distant metastasis cannot be assessed
[ ] pM0 No distant metastasis
[ ] pM1 Distant metastasis
   [ ] pM1a Metastasis in skin or subcutaneous tissue or lymph node(s) beyond the regional lymph nodes
   [ ] pM1b Visceral metastasis

Note: In-transit metastasis involves skin or subcutaneous tissue more than 2 cm from the primary tumor not beyond the regional lymph nodes.

Stage Grouping

[ ]	I	T1	N0	M0
		T2	N0	M0
[ ]	II	T3	N0	M0
[ ]	III	T4	N0	M0
		Any T	N1	M0
[ ]	IV	Any T	Any N	M1

Histopathologic Type

This classification is only for melanoma of the skin.

Sites of Distant Metastasis

Pulmonary PUL
Osseous OSS
Hepatic HEP
Brain BRA
Lymph nodes LYM
Bone marrow MAR
Pleura PLE
Peritoneum PER
Skin SKI
Other OTH

Staged by _____ M.D.
_____ Registrar
Date _____

Carcinoma of the Conjunctiva

ANATOMY

Primary Site. The conjunctiva (ICD-O 190.3) consists of stratified epithelium that contains mucus-secreting goblet cells; these cells are most numerous in the fornices. Palpebral conjunctiva lines the eyelid; bulbar conjunctiva covers the eyeball. Conjunctival epithelium merges with that of the cornea at the limbus. It is at this site, particularly at the temporal limbus, that carcinoma is most likely to arise. Conjunctival intraepithelial neoplasia (C.I.N.) embraces all forms of intraepithelial dysplasia, including *in situ* carcinoma. Mucinous adenocarcinoma is a rare form of adenocarcinoma of the conjunctival goblet cells.

Regional Lymph Nodes. The regional lymph nodes are the preauricular, submandibular, and cervical nodes.

Metastatic Sites. Tumors of the conjunctiva, in addition to spread by way of regional lymphatics, may also involve the eyelid proper, the orbit, lacrimal gland and brain.

RULES FOR CLASSIFICATION

Clinical Staging. The assessment of the cancer is based on inspection, slit-lamp examination, palpation of the regional lymph nodes, and, when indicated, radiologic examination (including computed tomography [CT]) and ultrasonographic examination of the orbit, paranasal sinuses, and chest.

Pathologic Staging. Complete resection of the primary site is indicated. Extensive local involvement of orbital spread requires exenteration. Histologic study of the margins of the deep aspect of resected tissues is necessary.

DEFINITION OF TNM

These definitions apply to both clinical and pathologic staging.

Primary Tumor (T)

- TX Primary tumor cannot be assessed
- T0 No evidence of primary tumor
- Tis Carcinoma *in situ*
- T1 Tumor 5 mm or less in greatest dimension
- T2 Tumor more than 5 mm in greatest dimension, without invasion of adjacent structures
- T3 Tumor invades adjacent structures, excluding the orbit
- T4 Tumor invades the orbit

Regional Lymph Nodes (N)

- NX Regional lymph nodes cannot be assessed
- N0 No regional lymph node metastasis
- N1 Regional lymph node metastasis

Distant Metastasis (M)

- MX Presence of distant metastasis cannot be assessed
- M0 No distant metastasis
- M1 Distant metastasis

STAGE GROUPING

No stage grouping is presently recommended.

DIFFERENCES BETWEEN THE 2ND AND 3RD EDITIONS

This classification is the same as that published in the second edition of the *Manual.*

HISTOPATHOLOGIC TYPE

This classification applies only to carcinoma of the conjunctiva.

HISTOPATHOLOGIC GRADE (G)

- GX Grade cannot be assessed
- G1 Well differentiated
- G2 Moderately well differentiated
- G3 Poorly differentiated
- G4 Undifferentiated

CARCINOMA OF THE CONJUNCTIVA

Data Form for Cancer Staging

Patient identification
Name _____
Address _____
Hospital or clinic number _____
Age _____ Sex _____ Race _____

Institution identification
Hospital or clinic _____
Address _____

Oncology Record

Anatomic site of cancer _____
Histologic type _____
Grade (G) _____
Date of classification _____

Chronology of classification
 (use separate form for each time staged)
[ ] Clinical (use all data prior to first treatment)
[ ] Pathologic (if definitively resected specimen available)

Definitions

Primary Tumor (T)

[ ] TX   Primary tumor cannot be assessed
[ ] T0   No evidence of primary tumor
[ ] Tis Tumor in situ
[ ] T1   Tumor 5 mm or less in greatest dimension
[ ] T2   Tumor more than 5 mm in greatest dimension, without invasion of adjacent structures
[ ] T3   Tumor invades adjacent structures, excluding the orbit
[ ] T4   Tumor invades the orbit

Lymph Node (N)

[ ] NX   Regional lymph nodes cannot be assessed
[ ] N0   No regional lymph node metastasis
[ ] N1   Regional lymph node metastasis

Distant Metastasis (M)

[ ] MX   Presence of distant metastasis cannot be assessed
[ ] M0   No distant metastasis
[ ] M1   Distant metastasis

Stage Grouping

No stage grouping is presently recommended.

Histopathologic Grade (G)

[ ] GX   Grade cannot be assessed
[ ] G1   Well differentiated
[ ] G2   Moderately well differentiated
[ ] G3   Poorly differentiated
[ ] G4   Undifferentiated

Illustration

Indicate on diagram and describe exact location and characteristics of tumor.

Sites of Distant Metastasis

Pulmonary   PUL
Osseous   OSS
Hepatic   HEP
Brain   BRA
Lymph nodes LYM
Bone marrow MAR
Pleura   PLE
Peritoneum   PER
Skin   SKI
Other   OTH

Staged by _____ M.D.
_____ Registrar
Date _____

39

Melanoma of the Conjunctiva

ANATOMY

Primary Site (ICD-O 190.3). In addition to mucus-secreting goblet cells within the stratified epithelium, melanocytic cells exist in the basal layer. These are of neuroectodermal origin, and melanocytic tumors may arise from these cells. Melanomas may arise from junctional and compound nevi, from primary acquired melanosis, or de novo. Tumors must be distinguished from nontumorous pigmentation.

Regional Lymph Nodes. The regional lymph nodes are the preauricular, submandibular, and cervical nodes.

Metastatic Sites. In addition to spread by lymphatics and the bloodstream, direct extension to the eyeball and orbit occur.

RULES FOR CLASSIFICATION

The classification applies only to melanoma. There should be histologic verification of the melanocytic lesion.

Clinical Staging. The assessment of the cancer is based on inspection, slit-lamp examination, palpation of the regional lymph nodes, and, when indicated, radiologic (including computed tomography [CT]) and ultrasonographic examination of the orbit, paranasal sinuses, and chest.

Pathologic Staging. Complete resection of the primary site is indicated. Histologic study of the margins and the deep aspect of resected tissues is necessary. Resection or needle biopsy of enlarged regional lymph nodes or orbital masses is desirable.

DEFINITION OF TNM

Clinical Classification

Primary Tumor (T)

TX   Primary tumor cannot be assessed
T0   No evidence of primary tumor
T1   Tumor(s) of bulbar conjunctiva occupying one quadrant or less
T2   Tumor(s) of bulbar conjunctiva occupying more than one quadrant
T3   Tumor(s) of conjunctival fornix and/or palpebral conjunctiva and/or caruncle
T4   Tumor invades eyelid, cornea, and/or orbit

Regional Lymph Nodes (N)

NX   Regional lymph nodes cannot be assessed
N0   No regional lymph node metastasis
N1   Regional lymph node metastasis

Distant Metastasis (M)

MX   Presence of distant metastasis cannot be assessed
M0   No distant metastasis
M1   Distant metastasis

Pathologic Classification (pTNM)

Primary Tumor (pT)

pTX   Primary tumor cannot be assessed
pT0   No evidence of primary tumor
pT1   Tumor(s) of bulbar conjunctiva occupying one quadrant or less and 2 mm or less in thickness
pT2   Tumor(s) of bulbar conjunctiva occupying more than one quadrant and 2 mm or less in thickness
pT3   Tumor(s) of the conjunctival fornix and/or palpebral conjunctiva and/or caruncle or tumor(s) of the bulbar conjunctiva, more than 2 mm in thickness
pT4   Tumor invades eyelid, cornea, and/or orbit

Regional Lymph Nodes (pN)

pNX   Regional lymph nodes cannot be assessed
pN0   No regional lymph node metastasis
pN1   Regional lymph node metastasis

Distant Metastasis (pM)

pMX   Presence of distant metastasis cannot be assessed
pM0   No distant metastasis
pM1   Distant metastasis

STAGE GROUPING

No stage grouping is presently recommended.

DIFFERENCES BETWEEN THE 2ND AND 3RD EDITIONS

This classification is the same as that published in the second edition of the *Manual.*

HISTOPATHOLOGIC TYPE

This categorization applies only to melanoma of the conjunctiva.

HISTOPATHOLOGIC GRADE (G)

Histopathologic grade represents the origin of the primary tumor.

GX   Origin cannot be assessed
G0   Primary acquired melanosis
G1   Malignant melanoma arises from a nevus
G2   Malignant melanoma(s) arises from primary acquired melanosis
G3   Malignant melanoma(s) arises de novo

BIBLIOGRAPHY

1. Liesegang TJ, Campbell RJ: Mayo Clinic experience with conjunctival melanomas. Arch Ophthalmol 98: 1385–1389, 1980
2. Silvers DN, Jakobiec FA, Freeman TR et al: Melanoma of the conjunctiva: A clinicopathologic study. In Jakobiec FA (ed): Ocular and Adnexal Tumors. Birmingham, Aesculapius, 1978
3. Zimmerman LE: The histogenesis of conjunctival melanomas., The First Algernon B. Reese Lecture. In Jakobiec FA (ed): Ocular and Adnexal Tumors. Birmingham, Aesculapius, 1978

MELANOMA OF THE CONJUNCTIVA

Data Form for Cancer Staging

Patient identification
Name _____
Address _____
Hospital or clinic number _____
Age _____ Sex _____ Race _____

Institution identification
Hospital or clinic _____
Address _____

Oncology Record

Anatomic site of cancer _____
Histologic type _____
Grade (G) _____
Date of classification _____

Chronology of classification
(use separate form for each time staged)
[ ] Clinical (use all data prior to first treatment)
[ ] Pathologic (if definitively resected specimen available)

Definitions

Primary Tumor (T)

[ ] TX   Primary tumor cannot be assessed
[ ] T0   No evidence of primary tumor
[ ] T1   Tumor(s) of bulbar conjunctiva occupying one quadrant or less
[ ] T2   Tumor(s) of bulbar conjunctiva occupying more than one quadrant
[ ] T3   Tumor(s) of conjunctival fornix and/or palpebral conjunctiva and/or caruncle
[ ] T4   Tumor invades eyelid, cornea, and/or orbit

Lymph Node (N)

[ ] NX   Regional lymph nodes cannot be assessed
[ ] N0   No regional lymph node metastasis
[ ] N1   Regional lymph node metastasis

Distant Metastasis (M)

[ ] MX   Presence of distant metastasis cannot be assessed
[ ] M0   No distant metastasis
[ ] M1   Distant metastasis

Primary Tumor (pT)

[ ] pTX   Primary tumor cannot be assessed
[ ] pT0   No evidence of primary tumor
[ ] pT1   Tumor(s) of bulbar conjunctiva occupying one quadrant or less and 2 mm or less in thickness
[ ] pT2   Tumor(s) of bulbar conjunctiva occupying more than one quadrant and 2 mm or less in thickness
[ ] pT3   Tumor(s) of conjunctival fornix or palpebral conjunctiva and/or caruncle and/or tumor of the bulbar conjunctiva, more than 2 mm in thickness
[ ] pT4   Tumor invades eyelid, cornea, and/or orbit

Lymph Node (pN)

[ ] pNX   Regional lymph nodes cannot be assessed
[ ] pN0   No regional lymph node metastasis
[ ] pN1   Regional lymph node metastasis

Distant Metastasis (pM)

[ ] pMX   Presence of distant metastasis cannot be assessed
[ ] pM0   No distant metastasis
[ ] pM1   Distant metastasis

Stage Grouping

No stage grouping is presently recommended.

Illustration

Indicate on diagram and describe exact location and characteristics of tumor.

Histopathologic Grade (G)

[ ] GX   Grade cannot be assessed
[ ] G0   Primary acquired melanosis
[ ] G1   Malignant melanoma arising in a nevus
[ ] G2   Malignant melanoma(s) arising from primary acquired melanosis
[ ] G3   Malignant melanoma(s) arising de novo

Sites of Distant Metastasis

Pulmonary   PUL
Osseous   OSS
Hepatic   HEP
Brain   BRA
Lymph nodes   LYM
Bone marrow   MAR
Pleura   PLE
Peritoneum   PER
Skin   SKI
Other   OTH

Staged by _____ M.D.
_____ Registrar
Date _____

40

Melanoma of the Uvea

The classification applies only to melanoma (ICD-O: M. 8720/3).

ANATOMY

Primary Site. The uvea (uveal tract) (ICD-O 190.0, 190.6) is the middle layer of the eyeball, situated between the cornea and sclera externally and the retina and its analogues internally. The uveal tract is divided into three regions: iris, ciliary body, and choroid. It is a highly vascular structure, with the choroid in particular being composed of large blood vessels with little intervening connective tissue. There are no lymphatic channels in the uvea. Systemic metastasis from uveal melanomas occurs by hematogenous routes. Uveal melanomas are believed to arise from uveal melanocytes and are, therefore, of neural crest origin. Melanomas may spread by local extension through Bruch's membrane to involve the retina and vitreous, or by extension through the sclera or optic nerve into the orbit.

Most uveal melanomas occur in the choroid. The ciliary body is less commonly the site of origin, and the iris is least commonly involved. Iris melanomas are relatively benign and slow growing, and they rarely metastasize. Melanomas of the ciliary body and choroid are cytologically more malignant and metastasize more frequently.

Regional Lymph Nodes. Since there are no intraocular lymphatics, this category applies only to extrascleral extension anteriorly. The regional lymph nodes are the preauricular, submandibular, and cervical nodes; involvement implies subconjunctival extension of the primary tumor.

Metastatic Sites. Uveal melanomas can metastasize through hematogenous routes to various organs. The liver is most commonly involved and is usually the first site of clinically detectable metastasis. Less commonly, the lung, pleura, subcutaneous tissues, bone, and other sites may be involved.

RULES FOR CLASSIFICATION

There should be histologic verification of the disease. Any unconfirmed case must be reported separately.

Clinical Staging. The assessment of the tumor is based on clinical examination including slit-lamp examination and direct and indirect ophthalmoscopy. Additional methods such as fluorescein angiography and isotope examination may enhance the accuracy of appraisal.

Pathologic Staging. Complete resection of the primary site is indicated. Histologic study of the margins and the deep aspect of resected tissues is necessary. Resection or needle biopsy of enlarged regional lymph nodes or orbital masses is desirable.

DEFINITION OF TNM

These definitions apply to both clinical and pathologic staging.

ANATOMIC SITES

Iris
Ciliary body
Choroid

Iris
Primary Tumor (T)

- TX Primary tumor cannot be assessed
- T0 No evidence of primary tumor
- T1 Tumor limited to the iris
- T2 Tumor involves one quadrant or less, with invasion into the anterior chamber angle
- T3 Tumor involves more than one quadrant, with invasion into the anterior chamber angle
- T4 Tumor with extraocular extension

Regional Lymph Nodes (N)

- NX Regional lymph nodes cannot be assessed
- N0 No regional lymph node metastasis
- N1 Regional lymph node metastasis

Distant Metastasis (M)

- MX Presence of distant metastasis cannot be assessed
- M0 No distant metastasis
- M1 Distant metastasis

Ciliary Body
Primary Tumor (T)

- TX Primary tumor cannot be assessed
- T0 No evidence of primary tumor
- T1 Tumor limited to the ciliary body
- T2 Tumor invades into anterior chamber and/or iris
- T3 Tumor invades choroid
- T4 Tumor with extraocular extension

Regional Lymph Nodes (N)

- NX Regional lymph nodes cannot be assessed
- N0 No regional lymph node metastasis
- N1 Regional lymph node metastasis

Distant Metastasis (M)

- MX Presence of distant metastasis cannot be assessed
- M0 No distant metastasis
- M1 Distant metastasis

Choroid
Primary Tumor (T)

- TX Primary tumor cannot be assessed
- T0 No evidence of primary tumor
- T1*† Tumor 10 mm or less in greatest dimension with an elevation 3 mm or less
  - T1a Tumor 7 mm or less in greatest dimension with an elevation 2 mm or less
  - T1b Tumor more than 7 mm but not more than 10 mm in greatest dimension with an elevation more than 2 mm but not more than 3 mm
- T2* Tumor more than 10 mm but not more than 15 mm in greatest dimension with an elevation of more than 3 mm but not more than 5 mm
- T3* Tumor more than 15 mm in greatest dimension or with an elevation more than 5 mm
- T4 Tumor with extraocular extension

Note: When dimension and elevation show a difference in classification, the highest category should be used for classification.

*Note: In clinical practice the tumor base may be estimated in optic disc diameters (dd) (average: 1 dd = 1.5 mm). The elevation may be estimated in diopters (average: 3 diopters = 1 mm). Other techniques used, such as ultrasonography and computerized stereometry, may provide a more accurate measurement.
†Note: It may be impossible to distinguish a large nevus from a small melanoma.

Melanoma of the Uvea

Regional Lymph Nodes (N)

NX Regional lymph nodes cannot be assessed
N0 No regional lymph node metastasis
N1 Regional lymph node metastasis

Distant Metastasis (M)

MX Presence of distant metastasis cannot be assessed
M0 No distant metastasis
M1 Distant metastasis

STAGE GROUPING

The classification of the structure most affected is used when more than one of the uveal structures is involved by tumor.

Iris and Ciliary Body

Stage	T	N	M
Stage I	T1	N0	M0
Stage II	T2	N0	M0
Stage III	T3	N0	M0
Stage IVA	T4	N0	M0
Stage IVB	Any T	N1	M0
	Any T	Any N	M1

Choroid

Stage	T	N	M
Stage IA	T1a	N0	M0
Stage IB	T1b	N0	M0
Stage II	T2	N0	M0
Stage III	T3	N0	M0
Stage IVA	T4	N0	M0
Stage IVB	Any T	N1	M0
	Any T	Any N	M1

DIFFERENCES BETWEEN THE 2ND AND 3RD EDITIONS

This classification is the same as that published in the second edition of the *Manual.*

HISTOPATHOLOGIC TYPE

The histopathologic types are:

Spindle cell melanoma
Mixed cell melanoma
Epithelioid cell melanoma

HISTOPATHOLOGIC GRADE (G)

GX Grade cannot be assessed
G1 Spindle cell melanoma
G2 Mixed cell melanoma
G3 Epithelioid cell melanoma

Venous Invasion (V)

VX Venous invasion cannot be assessed
V0 Veins do not contain tumor
V1 Veins in melanoma contain tumor
V2 Vortex veins contain tumor

Scleral Invasion (S)

SX Scleral invasion cannot be assessed
S0 Sclera does not contain tumor
S1 Intrascleral* invasion of tumor
S2 Extrascleral extension of tumor

Note: Includes perineural and perivascular invasion of scleral canals.

MELANOMA OF THE UVEA

Data Form for Cancer Staging

Patient identification
Name _____
Address _____
Hospital or clinic number _____
Age _____ Sex _____ Race _____

Institution identification
Hospital or clinic _____
Address _____

Oncology Record

Anatomic site of cancer _____
Histologic type _____
Grade (G) _____
Date of classification _____

Chronology of classification
(use separate form for each time staged)
[ ] Clinical (use all data prior to first treatment)
[ ] Pathologic (if definitively resected specimen available)

Definitions

Iris

Primary Tumor (T)

[ ] TX   Primary tumor cannot be assessed
[ ] T0   No evidence of primary tumor
[ ] T1   Tumor limited to the iris
[ ] T2   Tumor involves one quadrant or less, with invasion into the anterior chamber angle
[ ] T3   Tumor involves more than one quadrant, with invasion into the anterior chamber angle
[ ] T4   Tumor with extraocular extension

Lymph Node (N)

[ ] NX   Regional lymph nodes cannot be assessed
[ ] N0   No regional lymph node metastasis
[ ] N1   Regional lymph node metastasis

Distant Metastasis (M)

[ ] MX   Presence of distant metastasis cannot be assessed
[ ] M0   No distant metastasis
[ ] M1   Distant metastasis

Ciliary Body

Primary Tumor (T)

[ ] TX   Primary tumor cannot be assessed
[ ] T0   No evidence of primary tumor
[ ] T1   Tumor limited to ciliary body
[ ] T2   Tumor invades into anterior chamber and/or iris
[ ] T3   Tumor invades choroid
[ ] T4   Tumor with extraocular extension

Lymph Node (N)

[ ] NX   Regional lymph nodes cannot be assessed
[ ] N0   No regional lymph node metastasis
[ ] N1   Regional lymph node metastasis

Distant Metastasis (M)

[ ] MX   Presence of distant metastasis cannot be assessed
[ ] M0   No distant metastasis
[ ] M1   Distant metastasis

Choroid

Primary Tumor (T)

[ ] TX   Primary tumor cannot be assessed
[ ] T0   No evidence of primary tumor
[ ] T1   Tumor 10 mm or less in greatest dimension with an elevation 3 mm or less
[ ] T1a Tumor 7 mm or less in greatest dimension with an elevation 2 mm or less
[ ] T1b Tumor more than 7 mm but not more than 10 mm in greatest dimension with an elevation more than 2 mm but not more than 3 mm
[ ] T2   Tumor more than 10 mm but not more than 15 mm in greatest dimension with an elevation of more than 3 mm but not more than 5 mm
[ ] T3   Tumor more than 15 mm in greatest dimension or with an elevation more than 5 mm
[ ] T4   Tumor with extraocular extension

Lymph Node (N)

[ ] NX   Regional lymph nodes cannot be assessed
[ ] N0   No regional lymph node metastasis
[ ] N1   Regional lymph node metastasis

Distant Metastasis (M)

[ ] MX   Presence of distant metastasis cannot be assessed
[ ] M0   No distant metastasis
[ ] M1   Distant metastasis

Stage Grouping

Iris and Ciliary Body

[ ]	I	T1	N0	M0
[ ]	II	T2	N0	M0
[ ]	III	T3	N0	M0
[ ]	IVA	T4	N0	M0
[ ]	IVB	Any T	N1	M0
		Any T	Any N	M1

Choroid

[ ]	IA	T1a	N0	M0
[ ]	IB	T1b	N0	M0
[ ]	II	T2	N0	M0
[ ]	III	T3	N0	M0
[ ]	IVA	T4	N0	M0
[ ]	IVB	Any T	N1	M0
		Any T	Any N	M1

Staged by _____ M.D.
_____ Registrar
Date _____

American Joint Committee on Cancer—1988

Illustrations

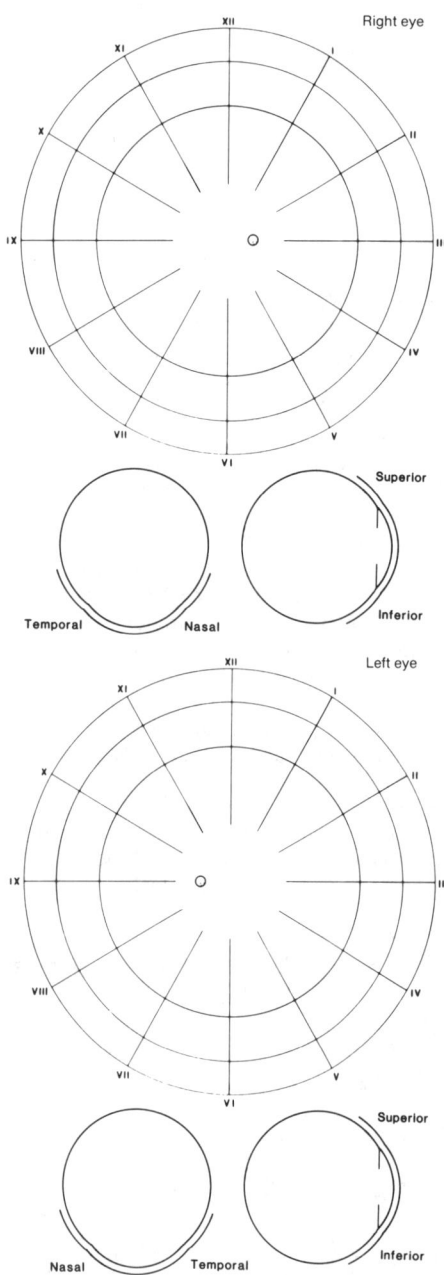

Indicate on diagrams and describe exact location and characteristics of tumor.

Histopathologic Type

Spindle cell melanoma
Mixed cell melanoma
Epithelioid cell melanoma

Histopathologic Grade (G)

[ ] GX Grade cannot be assessed
[ ] G0 Primary acquired melanosis
[ ] G1 Malignant melanoma arising in a nevus
[ ] G2 Malignant melanoma arising from primary acquired melanosis
[ ] G3 Malignant melanoma arising de novo

Sites of Distant Metastasis

Pulmonary   PUL
Osseous   OSS
Hepatic   HEP
Brain   BRA
Lymph nodes   LYM
Bone marrow   MAR
Pleura   PLE
Peritoneum   PER
Skin   SKI
Other   OTH

41

Retinoblastoma

ANATOMY

Primary Site. The retina (ICD-O 190.5) is composed of neurons and glial cells. The neurons give rise to retinoblastoma, whereas the glial cells give rise to astrocytomas, which in the retina are benign and extremely rare. The retina is limited internally by a membrane that separates it from the vitreous cavity. Externally it is limited by the retinal pigment epithelium and Bruch's membrane, which separate it from the choroid and act as natural barriers to extension of retinal tumors into the choroid. The continuation of the retina with the optic nerve allows direct extension of retinoblastomas into the optic nerve and then to the subarachnoid space. Since the retina has no lymphatics, spread of retinal tumors is either by direct extension into adjacent structures or by distant metastasis through hematogenous routes.

Regional Lymph Nodes. Since there are no intraocular lymphatics, the category applies only to anterior extrascleral extension. The regional lymph nodes are the preauricular, submandibular, and cervical nodes; involvement implies subconjunctival extension of the tumor.

Metastatic Sites. Retinoblastoma can metastasize through hematogenous routes to various sites, most notably the skull, long bones, brain, lymph nodes, and viscera.

RULES FOR CLASSIFICATION

Clinical Staging. Each eye must be classified separately. The classification does not apply to complete spontaneous regression of the tumor. There should be histologic verification of the disease in an enucleated eye. Any unconfirmed case must be reported separately. The extent of retinal involvement is indicated as a percentage. In bilateral cases, the extent of involvement of the more affected eye determines the T category.

Pathologic Staging. All clinical and pathologic data from the resected specimen are to be used.

DEFINITION OF TNM

Clinical Classification (cTNM)
Primary Tumor (T)

- TX Primary tumor cannot be assessed
- T0 No evidence of primary tumor
- T1 Tumor(s) limited to 25% or less of the retina
- T2 Tumor(s) involve(s) more than 25% but not more than 50% of the retina
- T3 Tumor(s) involve(s) more than 50% of the retina and/or invade(s) beyond the retina but remain(s) intraocular
  - T3a Tumor(s) involve(s) more than 50% of the retina and/or tumor cells in the vitreous
  - T3b Tumor(s) involve(s) optic disc
  - T3c Tumor(s) involve(s) anterior chamber and/or uvea
- T4 Tumor with extraocular invasion
  - T4a Tumor invades retrobulbar optic nerve
  - T4b Extraocular extension other than invasion of optic nerve

Note: The following suffixes may be added to the appropriate T categories: "m" indicates multiple tumors (e.g., T2 [m2]); "f" indicates cases with a known family history; and "d" indicates diffuse retinal involvement without the formation of discrete masses.

Regional Lymph Nodes (N)

- NX Regional lymph nodes cannot be assessed
- N0 No regional lymph node metastasis
- N1 Regional lymph node metastasis

Distant Metastasis (M)

- MX Presence of distant metastasis cannot be assessed
- M0 No distant metastasis
- M1 Distant metastasis

Pathologic Classification (pTNM)
Primary Tumor (pT)

- pTX Primary tumor cannot be assessed
- pT0 No evidence of primary tumor
- pT1 Tumor(s) limited to 25% or less of the retina
- pT2 Tumor(s) involve(s) more than 25% but not more than 50% of the retina
- pT3 Tumor(s) involve(s) more than 50% of the retina and/or invade(s) beyond the retina but remain(s) intraocular
  - pT3a Tumor(s) involve(s) more than 50% of the retina and/or tumor cells in the vitreous
  - pT3b Tumor invades optic nerve as far as the lamina cribrosa
  - pT3c Tumor in anterior chamber and/or invasion with thickening of the uvea and/or intrascleral invasion
- pT4 Tumor with extraocular invasion
  - pT4a Intraneural tumor beyond the lamina cribrosa but not at the line of resection
  - pT4b Tumor at the line of resection or other extraocular extension

Regional Lymph Nodes (pN)

- pNX Regional lymph nodes cannot be assessed
- pN0 No regional lymph node metastasis
- pN1 Regional lymph node metastasis

Distant Metastasis (pM)

- pMX Presence of distant metastasis cannot be assessed
- pM0 No distant metastasis
- pM1 Distant metastasis

STAGE GROUPING

In cases of bilateral disease the more affected eye is used for the stage grouping.

Stage	T	N	M
Stage IA	T1	N0	M0
Stage IB	T2	N0	M0
Stage IIA	T3a	N0	M0
Stage IIB	T3b	N0	M0
Stage IIC	T3c	N0	M0
Stage IIIA	T4a	N0	M0
Stage IIIB	T4b	N0	M0
Stage IV	Any T	N1	M0
	Any T	Any N	M1

Note: Pathologic stage grouping corresponds to the clinical stage grouping.

DIFFERENCES BETWEEN THE 2ND AND 3RD EDITIONS

Note minor difference in grading of Stage IV in this edition of the *Manual.*

HISTOPATHOLOGIC TYPE

This classification applies only to retinoblastoma.

HISTOPATHOLOGIC GRADE (G)

For the purpose of TNM, grading is not considered appropriate at present.

RETINOBLASTOMA

Data Form for Cancer Staging

Patient identification
Name _____
Address _____
Hospital or clinic number _____
Age _____ Sex _____ Race _____

Institution identification
Hospital or clinic _____
Address _____

Oncology Record

Anatomic site of cancer _____
Histologic type _____
Grade (G) _____
Date of classification _____

Chronology of classification
(use separate form for each time staged)
[ ] Clinical (use all data prior to first treatment)
[ ] Pathologic (if definitively resected specimen available)

Definitions

Primary Tumor (T)
[ ] TX   Primary tumor cannot be assessed
[ ] T0   No evidence of primary tumor
[ ] T1   Tumor(s) limited to 25% or less of the retina
[ ] T2   Tumor(s) involve(s) more than 25% but not more than 50% of the retina
[ ] T3   Tumor(s) involve(s) more than 50% of the retina and/or invade(s) beyond the retina but remain(s) intraocular
  [ ] T3a   Tumor(s) involve(s) more than 50% of the retina and/or tumor cells in the vitreous
  [ ] T3b   Tumor(s) involve(s) optic disc
  [ ] T3c   Tumor(s) involve(s) anterior chamber and/or uvea
[ ] T4   Tumor with extraocular invasion
  [ ] T4a   Tumor invades retrobulbar optic nerve
  [ ] T4b   Extraocular extension other than invasion of optic nerve

Lymph Node (N)
[ ] NX   Regional lymph nodes cannot be assessed
[ ] N0   No regional lymph node metastasis
[ ] N1   Regional lymph node metastasis

Distant Metastasis (M)
[ ] MX   Presence of distant metastasis cannot be assessed
[ ] M0   No distant metastasis
[ ] M1   Distant metastasis

Primary Tumor (pT)
[ ] pTX   Primary tumor cannot be assessed
[ ] pT0   No evidence of primary tumor
[ ] pT1   Tumor(s) limited to 25% or less of the retina
[ ] pT2   Tumor(s) involve(s) more than 25% but not more than 50% of the retina
[ ] pT3   Tumor(s) involve(s) more than 50% of the retina and/or invade(s) beyond the retina but remain(s) intraocular
  [ ] pT3a   Tumor(s) involve(s) more than 50% of the retina and/or tumor cells in the vitreous
  [ ] pT3b   Tumor invades optic nerve as far as the lamina cribrosa
  [ ] pT3c   Tumor in anterior chamber and/or invasion with thickening of the uvea and/or intrascleral invasion
[ ] pT4   Tumor with extraocular invasion
  [ ] pT4a   Intraneural tumor beyond the lamina cribrosa but not at the line of resection
  [ ] pT4b   Tumor at the line of resection or other extraocular extension

Lymph Node (pN)
[ ] pNX   Regional lymph nodes cannot be assessed
[ ] pN0   No regional lymph node metastasis
[ ] pN1   Regional lymph node metastasis

Distant Metastasis (pM)
[ ] pMX   Presence of distant metastasis cannot be assessed
[ ] pM0   No distant metastasis
[ ] pM1   Distant metastasis

Stage Grouping

[ ] IA	T1	N0	M0
[ ] IB	T2	N0	M0
[ ] IIA	T3a	N0	M0
[ ] IIB	T3b	N0	M0
[ ] IIC	T3c	N0	M0
[ ] IIIA	T4a	N0	M0
[ ] IIIB	T4b	N0	M0
[ ] IV	Any T	N1	M0
	Any T	Any N	M1

Histopathologic Type

This classification applies only to retinoblastoma.

Sites of Distant Metastasis

Pulmonary	PUL
Osseous	OSS
Hepatic	HEP
Brain	BRA
Lymph nodes	LYM
Bone marrow	MAR
Pleura	PLE
Peritoneum	PER
Skin	SKI
Other	OTH

Staged by _____ M.D.
_____ Registrar
Date _____

Illustrations

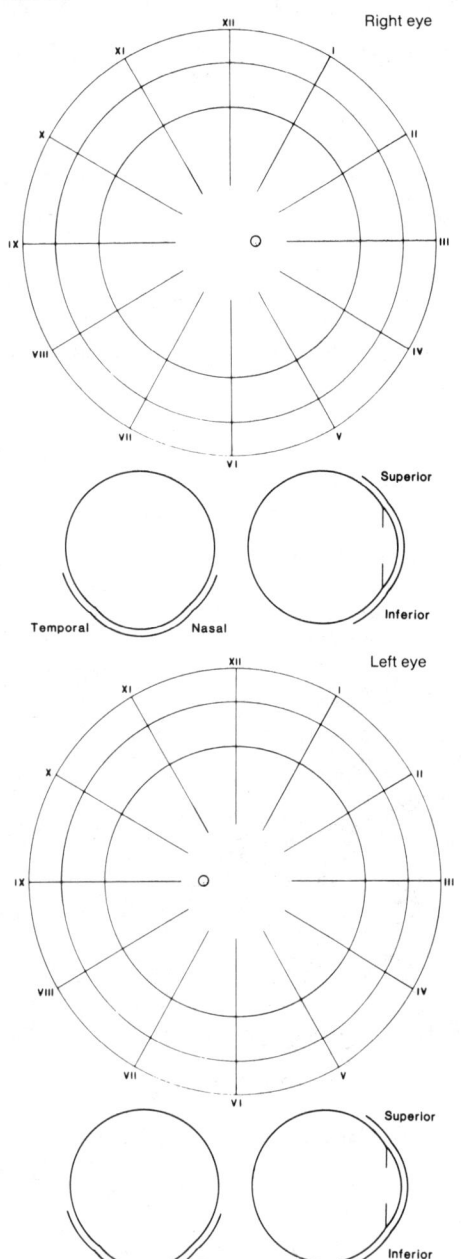

Indicate on diagrams and describe exact location and characteristics of tumor.

_____
_____
_____
_____

42 Sarcoma of the Orbit

Sarcomas of the orbit include a broad spectrum of soft-tissue tumors and sarcomas of bone.

ANATOMY

Primary Site. Sarcoma of the orbit (ICD-O 190.1) occurs in the soft tissues and bone of the orbital fossa.

Regional Lymph Nodes. Anterior spread of the tumor to involve the eyelids and conjunctiva may gain access to the lymphatic circulation.

Metastatic Sites. Metastatic spread occurs by way of the bloodstream to distant sites.

RULES FOR CLASSIFICATION

Clinical Classification. Clinical classification is based on symptoms and signs relating to visual loss, degree of proptosis or displacement, papilledema, and optic atrophy. Diagnostic tests include radiographs of the orbit, computed tomography (CT), and angiography.

Pathologic Classification. Pathologic classification is based on the histopathology of the tumor, its grade, and the extent of removal.

DEFINITION OF TNM

Primary Tumor (T)

TX Primary tumor cannot be assessed
T0 No evidence of primary tumor
T1 Tumor 15 mm or less in greatest dimension
T2 Tumor more than 15 mm in greatest dimension
T3 Tumor of any size with diffuse invasion of orbital tissues and/or bony walls
T4 Tumor invades beyond the orbit to adjacent sinuses and/or to cranium

Regional Lymph Nodes (N)

NX Regional lymph nodes cannot be assessed
N0 No regional lymph node metastasis
N1 Regional lymph node metastasis

Distant Metastasis (M)

MX Presence of distant metastasis cannot be assessed
M0 No distant metastasis
M1 Distant metastasis

STAGE GROUPING

No stage grouping is presently recommended.

DIFFERENCES BETWEEN THE 2ND AND 3RD EDITIONS

This classification is the same as that published in the second edition of the *Manual.*

HISTOPATHOLOGIC TYPE

Sarcomas of the orbit include a broad spectrum of soft-tissue tumors and sarcomas of bone.

HISTOPATHOLOGIC GRADE (G)

GX Grade cannot be assessed
G1 Well differentiated
G2 Moderately well differentiated
G3 Poorly differentiated
G4 Undifferentiated

BIBLIOGRAPHY

1. Backwinkel KD, Diddams JA: Hemangiopericytoma: Report of a case and comprehensive review of the literature. Cancer 25:896, 1970
2. Croxatto JO, Font RL: Hemangiopericytoma of the orbit: A clinicopathologic study of 30 cases. Hum Pathol 13:210–218, 1982
3. Ellsworth RM: Rhabdomyosarcoma of the orbit. New Orleans, Academy of Ophthalmology Symposium on Surgery of the Orbit and Adnexa. St. Louis, CV Mosby, 1974
4. Enzinger FM, Lattes R, Torioni H: Histologic typing of soft tissue tumours. International Histological Classification of Tumours, No. 3. Geneva, World Health Organization, 1969
5. Font RL, Hidayat A: Fibrous histiocytoma of the orbit: A clinicopathologic study of 150 cases. Hum Pathol 13:199–209, 1982
6. Foos R: Fibrosarcoma of the orbit. Am J Ophthalmol 57:244, 1969
7. Guccion JG, Font RL, Enzinger FM et al: Extraskeletal mesenchymal chondrosarcoma. Arch Pathol 95:336–340, 1973
8. Henderson JW, Farrow GM: Primary orbital hemangiopericytoma: An aggressive and potentially malignant neoplasm. Arch Ophthalmol 96:666–673, 1978
9. Jaffe N, Filler RM, Farber S et al: Rhabdomyosarcoma in children: Improved outlook with a multidisciplinary approach. Am J Surg 125:482, 1973
10. Jones IS, Reese AB, Krout J: Orbital rhabdomyosarcoma: An analysis of sixty-two cases. Trans Am Ophthalmol Soc 63:223–255, 1965
11. Knowles DM, Jakobiec FA, Potter GD et al: Ophthalmic striated muscle neoplasms. Surv Ophthalmol 21:219–261, 1976
12. Porterfield JF, Zimmerman LE: Rhabdomyosarcoma of the orbit: A clinicopathologic study of 55 cases. Virchows Arch (Path Anat) 335:329–344, 1962
13. Russell WO, Cohen J, Enzinger F et al: A clinical and pathological staging system for soft tissue sarcomas. Cancer 40:1562–1570, 1977
14. Suit HD, Russell WO, Martin RG: Sarcoma of soft tissue: Clinical and histopathologic parameters and response to treatment. Cancer 35:1478–1483, 1975
15. Zimmerman LE, Sobin LH: Histological typing of tumours of the eye and its adnexa. International Histological Classification of Tumours, No. 24. Geneva, World Health Organization, 1981

SARCOMA OF THE ORBIT

Data Form for Cancer Staging

Patient identification
Name _____
Address _____
Hospital or clinic number _____
Age _____ Sex _____ Race _____

Institution identification
Hospital or clinic _____
Address _____

Oncology Record

Anatomic site of cancer _____
Histologic type _____
Grade (G) _____
Date of classification _____

Chronology of classification
(use separate form for each time staged)
[ ] Clinical (use all data prior to first treatment)
[ ] Pathologic (if definitively resected specimen available)

Definitions

Primary Tumor (T)
[ ] TX Primary tumor cannot be assessed
[ ] T0 No evidence of primary tumor
[ ] T1 Tumor 15 mm or less in greatest dimension
[ ] T2 Tumor more than 15 mm in greatest dimension
[ ] T3 Tumor of any size with diffuse invasion of orbital tissues and/or bony walls
[ ] T4 Tumor invades beyond the orbit to adjacent sinuses and/or to cranium

Lymph Node (N)
[ ] NX Regional lymph nodes cannot be assessed
[ ] N0 No regional lymph node metastasis
[ ] N1 Regional lymph node metastasis

Distant Metastasis (M)
[ ] MX Presence of distant metastasis cannot be assessed
[ ] M0 No distant metastasis
[ ] M1 Distant metastasis

Stage Grouping

No stage grouping is presently recommended.

Histopathologic Type

Sarcomas of the orbit include a broad spectrum of soft-tissue tumors and sarcomas of bone.

Histopathologic Grade (G)

[ ] GX Grade cannot be assessed
[ ] G1 Well differentiated
[ ] G2 Moderately well differentiated
[ ] G3 Poorly differentiated
[ ] G4 Undifferentiated

Illustration

Indicate on diagram and describe exact location and characteristics of tumor.

_____
_____
_____
_____
_____
_____

Sites of Distant Metastasis

Pulmonary   PUL
Osseous   OSS
Hepatic   HEP
Brain   BRA
Lymph nodes LYM
Bone marrow MAR
Pleura   PLE
Peritoneum   PER
Skin   SKI
Other   OTH

Staged by _____ M.D.
_____ Registrar
Date _____

43

Carcinoma of the Lacrimal Gland

A retrospective study of 265 epithelial tumors of the lacrimal gland has been completed from material on file in the Registry of Ophthalmic Pathology at the Armed Forces Institute of Pathology. The histologic classification used is a modification of the WHO classification of salivary gland tumors. The lacrimal gland includes both lobules: the superficial (palpebral lobe) portion and the deep intraorbital portion.

ANATOMY

Primary Site. The lacrimal gland (ICD-O 190.2) lies in a bony excavation that is covered by periosteum. It is located in the lateral orbital wall (the fossa of the lacrimal gland). The smaller palpebral portion projects into the lateral portion of the upper lid between the palpebral fascia and the conjunctiva.

Regional Lymph Nodes. The regional lymph nodes include the preauricular, submandibular, and cervical nodes.

Metastatic Sites. The lung is the most common metastatic site, followed by bone and remote viscera.

RULES FOR CLASSIFICATION

Clinical Staging. A complete physical examination, x-ray films of the orbit, including computed tomography (CT) scans, ultrasonograms, and plain films, and tomograms of the adjacent paranasal sinuses should be carried out. Chest x-ray films, radionuclide bone scans, and blood chemistries (SMA-12) should also be available.

Pathologic Staging. After complete resection of the mass, the entire specimen should be evaluated to determine the type of tumor and the grade of malignancy.

DEFINITION OF TNM

This classification applies to both clinical and pathologic staging.

Primary Tumor (T)

- TX Primary tumor cannot be assessed
- T0 No evidence of primary tumor
- T1 Tumor 2.5 cm or less in greatest dimension limited to the lacrimal gland and mobile within the lacrimal fossa
- T2 Tumor 2.5 cm or less in greatest dimension invading the periosteum of the fossa of the lacrimal gland
- T3 Tumor more than 2.5 cm but not more than 5 cm in greatest dimension
  - T3a Tumor limited to the lacrimal gland and mobile within the fossa
  - T3b Tumor invades the periosteum of the fossa of the lacrimal gland
- T4 Tumor more than 5 cm in greatest dimension
  - T4a Tumor invades the orbital soft tissues, optic nerve, or globe *without* bone invasion
  - T4b Tumor invades the orbital soft tissues, optic nerve, or globe *with* bone invasion

Regional Lymph Nodes (N)

- NX Regional lymph nodes cannot be assessed
- N0 No regional lymph node metastasis
- N1 Regional lymph node metastasis

Distant Metastasis (M)

- MX Presence of distant metastasis cannot be assessed
- M0 No distant metastasis
- M1 Distant metastasis

STAGE GROUPING

No stage grouping is presently recommended.

DIFFERENCES BETWEEN THE 2ND AND 3RD EDITIONS

This classification is the same as that published in the second edition of the *Manual.*

HISTOPATHOLOGIC TYPE

The major malignant primary epithelial tumors include the following:

Carcinoma in pleomorphic adenoma (malignant mixed tumor), which includes adenocarcinoma and adenoid cystic carcinoma arising in benign mixed tumor (BMT)

Adenoid cystic carcinoma (cylindroma), arising de novo

Adenocarcinoma, arising de novo

Mucoepidermoid carcinoma

Squamous cell carcinoma

HISTOPATHOLOGIC GRADE (G)

- GX Grade cannot be assessed
- G1 Well differentiated
- G2 Moderately well differentiated: Includes adenoid cystic carcinoma without baseloid (solid) pattern
- G3 Poorly differentiated: Includes adenoid cystic carcinoma with baseloid (solid) pattern
- G4 Undifferentiated

BIBLIOGRAPHY

1. Font RL, Gamel JW: Epithelial tumors of the lacrimal gland: An analysis of 265 cases. In Jakobiec FA (ed): Ocular and Adnexal Tumors, pp 787–805. Birmingham, Aesculapius, 1978
2. Font RL, Gamel JW: Adenoid cystic carcinoma of the lacrimal gland: A clinicopathologic study of 79 cases. In Nicholson D (ed): Ocular Pathology Update, pp 277–283. New York, Masson, 1980
3. Foote FW Jr, Frazell EL: Tumors of the major salivary glands. Atlas of Tumor Pathology, Sect. IV, Fasc. 11. Washington, Armed Forces Institute of Pathology, 1954
4. Forrest A: Pathologic criteria for effective management of epithelial lacrimal gland tumors. Am J Ophthalmol (Suppl) 71:178, 1971
5. Forrest AW: Epithelial lacrimal gland tumors: Pathology as a guide to prognosis. Trans Am Acad Ophthalmol Otolaryngol 58:848, 1954
6. Thackray AC, Sobin LH: Histological typing of salivary gland tumours. International Histological Classification of Tumours, Vol. 7. Geneva, World Health Organization, 1972
7. Zimmerman LE, Sanders TE, Ackerman LV: Epithelial tumors of the lacrimal gland: Prognostic and therapeutic significance of histologic types. In Zimmerman LE (ed): Tumors of the Eye and Adnexa, Vol. 2, No. 2, p 337. International Ophthalmology Clinics. Boston, Little, Brown & Co, 1962

LACRIMAL GLAND

Data Form for Cancer Staging

Patient identification
Name _____
Address _____
Hospital or clinic number _____
Age _____ Sex _____ Race _____

Institution identification
Hospital or clinic _____
Address _____

Oncology Record

Anatomic site of cancer _____
Histologic type _____
Grade (G) _____
Date of classification _____

Chronology of classification
(use separate form for each time staged)
[ ] Clinical (use all data prior to first treatment)
[ ] Pathologic (if definitively resected specimen available)

Definitions

Primary Tumor (T)

[ ] TX   Primary tumor cannot be assessed
[ ] T0   No evidence of primary tumor
[ ] T1   Tumor 2.5 cm or less in greatest dimension limited to the lacrimal gland
[ ] T2   Tumor 2.5 cm or less in greatest dimension invading the periosteum of the fossa of the lacrimal gland
[ ] T3   Tumor more than 2.5 cm but not more than 5 cm in greatest dimension
  [ ] T3a   Tumor limited to the lacrimal gland and mobile within the fossa
  [ ] T3b   Tumor invades the periosteum of the fossa of the lacrimal gland
[ ] T4   Tumor more than 5 cm in greatest dimension
  [ ] T4a   With invasion of orbital soft tissues, optic nerve, or globe, *without* bone invasion
  [ ] T4b   With invasion of the orbital soft tissues, optic nerve, or globe, *with* bone invasion

Lymph Node (N)

[ ] NX   Regional lymph nodes cannot be assessed
[ ] N0   No regional lymph node metastasis
[ ] N1   Regional lymph node metastasis

Distant Metastasis (M)

[ ] MX   Presence of distant metastasis cannot be assessed
[ ] M0   No distant metastasis
[ ] M1   Distant metastasis

Stage Grouping

No stage grouping is presently recommended.

Histopathologic Type

The major malignant primary epithelial tumors include the following:

Carcinoma in pleomorphic adenoma (malignant mixed tumor), which includes adenocarcinoma and adenoid cystic carcinoma arising in benign mixed tumor (BMT)
Adenoid cystic carcinoma (cylindroma) arising de novo
Adenocarcinoma (arising de novo)
Mucoepidermoid carcinoma
Squamous cell carcinoma

Illustration

Indicate on diagram and describe exact location and characteristics of tumor.

_____
_____

Histopathologic Grade (G)

[ ] GX   Grade cannot be assessed
[ ] G1   Well differentiated
[ ] G2   Moderately well differentiated: includes adenoid cystic carcinoma without baseloid (solid) pattern
[ ] G3   Poorly differentiated: includes adenoid cystic carcinoma with baseloid (solid) pattern
[ ] G4   Undifferentiated

Staged by _____ M.D.
_____ Registrar
Date _____

Sites of Distant Metastasis

Pulmonary	PUL
Osseous	OSS
Hepatic	HEP
Brain	BRA
Lymph nodes	LYM
Bone marrow	MAR
Pleura	PLE
Peritoneum	PER
Skin	SKI
Other	OTH

BRAIN

44

The most critical feature in the classification of brain tumors is histopathology. Accurate pathologic criteria and classification are essential to an understanding of the clinical and biologic behavior of the gliomas in particular, and most other tumors as well. The anatomic location and extent of tumors within the brain are also of clinical and prognostic significance. Neuroradiologic-diagnostic procedures have become increasingly more accurate and reliable in providing topographic and morphologic information on tumors of the brain and are useful at various points in diagnosis and management.

ANATOMY

Primary Site. A variety of tissues within the brain (ICD-O 191) can give rise to neoplasms. These include astrocytes and other glial cells, meninges (ICD-O 192.1), blood vessels, pituitary and pineal cells, and neural elements proper. The major structural sites involved are the various lobes of the cerebral hemispheres; the midline structures, including midbrain, pons, and medulla; and the posterior fossa.

Regional Lymph Nodes. There are no lymphatic structures draining the brain.

Metastatic Sites. Certain brain tumors can seed into the subarachnoid space. Hematogenous spread is very uncommon but on rare occasions has occurred in bone and other sites.

RULES FOR CLASSIFICATION

Clinical Staging. This staging is based on neurologic symptoms and signs and neurologic diagnostic tests, including skull radiographs, electroencephalograms, isotopic brain scans, cerebral angiography, pneumoencephalography, and computed tomographic scanning. All diagnostic information available prior to first definitive treatment may be used.

Pathologic Staging. This staging is based on histopathology, grade, and microscopic evidence of completeness of removal of a resected tumor.

DEFINITION OF TNM
Primary Tumor (T)

TX Primary tumor cannot be assessed
T0 No evidence of primary tumor

Supratentorial Tumor

T1 Tumor 5 cm or less in greatest dimension; limited to one side
T2 Tumor more than 5 cm in greatest dimension; limited to one side
T3 Tumor invades or encroaches upon the ventricular system
T4 Tumor crosses the midline, invades the opposite hemisphere, or invades infratentorially

Infratentorial Tumor

T1 Tumor 3 cm or less in greatest dimension; limited to one side
T2 Tumor more than 3 cm in greatest dimension; limited to one side
T3 Tumor invades or encroaches upon the ventricular system
T4 Tumor crosses the midline, invades the opposite hemisphere, or invades supratentorially

Regional Lymph Nodes (N)

This category does not apply to this site.

Distant Metastasis (M)

MX Presence of distant metastasis cannot be assessed
M0 No distant metastasis
M1 Distant metastasis

HISTOPATHOLOGIC GRADE (G)

GX Grade cannot be assessed
G1 Well differentiated
G2 Moderately well differentiated
G3 Poorly differentiated
G4 Undifferentiated

STAGE GROUPING

Stage	G	T	M
Stage IA	G1	T1	M0
Stage IB	G1	T2	M0
	G1	T3	M0
Stage IIA	G2	T1	M0
Stage IIB	G2	T2	M0
	G2	T3	M0
Stage IIIA	G3	T1	M0
Stage IIIB	G3	T2	M0
	G3	T3	M0
Stage IV	G1, 2, 3	T4	M0
	G4	Any T	M0
	Any G	Any T	M1

DIFFERENCES BETWEEN THE 2ND AND 3RD EDITIONS

This classification is the same as that published in the second edition of the *Manual.*

HISTOPATHOLOGIC TYPE

Tumors that are included in the analysis and evaluation are as follows:

1. Astrocytomas
2. Oligodendrogliomas
3. Ependymal and choroid plexus tumors
4. Glioblastomas
5. Medulloblastomas
6. Meningiomas, malignant
7. Neurilemmomas (neurinomas, schwannomas), malignant
8. Hemangioblastomas
9. Neurosarcomas
10. Sarcomas

Histologic grade usually correlates with biologic activity of the tumor. This is particularly the case with malignant astrocytomas, the most common form of glioma. The age of the patient at the time of diagnosis is also of major importance for prognosis.

BRAIN

Data Form for Cancer Staging

Patient identification
Name _____
Address _____
Hospital or clinic number _____
Age _____ Sex _____ Race _____

Institution identification
Hospital or clinic _____
Address _____

Oncology Record

Anatomic site of cancer _____
Histologic type _____
Grade (G) _____
Date of classification _____

Chronology of classification
(use separate form for each time staged)
[ ] Clinical (use all data prior to first treatment)
[ ] Pathologic (if definitively resected specimen available)

Definitions

Primary Tumor (T)
[ ] TX   Primary tumor cannot be assessed
[ ] T0   No evidence of primary tumor

Supratentorial tumor
[ ] T1   Tumor 5 cm or less in greatest dimension; limited to one side
[ ] T2   Tumor more than 5 cm in greatest dimension; limited to one side
[ ] T3   Tumor invades or encroaches upon the ventricular system
[ ] T4   Tumor crosses the midline, invades the opposite hemisphere, or extends infratentorially

Infratentorial tumor
[ ] T1   Tumor 3 cm or less in greatest dimension; limited to one side
[ ] T2   Tumor more than 3 cm in greatest dimension; limited to one side
[ ] T3   Tumor invades or encroaches upon the ventricular system
[ ] T4   Tumor crosses the midline, invades the opposite hemisphere, or invades supratentorially

Lymph Node (N)
This category does not apply to this site.

Distant Metastasis (M)
[ ] MX   Presence of distant metastasis cannot be assessed
[ ] M0   No distant metastasis
[ ] M1   Distant metastasis

Illustrations

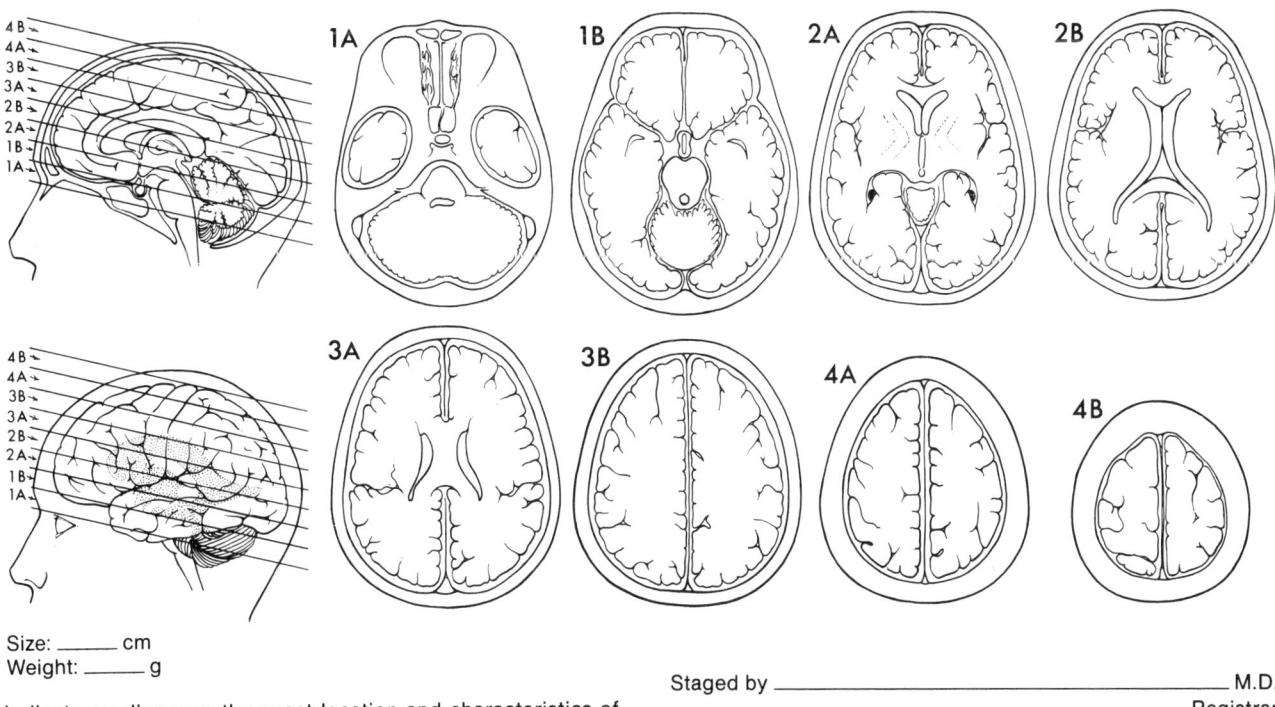

Size: _____ cm
Weight: _____ g

Indicate on diagrams the exact location and characteristics of tumor.

Staged by _____ M.D.
_____ Registrar
Date _____

American Joint Committee on Cancer—1988

Stage Grouping

[ ]	IA	G1	T1	M0
[ ]	IB	G1	T2	M0
		G1	T3	M0
[ ]	IIA	G2	T1	M0
[ ]	IIB	G2	T2	M0
		G2	T3	M0
[ ]	IIIA	G3	T1	M0
[ ]	IIIB	G3	T2	M0
		G3	T3	M0
[ ]	IV	G1	T4	M0
		G2	T4	M0
		G3	T4	M0
		G4	Any T	M0
		Any G	Any T	M1

Histopathologic Grade (G)

[ ] GX Grade cannot be assessed
[ ] G1 Well differentiated
[ ] G2 Moderately well differentiated
[ ] G3 Poorly differentiated
[ ] G4 Undifferentiated

Histopathologic Type

Tumors that are included in the analysis and evaluation are as follows:

1. Astrocytomas
2. Oligodendrogliomas
3. Ependymal and choroid plexus tumors
4. Glioblastomas
5. Medulloblastomas
6. Meningiomas, malignant
7. Neurilemmomas (neurinomas, schwannomas), malignant
8. Hemangioblastomas
9. Neurosarcomas
10. Sarcomas

Sites of Distant Metastasis

Pulmonary	PUL
Osseous	OSS
Hepatic	HEP
Brain	BRA
Lymph nodes	LYM
Bone marrow	MAR
Pleura	PLE
Peritoneum	PER
Skin	SKI
Other	OTH

APPENDIX

Histologic Grading of Tumors of the Central Nervous System

Criteria for the Diagnosis of Malignancy in Tumors of the Central Nervous System and Allied Structures

The uncritical application, to tumors of the central nervous system and allied structures, of those criteria for histologic and biologic malignancy that generally pertain to other neoplasms is inadequate for the following reasons:

1. Irrespective of the histologic malignancy of the tumor, its unimpeded growth within the confines of the skull as a space-occupying and expanding lesion inevitably leads to a fatal termination, which by definition is equated with clinical malignancy.
2. Similarly, the local pressure caused by an intracranial tumor upon vital neural structures may result in the clinical effects of malignancy, irrespective of the histologic type of tumor.
3. The obstructive effect of a growing tumor leads to the production of secondary occlusive hydrocephalus.
4. Certain criteria of malignancy of neoplasms that in other body systems pertain to their growth and spread (especially the characteristic of infiltrative growth and the capacity to metastasize, either within or outside the central nervous system) do not necessarily pertain to, or have to be modified to, the evaluation of the malignant behavior of central nervous system tumors.

Thus, tumors of the central nervous system and allied structures, in addition to their intrinsic benign or malignant histologic character that to a considerable extent determines their biologic behavior, may by their specific localization acquire certain characteristics that collectively will add up to the picture of what is regarded as benign, semibenign, relatively malignant, or highly malignant.

The numerical grading used in this classification is based upon histologic criteria of malignancy and should be considered as an estimate of the usual behavior of each type of tumor. Numerical grade 1 is considered to be the least malignant and grades 2, 3, and 4 indicate increasing degrees of malignancy.

In this general evaluation, the pathologist confronted with the problem of malignancy and prognosis is faced with two sets of data. In the first analysis the evaluation of malignancy must clearly be based on a retrospective assessment of the postoperative prognosis and survival rates of other known similar examples, so that a final and reasonably accurate clinicopathologic correlation is arrived at that both reinforces the purely histopathologic evaluation of malignancy and is reinforced by it.

Second, the pathologist deduces malignancy from a number of purely histologic and cytologic data. These include increase of cellularity, the presence and rate of mitotic figures, the presence of atypical mitotic figures, pleomorphism of tumor cells, pleomorphism of tissue architecture—particularly necroses, abnormally prominent stromal reaction, disorderly stromal reaction, and overgrowth—and the formation of pathologic blood vessels (corresponding to the angiographic appearance of arteriovenous fistulas).

On the other hand, other features that are usually regarded as indicative of or synonymous with malignancy need not necessarily be recognized in the case of tumors of the central nervous system, especially those of neuroectodermal origin. For instance, lack of circumscription and focal parenchymatous invasion is not a necessary accompaniment of cellular anaplasia or ultimate clinical malignancy. Also, the actual presence of mitotic figures (as in oligodendroglioma) does not necessarily imply a particularly malignant behavior; the overall number of mitoses and the presence of abnormal mitotic figures are more important in evaluation. Similarly, local invasion of the leptomeninges is often clearly dissociated from either of the two features just quoted. This is the case, for example, in the pilocytic astrocytoma that involves the wall of the third ventricle, the optic nerve, the cerebellum, and so on.

Although distant meningeal and ventricular metastases are often characteristic of highly malignant tumors such as medulloblastoma, this phenomenon again is not always to be correlated with the highest degrees of cytologic malignancy, as seen in some oligodendrogliomas.

The Question of Grading

Following Broders' classification of epithelial tumors elsewhere in the body, an attempt has been made by Kernohan and his school to apply a system of grading by ascending degrees of malignancy, numbered 1 to 4, to certain tumors of neuroectodermal origin, namely astrocytoma, oligodendroglioma, ependymoma, and neuroastrocytoma. This attempt stemmed both from a desire to simplify the then current classification of tumors of the central nervous system and from a need to offer to the neurosurgeon a prognostic evaluation of the tumor removed at surgery, based on certain definite histologic and cytologic criteria. Attractive though this attempt at simplification might be, however, it has to meet with a number of objections:

1. The sample of tissue so analyzed may from surgical necessity not be representative of the tumor as a whole.
2. The specific evolution of the particular tumor in terms of its anaplastic potentialities is not fully expressed by such a scheme of grading. For example, a cerebellar pilocytic astrocytoma graded 1 does not have the same anaplastic potential as a cerebral astrocytoma or some other tumors also graded 1.
3. The pleomorphism of cell and tissue structures so frequently inherent in primary neuroectodermal tumors poses additional difficulties to the application of a simplified system of grading.
4. This cytologic grading makes it extremely difficult to place tumors with mixed cell populations into an already predetermined tumor category.

Nevertheless, the above remarks should not be regarded as basically antagonistic to some attempts at expressing the degree of malignancy of a particular tumor of the central nervous system. Indeed, from the clinical and therapeutic points of view, no classification based on purely histologic entities is satisfactory unless adequate cognizance is taken of, and information provided on, the degree of malignancy of a particular tumor submitted for examination. Thus, it is the duty and prerogative of the pathologist to provide his clinical colleagues with an informed opinion on the likely evolution of a particular tumor, and to some extent this prognostic opinion is embodied in the recognition of specific clinicopathologic neuro-oncologic entities. As an illustration, it might be pointed out that two tumors of similar cellularity, isomorphous appearance, and mitotic rate, such as the medulloblastomas and some oligodendrogliomas, usually do not exhibit the same biologic behavior. This acquired body of knowledge is clearly the result of previous collaboration among clinicians and pathologists in the field of neuro-oncology.

BIBLIOGRAPHY

1. Jelsma R, Bucy PC: Glioblastoma multiforme: Its treatment and some factors affecting survival. Arch Neurol 20:161–171, 1969
2. Salcman M: Survival in glioblastoma: Historical perspective. Neurosurgery 7:435–439, 1980
3. Scanlon PW, Taylor WF: Radiotherapy of intracranial astrocytomas: Analysis of 417 cases treated from 1960 through 1969. Neurosurgery 5:301–308, 1979
4. Walker MD, Alexander E Jr, Hunt WE et al: Evaluation of BCNU and/or radiotherapy in the treatment of anaplastic gliomas: A cooperative clinical trial. J Neurosurg 49:333–343, 1978
5. Wilson CB, Gutin P, Boldrey EB et al: Single-agent chemotherapy of brain tumors: A five-year review. Arch Neurol 33:739–744, 1976
6. Zulch KJ: Histologic typing of tumours of the central nervous system. International Histological Classification of Tumours, No. 21. Geneva, World Health Organization, 1979

HODGKIN'S AND NON-HODGKIN'S LYMPHOMA

45

Hodgkin's Disease

A distinctive form of lymphoma, Hodgkin's disease has served as a model for treatment trials, for great strides have been made in the therapy of this disease. Staging of Hodgkin's lymphoma is not based on the local extent of disease but on its distribution and symptomatology. The classic TNM system is not useful for staging Hodgkin's disease. It is usually not possible to determine the primary tumor site. When the patient presents, the disease is often widely disseminated. Important for staging is the evaluation of many organs and groups of lymph nodes for tumor involvement. The disease is often associated with unusual immunologic abnormalities and a diversity of histologic changes. Staging is considered critical for patient management.

ANATOMY

The major lymphatic structures include groups and chains of lymph nodes, the spleen, and the thymus gland. The digestive system is also an important lymphoid organ that has collections of lymphoid tissue known as Waldeyer's ring in the oropharynx, Peyer's patches in the ileum, and lymphoid nodules in the appendix. Hodgkin's disease can involve almost any organ or tissue, especially the liver, bone marrow, and spleen, in addition to the lymph nodes.

RULES FOR CLASSIFICATION

Clinical Staging. The clinical stage is determined by physical examination, history, imaging studies, blood tests, and initial biopsy. Such studies usually establish the diagnosis and histologic type of Hodgkin's disease. Histologic confirmation is essential. All symptoms should be recorded.

Pathologic Staging. Pathologic staging depends on laparotomy, multiple biopsies to assess the distribution of the disease, including liver biopsy, and splenectomy. Involved organs or sites should be listed.

STAGE GROUPING

Stage I Involvement of single lymph node region (I) or localized involvement of a single extralymphatic organ or site (I_E).

Stage II Involvement of two or more lymph node regions on the same side of the diaphragm (II) or localized involvement of a single associated extralymphatic organ or site and its regional lymph node(s) with or without involvement of other lymph node regions on the same side of the diaphragm (II_E).

Note: The number of lymph node regions involved may be indicated by a subscript (e.g., II_3).

Stage III Involvement of lymph node regions on both sides of the diaphragm (III), which may also be accompanied by localized involvement of an associated extralymphatic organ or site (III_E), by involvement of the spleen (III_S), or both (III_{E+S}).

Stage IV Disseminated (multifocal) involvement of one or more extralymphatic organs, with or without associated lymph node involvement, or isolated extralymphatic organ involvement with distant (non-regional) nodal involvement.

DIFFERENCES BETWEEN THE 2ND AND 3RD EDITIONS

This classification is the same as that published in the second edition of the *Manual*.

SYSTEMIC SYMPTOMS

Each stage is subdivided into "A" and "B" categories, "B" for those with defined systemic symptoms and "A" for those without. The B designation is given to those patients with (1) unexplained loss of more than 10% of body weight in the 6 months before admission; (2) unexplained fever with temperatures above 38°C; and (3) drenching night sweats. Pruritus alone does not qualify for B classification,* nor does a short febrile illness associated with an infection.

Note: Pruritus as a systemic symptom remains controversial. This symptom is hard to define quantitatively and uniformly, but when it is recurrent, generalized, and otherwise unexplained, and when it ebbs and flows parallel to disease activity, it may be the equivalent of a B symptom.

HISTOPATHOLOGIC TYPE

Hodgkin's disease is divided into four histologic types and "unclassified." These types should be recorded because they have prognostic significance. They are:

Nodular sclerosis
Lymphocyte predominance
Mixed cellularity
Lymphocyte depletion
Unclassified

Histologic classification should be based on paraffin-embedded hematoxylin and eosin-stained sections.

BIBLIOGRAPHY

1. Boyd NF, Feinstein AR: Symptoms as an index of growth rates and prognosis in Hodgkin's disease. Clin Invest Med 1:25–31, 1978
2. Carbonne PP, Kaplan HS, Musshoff K et al: Report of the committee on Hodgkin's disease staging classification. Cancer Res 31:1860–1861, 1971
3. Kaplan HS: *Hodgkin's Disease*, 2nd ed. Cambridge, Harvard University Press, 1980
4. Symposium: "Staging of Hodgkin's Disease." Ann Arbor, Michigan. Cancer Res 31: 1971.

HODGKIN'S DISEASE

Data Form for Cancer Staging

Patient identification
Name _____
Address _____
Hospital or clinic number _____
Age _____ Sex _____ Race _____

Institution identification
Hospital or clinic _____
Address _____

Oncology Record

Anatomic site of cancer _____
Histologic type _____
Grade (G) _____
Date of classification _____

Chronology of classification
  (use separate form for each time staged)
[ ] Clinical (use all data prior to first treatment)
[ ] Pathologic (if definitively resected specimen available)

Definitions

Stage Grouping

Stage I   Involvement of single lymph node region (I) or localized involvement of a single extralymphatic organ or site (I_E).

Stage II Involvement of two or more lymph node regions on the same side of the diaphragm (II) or localized involvement of a single associated extralymphatic organ or site and its regional lymph node(s) with or without involvement of other lymph node regions on the same side of the diaphragm (II_E).
NOTE: The number of lymph node regions involved may be indicated by a subscript (e.g., II_3).

Stage III Involvement of lymph node regions on both sides of the diaphragm (III), which may also be accompanied by localized involvement of an associated extralymphatic organ or site (III_E), by involvement of the spleen (III_S), or both (III_{E+S}).

Stage IV Disseminated (multifocal) involvement of one or more extralymphatic organs, with or without associated lymph node involvement, or isolated extralymphatic organ involvement with distant (non-regional) nodal involvement.

Histopathologic Type

Hodgkin's disease is divided into four histologic types and "unclassified." These types should be recorded because they have prognostic significance. They are:

Nodular sclerosis
Lymphocyte predominance
Mixed cellularity
Lymphocyte depletion
Unclassified

Histologic classification should be based on paraffin-embedded hematoxylin and eosin-stained sections.

Staged by _____ M.D.
         _____ Registrar
Date _____

46

Non-Hodgkin's Lymphoma

The histologic classification of the non-Hodgkin's lymphomas has been an area of considerable controversy. At present a number of competing classifications are in use, including those of Rappaport, Lukes and Collins, the WHO, Dorfman, Kiel, and the British National Lymphoma Investigation Group. In an effort to bring some uniformity to the classification of these disorders, an international panel of expert pathologists has generated a *Working Formulation*, which attempts to provide a means of interpretation of these somewhat divergent classification schemes. Although this formulation may still be in an evolutionary state, it does provide a useful format in which to discuss the staging and workup of these lymphomas.

The anatomic staging system currently employed was developed for Hodgkin's disease and has been extended to the non-Hodgkin's lymphomas, although it is more directly applicable to Hodgkin's disease. As a result, some difficulties arise in some instances when attempting to apply traditional staging systems to non-Hodgkin's lymphomas. However, in the main it has proved to be a workable system and has the advantage of being familiar and similar to that used in Hodgkin's disease.

The TNM classification, however, is not a workable system for staging the malignant lymphomas. The site of origin of these diseases is often unclear, and there is no way to differentiate T, N, and M from each other. In the non-Hodgkin's lymphomas, the pattern of node involvement (follicular versus diffuse), the degree of cellular differentiation (well-differentiated vs. lymphoblastic), and the bulk of disease at individual sites is often more important than anatomic considerations.

ANATOMY

The major lymphatic structures include groups and chains of lymph nodes, the spleen, thymus, Waldeyer's ring, appendix, and Peyer's patches. Minor lymphoid collections are widely dispersed in other viscera and tissues, such as the bone marrow, liver, skin, bone, lung, pleura, and gonads. Involvement of extranodal sites is more commonly seen in the non-Hodgkin's lymphomas than in Hodgkin's disease.

RULES FOR CLASSIFICATION

The diagnosis of malignant lymphoma requires the biopsy of lymph nodes or of an extranodal lymphoid tumor. Frozen sections are never to be used as a definitive diagnostic source, and confirmation rests on the review of the fixed specimen.

Clinical Staging. Staging generally involves the use of a combination of clinical, radiologic, and surgical procedures, progressing sequentially from less invasive to more invasive, necessary to define final stage and to provide a sound basis for planning therapy. Clinical staging includes a carefully recorded medical history, a physical examination, urinalysis, chest roentgenograms, blood chemistry determinations, a complete blood examination, and bilateral biopsies of the bone marrow. In addition, most investigators use a bilateral lower-extremity lymphangiogram and an abdominal CAT scan to fulfill the mandatory staging requirements. Other procedures often useful in full staging of patients include bone roentgenograms, technetium 99m-labeled polyphosphate bone scans, CAT scans, or tomography of the thorax (if the initial chest x-ray is abnormal). Additional procedures helpful under certain circumstances include upper GI series (if Waldeyer's ring is involved or if patients have GI symptoms), lumbar puncture (if patients have diffuse histologies and bone marrow involvement), ultrasound, gallium scans, and radioisotopic scans of the spleen and liver. Surface marker studies and studies of immunoglobulin gene rearrangement have been increasingly used to characterize these lymphomas, although these presently must be thought of as research tools.

Pathologic Staging. Initial diagnosis is almost always made by surgical biopsy. In addition, biopsy of accessible extranodal primary tumors is desirable. Extranodal sites of disease at presentation are seen in about 30% of patients. About 25% of patients with non-Hodgkin's lymphomas present with evidence of abdominal disease requiring laparotomy for diagnosis. However, staging laparotomy is not routinely used in this disease and should only be used when treatment changes would result from the results of the surgery. If liver involvement is suspected, it may be biopsied by a percutaneous needle procedure, or multiple directed biopsies of both lobes may be obtained using peritoneoscopy. Although a staging laparotomy is employed selectively and only after careful consideration of its impact on both staging and subsequent therapy, when employed it should include splenectomy, wedge liver biopsy, and biopsies of the perisplenic, mesenteric, porta-hepatic, para-aortic, and bilateral iliac nodes, unless underlying medical problems prohibit such biopsies.

Retreatment Staging. Suspected recurrence or relapses require biopsy confirmation, particularly if a complete remission of greater than one year has occurred. Patients may be restaged at this juncture using the procedures previously outlined.

STAGE GROUPING

Stage I Involvement of a single lymph node region (I) or localized involvement of a single extralymphatic organ or site (I_E).

Stage II Involvement of two or more lymph node regions on the same side of the diaphragm (II), or localized involvement of a single associated extralymphatic organ or site and its regional nodes with or without other lymph node regions on the same side of the diaphragm (II_E).
Note: The number of lymph node regions involved may be indicated by a subscript (e.g., II_3).

Stage III Involvement of lymph node regions on both sides of the diaphragm (III) that may also be accompanied by localized involvement of an extralymphatic organ or site (III_E), by involvement of the spleen (III_S), or both (III_{E+S}).

Stage IV Disseminated (multifocal) involvement of one or more extralymphatic organs with or without associated lymph node (involvement, or isolated extralymphatic organ involvement with distant (non-regional) nodal involvement.

DIFFERENCES BETWEEN THE 2ND AND 3RD EDITIONS

In the second edition of the *Manual*, all lymphomas were staged following the classification for Hodgkin's disease. In this edition, separate classifications were developed for the Hodgkin's and non-Hodgkin's lymphomas.

SYSTEMIC SYMPTOMS

Systemic symptoms are not as commonly associated with the non-Hodgkin's lymphomas as with Hodgkin's disease, and patients with non-Hodgkin's lymphomas often have remarkably few symptoms, even though many node areas and/or extranodal sites are involved. However, when systemic symptoms are seen, they do have prognostic significance.

Each stage is subdivided into "A" and "B" categories: "B" for those with defined systematic symptoms and "A" for those without. The B designation is given to those patients with (1) unexplained loss of more than 10% of body weight in the 6 months before admission; (2) unexplained fever with temperatures above 38°C; and (3) drenching night sweats. Pruritus alone does not qualify for B classification,* nor does a short febrile illness associated with an infection. In addition, an accurate assessment of the performance status (ECOG, Karnofsky, or AJCC) with allowances for unrelated diseases is most important.

Note: Pruritus as a systemic symptom remains controversial. This symptom is hard to define quantitatively and uniformly, but when it is recurrent, generalized, and otherwise unexplained, and when it ebbs and flows parallel to disease activity, it may be the equivalent of a B symptom.

GENERAL CONSIDERATIONS

The anatomic extent of disease in the non-Hodgkin's lymphomas is defined by the appropriate sequence of diagnostic procedures selected for a given histologic subset and a particular individual. The exact sequence of staging procedures and the magnitude of invasive staging will rest upon the patient's histology, the therapeutic approach contemplated, as well as the stage of disease. No invasive staging procedure should be employed merely to change the patient's stage, if that change of stage will not alter the therapy selected or the outcome of treatment. There is always some variation, often with good reason, in the degree of completeness and adequacy of the data used for final staging.

In general, the yield from particular staging procedures is dependent upon the histology of the patient's lymphoma. For instance, in the low grade or indolent follicular lymphomas (see Histopathology) some 80% to 90% of patients will have positive lymphangiograms, 40% will have liver involvement, and approximately 40% will have bone marrow involvement as well. When comprehensive staging is done on these patients, over 90% have Stage III–IV disease. This high frequency of advanced disease makes staging laparotomy rarely, if ever, required in the workup of follicular lymphoma because treatment decisions are rarely influenced by the findings in the majority of patients.

In contrast, in the intermediate or high grade lymphomas (the diffuse large cell varieties) (see Histopathology), a much lower incidence of visceral disease is generally found at initial staging. As an example, some 30% to 40% of patients have positive lymphangiograms, the frequency of positive bone marrows is about 15% to 20%, and about 15% to 20% of liver biopsies are positive. After final comprehensive staging, about 25% to 30% of patients with diffuse aggressive lymphoma appear to have localized (Stage I and II) disease. Again, the importance of the extent of staging rests upon the subsequent therapeutic approaches taken and the success of that therapy. Comprehensive staging is required if a localized form of therapy (*i.e.,* involved field irradiation) is being considered.

CAT scanners have the ability to define enlarged nodes in areas not filled by the dye during lymphangiography. Foci of lymphoreticular disease in the para-aortic region above the level of the second lumbar vertebra, in the porta-hepatic, splenic hilus, mesentery, gut wall, and retrocrural nodes and in other sites in the abdomen cannot be demonstrated by lymphangiography. In these and other instances, CAT scans are a useful addition to other staging procedures. On the other hand, CAT scanning is unable to detect small defects in otherwise normal-sized nodes. Thus, a complementary role of CAT scanning and lymphangiography is seen in the non-Hodgkin's lymphomas.

HISTOPATHOLOGIC TYPE

While individual institutions and particular pathologists may use one of the many classifications of these lymphomas mentioned earlier (see Introduction), the corresponding Working Formulation equivalent should be identified so that interinstitutional comparisons can be made and accurate staging approaches selected. The modified Working Formulation is listed below. It should be noted that the term non-Hodgkin's lymphoma is not used, follicular is employed rather than nodular, and surface markers are not required. The reader is referred to several references in the bibliography where cross comparisons are made between the various classifications.

HISTOPATHOLOGIC GRADE (G)

Working Formulation

I. Low-Grade Malignant Lymphoma
   A. Small lymphocytic
   B. Follicular, predominantly small cleaved cell
   C. Follicular mixed, small and large cell
II. Intermediate-Grade Malignant Lymphoma
   D. Follicular, predominantly large cell
   E. Diffuse small cleaved cell
   F. Diffuse mixed, small and large cell
   G. Diffuse large cell, cleaved or noncleaved
III. High-Grade Malignant Lymphoma
   H. Diffuse large cell immunoblastic
   I. Small noncleaved cell (Burkitt's or non-Burkitt's)
   J. Lymphoblastic (convoluted or nonconvoluted)
IV. Miscellaneous
   Composite
   Mycosis fungoides
   True histiocytic
   Other

BIBLIOGRAPHY

1. Bunn PA Jr, Lamberg SI: Report of the committee on staging and classification of cutaneous T-cell lymphomas. Cancer Treat Rep 63:725–728, 1979
2. Chabner BA, Johnson RE, Young RC et al: Sequential nonsurgical and surgical staging of non-Hodgkin's lymphoma. Cancer 42:922–925, 1978
3. Nathwani BN: A critical analysis of the classifications of non-Hodgkin's lymphoma. Cancer 44:347–384, 1979
4. Rosenberg SA: National Cancer Institute sponsored study of classifications of non-Hodgkin's lymphomas. Summary and description of a working formulation for clinical usage. Cancer 49:2112–2135, 1982

NON-HODGKIN'S LYMPHOMA

Data Form for Cancer Staging

Patient identification
Name _____
Address _____
Hospital or clinic number _____
Age _____ Sex _____ Race _____

Institution identification
Hospital or clinic _____
Address _____

Oncology Record

Anatomic site of cancer _____
Histologic type _____
Grade (G) _____
Date of classification _____

Chronology of classification
(use separate form for each time staged)
[ ] Clinical (use all data prior to first treatment)
[ ] Pathologic (if definitively resected specimen available)

Definitions

Stage Grouping

Stage I — Involvement of a single lymph node region (I) or localized involvement of a single extralymphatic organ or site (I_E).

Stage II — Involvement of two or more lymph node regions on the same side of the diaphragm (II), or localized involvement of a single associated extralymphatic organ or site and its regional nodes with or without other lymph node regions on the same side of the diaphragm (II_E).
NOTE: The number of lymph node regions involved may be indicated by a subscript (e.g., II_3).

Stage III — Involvement of lymph node regions on both sides of the diaphragm (III) that may also be accompanied by localized involvement of an extralymphatic organ or site (III_E), by involvement of the spleen (III_S), or both (III_{E+S}).

Stage IV — Disseminated (multifocal) involvement of one or more extralymphatic organs with or without associated lymph node involvement, or isolated extralymphatic organ involvement with distant (nonregional) nodal involvement.

Histopathologic Grade (G)

Working Formulation

I. Low-Grade Malignant Lymphoma
   A. Small lymphocytic
   B. Follicular, predominantly small cleaved cell
   C. Follicular mixed, small and large cell

II. Intermediate-Grade Malignant Lymphoma
   D. Follicular, predominantly large cell
   E. Diffuse small cleaved cell
   F. Diffuse mixed, small and large cell
   G. Diffuse large cell, cleaved/noncleaved

III. High-Grade Malignant Lymphoma
   H. Diffuse large cell immunoblastic
   I. Small noncleaved cell (Burkitt's/non-Burkitt's)
   J. Lymphoblastic (convoluted/nonconvoluted)

IV. Miscellaneous
Composite
Mycosis fungoides
True histiocytic
Other

Histopathologic Type

While individual institutions and particular pathologists may use one of the many classifications of these lymphomas mentioned earlier (see Introduction), the corresponding Working Formulation equivalent should be identified so that interinstitutional comparisons can be made and accurate staging approaches selected. The modified Working Formulation is listed below. It should be noted that the term *non-Hodgkin's lymphoma* is not used, *follicular* is employed rather than *nodular*, and surface markers are not required. The reader is referred to several references in the bibliography where cross comparisons are made between the various classifications.

Staged by _____ M.D.
_____ Registrar
Date _____

PEDIATRIC CANCERS

47

Nephroblastoma (Wilms' Tumor)

Pediatric tumors are classified according to the recommendations of the Societé Internationale d'Oncologie Pediatrique (SIOP). The TNM classification used in this edition of the *Manual* for pediatric tumors is the same as that published in the 1983 edition. However, the post-surgical evaluative staging sequence has been deleted. Tumors are staged clinically before definitive treatment and pathologically after examination of the resected specimen. The prognosis of childhood cancers has improved dramatically in the last 15 years. In clinical trials and cooperative group protocols, a different or modified staging classification may be used.

Malignant tumors of childhood include neuroblastomas, nephroblastomas or Wilms' tumor, and the soft tissue sarcomas, which include the rhabdomyosarcomas. Neuroblastomas are the most common tumor found at birth. Nephroblastomas have had over 75 synonyms, which will not be listed. Rhabdomyosarcoma is the most common soft tissue sarcoma found in childhood.

These pediatric cancers may be present at the time of birth or develop during the first several years of life. Some pediatric cancers, especially Wilms' tumor, may be associated with congenital anomalies in other organs.

Cancers in children are staged the same as in adults, except in one respect. For children, it is necessary to include a category for those cases in which a surgical exploration was carried out and a nonresectable tumor found. Such cases are designated with a "c" in the T category; for example, "pT3c" means that a nonresectable tumor was found on surgical exploration. The other two staging elements, that is, the "N" and "M," are completed and the stage assigned according to all three categories.

Nephroblastoma, or Wilms' tumor, is usually found in the kidney of young children. These tumors may be bilateral. Histologically, they are often mixed, that is, composed of stromal and epithelial derivatives in various stages of differentiation. Nephroblastomas are most commonly seen in children under 8 years of age, with the peak in the second year of life. Bilateral and familial nephroblastomas tend to occur at a younger age than nephroblastomas in general. The younger the child, the better the prognosis. Nephroblastomas usually present as an abdominal mass. Plasma and urine erythropoietin levels are often elevated. Treatment for these cancers has improved dramatically in the past 15 years. These tumors are staged clinically and pathologically.

ANATOMY

Primary Site. Nephroblastomas arise from the kidneys (ICD-O 189.0). These tumors may be bilateral and multiple.

Regional Lymph Nodes. The regional lymph nodes are the hilar nodes, the para-aortic nodes, and the paracaval nodes located between the diaphragm and the bifurcation of the aorta. All other lymph nodes involved are considered distant metastases and must be coded as M1.

Metastatic Sites. Distant metastases are most frequent in the lungs, liver, and regional lymph nodes. Tumor may also extend along the renal vein and the inferior vena cava. Involvement of the opposite kidney is usually considered as a second primary tumor and not as a metastasis.

RULES FOR CLASSIFICATION

This classification applies only to nephroblastoma (Wilms' tumor).

Clinical Staging. Clinical classification is based on the surface area of the primary tumor as revealed by imaging, whether bilateral or unilateral, and whether or not the tumor has broken through and ruptured its capsule. Extension of the tumor through its capsule worsens the prognosis.

Clinical classification is based on evidence acquired prior to the decision about definitive treatment. Such evidence arises from clinical, radiologic, endoscopic, and other relevant studies. When TNM is used without a prefix, it implies clinical classification (cTNM).

Pathologic Staging. Pathologic classification is based on regional extension beyond the confines of the kidney. It is based on evidence acquired prior to the decision about definitive treatment and is supplemented or modified by the additional evidence acquired from definitive surgery and from the examination of the resected specimen.

DEFINITION OF TNM

Clinical Classification (cTNM)
Primary Tumor (cT)

TX Primary tumor cannot be assessed
T0 No evidence of primary tumor
T1 Unilateral tumor 80 cm^2 or less in area (including kidney)[1]
T2 Unilateral tumor more than 80 cm^2 in area (including kidney)
T3 Unilateral tumor rupture before treatment
T4 Bilateral tumors

Note: The area is calculated by multiplying the vertical and horizontal dimensions of the radiologic shadow of the tumor and kidney.

Regional Lymph Nodes (cN)

NX Regional lymph nodes cannot be assessed
N0 No regional lymph node metastasis
N1 Regional lymph node metastasis

Distant Metastasis (cM)

MX Presence of distant metastasis cannot be assessed
M0 No distant metastasis
M1 Distant metastasis

Pathologic Classification (pTNM)
Primary Tumor (pT)

pTX Primary tumor cannot be assessed
pT0 No evidence of primary tumor
pT1 Intrarenal tumor completely encapsulated; excision complete and margins histologically free
pT2 Tumor invades beyond the capsule or renal parenchyma*; excision complete
pT3 Tumor invades beyond the capsule or renal parenchyma*; excision incomplete *or* preoperative or operative rupture
    pT3a Microscopic residual tumor limited to tumor bed
    pT3b Macroscopic residual tumor or spillage or malignant ascites
    pT3c Surgical exploration only; tumor not resected
pT4 Bilateral tumors

Nephroblastoma (Wilm's Tumor)

*Note: This includes breach of the renal capsule or tumor seen microscopically outside the capsule; tumor adhesions microscopically confirmed; infiltrations of, or tumor thrombus within, the renal vessels outside the kidney; infiltration of the renal pelvis or ureter, parapelvic, and pericaliceal fat.

Regional Lymph Nodes (pN)

pNX Regional lymph nodes cannot be assessed
pN0 No regional lymph node metastasis
pN1 Regional lymph node metastasis
    pN1a Regional lymph node metastasis completely resected
    pN1b Regional lymph node metastasis incompletely resected

Distant Metastasis (pM)

pMX Presence of distant metastasis cannot be assessed
pM0 No distant metastasis
pM1 Distant metastasis

CLINICAL STAGE GROUPING (cTNM)

Stage	T	N	M
Stage I	T1	N0	M0
Stage II	T2	N0	M0
Stage III	T1	N1	M0
	T2	N1	M0
	T3	Any N	M0
Stage IVA	T1	Any N	M1
	T2	Any N	M1
	T3	Any N	M1
Stage IVB	T4	Any N	Any M

PATHOLOGIC STAGE GROUPING (pTNM)

Stage	T	N	M
Stage I	T1	N0	M0
Stage II	T1	N1a	M0
	T2	N0, N1a	M0
Stage IIIA	T3a	N0, N1a	M0
Stage IIIB	T1	N1b	M0
	T2	N1b	M0
	T3a	N1b	M0
	T3b	Any N	M0
	T3c	Any N	M0
Stage IVA	T1	Any N	M1
	T2	Any N	M1
	T3a	Any N	M1
	T3b	Any N	M1
	T3c	Any N	M1
Stage IVB	T4	Any N	Any M

DIFFERENCES BETWEEN THE 2ND AND 3RD EDITIONS

This classification is the same as that published in the second edition of the *Manual*.

HISTOPATHOLOGIC TYPE

These are a distinctive group of tumors that show various histologies, differentiation, and components. A number of synonyms include angiomyosarcoma, adenosarcoma, mesoblastic nephroma, and embryoma. The various synonyms, of which there are over 75, reflect the different tissue components that may be present.

HISTOPATHOLOGIC GRADE (G)

Grading is usually not used.

BIBLIOGRAPHY

1. Bennington JL, Beckwith JB: Tumors of the Kidney, Renal Pelvis, and Ureter. Atlas of Tumor Pathology, Second Series, Fascicle 12. Washington, DC, Armed Forces Institute of Pathology, 1975
2. Hrabovsky EE, Othersen HB Jr, deLorimier A et al: Wilms' tumor in the neonate. J Pediatr Surg 21: 385–387, 1986
3. Jereb B, Sanstedt B: Structure and size versus prognosis in nephroblastoma. Cancer 31:1473–1481, 1973
4. Klapproth HJ: Wilms' tumor: A report of 45 cases and an analysis of 1,351 cases reported in the world literature from 1940 to 1958. J Urol 81:633–648, 1959
5. Kumar APM, Huster O, Fleming ID et al: Capsular and vascular invasion: Important prognostic factors in Wilms' tumor. J Pediatr Surg 10:301–309, 1975

NEPHROBLASTOMA

Data Form for Cancer Staging

Patient identification
Name _____
Address _____
Hospital or clinic number _____
Age _____ Sex _____ Race _____

Institution identification
Hospital or clinic _____
Address _____

Oncology Record

Anatomic site of cancer _____
Histologic type _____
Grade (G) _____
Date of classification _____

Chronology of classification
  (use separate form for each time staged)
[ ] Clinical (use all data prior to first treatment)
[ ] Pathologic (if definitively resected specimen available)

Definitions

Primary Tumor (T)

[ ] TX Primary tumor cannot be assessed
[ ] T0 No evidence of primary tumor
[ ] T1 Unilateral tumor 80 cm^2 or less in area (including kidney)
[ ] T2 Unilateral tumor more than 80 cm^2 in area (including kidney)[1]
[ ] T3 Unilateral tumor rupture before treatment
[ ] T4 Bilateral tumors

Lymph Node (N)

[ ] NX Regional lymph nodes cannot be assessed
[ ] N0 No regional lymph node metastasis
[ ] N1 Regional lymph node metastasis

Distant Metastasis (M)

[ ] MX Presence of distant metastasis cannot be assessed
[ ] M0 No distant metastasis
[ ] M1 Distant metastasis

Primary Tumor (pT)

[ ] pTX Primary tumor cannot be assessed
[ ] pT0 No evidence of primary tumor
[ ] pT1 Intrarenal tumor completely encapsulated; excision complete and margins histologically free
[ ] pT2 Tumor invades beyond the capsule or renal parenchyma; excision complete
[ ] pT3 Tumor invades beyond the capsule or renal parenchyma; excision incomplete or preoperative or operative rupture
  [ ] pT3a Microscopic residual tumor limited to tumor bed
  [ ] pT3b Macroscopic residual tumor or spillage or malignant ascites
  [ ] pT3c Surgical exploration only, tumor not resected
[ ] pT4 Bilateral tumors

Lymph Node (pN)

[ ] pNX Regional lymph nodes cannot be assessed
[ ] pN0 No regional lymph node metastasis
[ ] pN1 Regional lymph node metastasis
  [ ] pN1a Regional lymph node metastasis completely resected
  [ ] pN1b Regional lymph node metastasis incompletely resected

Distant Metastasis (pM)

[ ] pMX Presence of distant metastasis cannot be assessed
[ ] pM0 No distant metastasis
[ ] pM1 Distant metastasis

Clinical Stage Grouping (cTNM)

[ ] I	T1	N0	M0
[ ] II	T2	N0	M0
[ ] III	T1	N1	M0
	T2	N1	M0
	T3	Any N	M0
[ ] IVA	T1	Any N	M1
	T2	Any N	M1
	T3	Any N	M1
[ ] IVB	T4	Any N	Any M

Pathologic Stage Grouping (pTNM)

[ ] I	T1	N0	M0
[ ] II	T1	N1a	M0
	T2	N0	M0
	T2	N1a	M0
[ ] IIIA	T3a	N0	M0
	T3a	N1a	M0
[ ] IIIB	T1	N1b	M0
	T2	N1b	M0
	T3a	N1b	M0
	T3b	Any N	M0
	T3c	Any N	M0
[ ] IVA	T1	Any N	M1
	T2	Any N	M1
	T3a	Any N	M1
	T3b	Any N	M1
	T3c	Any N	M1
[ ] IVB	T4	Any N	Any M

Staged by _____ M.D.
_____ Registrar
Date _____

Histopathologic Type

These are a distinctive group of tumors that show various histologies, differentiation, and components. A number of synonyms include angiomyosarcoma, adenosarcoma, mesoblastic nephroma, and embryoma. The various synonyms, of which there are over 75, reflect the different tissue components that may be present.

Sites of Distant Metastasis

Pulmonary	PUL
Osseous	OSS
Hepatic	HEP
Brain	BRA
Lymph nodes	LYM
Bone marrow	MAR
Pleura	PLE
Peritoneum	PER
Skin	SKI
Other	OTH

48

Neuroblastoma

Neuroblastomas usually arise from the adrenal glands. These tumors are highly malignant with a 5-year survival of approximately 30% when discovered in the first year of life. Spontaneous regression of neuroblastomas does occur, especially in very young infants. For this reason, these tumors are of great interest to oncologists and medical scientists. Neuroblastomas are almost always found in children less than 8 years of age. These tumors may elaborate epinephrine and norepinephrine. Neuroblastomas can cause widespread and rapid metastases.

ANATOMY

Primary Site. Neuroblastomas usually originate in the adrenal medulla (ICD-O 194.0). However, they may be found at other sites, for example, in the posterior mediastinum. In fact, these tumors can be found at any location along the course of the sympathetic chain, from the cervical region to the pelvis. These tumors may be multicentric in origin.

Regional Lymph Nodes. The regional lymph nodes are defined as follows:

Cervical region	Cervical and supraclavicular nodes
Thoracic region	Intrathoracic and infraclavicular nodes
Abdominal and pelvic regions	Subdiaphragmatic, intra-abdominal, and pelvic nodes, including the external iliac nodes
Other regions	The appropriate regional lymph nodes

Metastatic Sites. Metastases are usually found in the liver, orbit, and bones, although nearly every organ can be affected. When the tumor develops in utero, the placenta may also be involved.

RULES FOR CLASSIFICATION

Clinical Staging. Because it is often impossible to differentiate between the primary tumor and the adjacent lymph nodes, the T assessment relates to the total mass. When there is doubt about multicentricity and metastasis, the latter is presumed. Size is estimated clinically or radiologically; for classification, the larger measurement should be used. There should be histologic confirmation of the disease and/or confirmation by biochemical tests.

Pathologic Staging. All clinical data and that found on examination of the surgically resected specimen is to be used. Definitions of pTNM differ from cTNM.

DEFINITION OF TNM

Clinical Classification (cTNM)
Primary Tumor (T)

- TX Primary tumor cannot be assessed
- T0 No evidence of primary tumor
- T1 Single tumor 5 cm or less in greatest dimension
- T2 Single tumor more than 5 cm but not more than 10 cm in greatest dimension
- T3 Single tumor more than 10 cm in greatest dimension
- T4 Multicentric tumors occurring simultaneously

Regional Lymph Nodes (N)

- NX Regional lymph nodes cannot be assessed
- N0 No regional lymph node metastasis
- N1 Regional lymph node metastasis

Distant Metastasis (M)

- MX Presence of distant metastasis cannot be assessed
- M0 No distant metastasis
- M1 Distant metastasis

Pathologic Classification (pTNM)
Primary Tumor (pT)

- pTX Primary tumor cannot be assessed
- pT0 No evidence of primary tumor
- pT1 Excision of tumor complete and margins histologically free
- pT2 The category does not apply to neuroblastoma
- pT3 Residual tumor
  - pT3a Microscopic residual tumor
  - pT3b Macroscopic residual tumor or grossly incomplete excision
  - pT3c Surgical exploration only, tumor not resected
- pT4 Multicentric tumors

Regional Lymph Nodes (pN)

- pNX Regional lymph nodes cannot be assessed
- pN0 No regional lymph node metastasis
- pN1 Regional lymph node metastasis
  - pN1a Regional lymph node metastases completely resected
  - pN1b Regional lymph node metastases incompletely resected

Distant Metastasis (pM)

- pMX Presence of distant metastasis cannot be assessed
- pM0 No distant metastasis
- pM1 Distant metastasis

CLINICAL STAGE GROUPING (cTNM)

Stage	T	N	M
Stage I	T1	N0	M0
Stage II	T2	N0	M0
Stage III	T1	N1	M0
	T2	N1	M0
	T3	Any N	M0
Stage IVA	T1	Any N	M1
	T2	Any N	M1
	T3	Any N	M1
Stage IVB	T4	Any N	Any M

PATHOLOGIC STAGE GROUPING (pTNM)

Stage	T	N	M
Stage I	T1	N0	M0
Stage II	T1	N1a	M0
Stage IIIA	T3a	N0, N1a	M0
Stage IIIB	T1	N1b	M0
	T3a	N1b	M0
	T3b	Any N	M0
	T3c	Any N	M0
Stage IVA	T1	Any N	M1
	T3a	Any N	M1
	T3b	Any N	M1
	T3c	Any N	M1
Stage IVB	T4	Any N	Any M

DIFFERENCES BETWEEN THE 2ND AND 3RD EDITIONS

This classification is the same as that published in the second edition of the *Manual*.

HISTOPATHOLOGIC TYPE

These tumors can be designated by several terms, including sympathicoblastomas, sympathicogoniomas, malignant ganglioneuromas, and gangliosympathicoblastomas, depending on the extent of cellular differentiation. Ganglioneuroma, which apparently is a well differentiated neuroblastoma, is also covered by this staging classification, even though it behaves in a benign fashion.

HISTOPATHOLOGIC GRADE (G)

GX Grade cannot be assessed
G1 Well differentiated
G2 Moderately well differentiated
G3 Poorly differentiated
G4 Undifferentiated

BIBLIOGRAPHY

1. Cohen MD, Weitman RM, Provisor AJ et al: Efficacy of magnetic resonance imaging in 139 children with tumors. Arch Surg 121:522–529, 1986
2. Gross RE, Farber S, Martin LW: Neuroblastoma sympatheticum. Pediatrics 23:1179–1191, 1959
3. Hughes M, Marsden HB, Palmer MK: Histologic patterns of neuroblastoma related to prognosis and clinical staging. Cancer 34:1706–1711, 1974
4. Jaffe N: Neuroblastoma: Review of the literature and an examination of factors contributing to its enigmatic character. Cancer Treat Rev 3:61–82, 1976
5. Massad M, Slim MS, Mansour A et al: Neuroblastoma: Report on a 21-year experience. J Pediatr Surg 21:388–391, 1986

NEUROBLASTOMA

Data Form for Cancer Staging

Patient identification
Name
Address
Hospital or clinic number
Age _____ Sex _____ Race _____

Institution identification
Hospital or clinic
Address

Oncology Record

Anatomic site of cancer
Histologic type
Grade (G)
Date of classification

Chronology of classification
(use separate form for each time staged)
[ ] Clinical (use all data prior to first treatment)
[ ] Pathologic (if definitively resected specimen available)

Definitions

Primary Tumor (T)

[ ] TX Primary tumor cannot be assessed
[ ] T0 No evidence of primary tumor
[ ] T1 Single tumor 5 cm or less in greatest dimension
[ ] T2 Single tumor more than 5 cm but not more than 10 cm in greatest dimension
[ ] T3 Single tumor more than 10 cm in greatest dimension
[ ] T4 Multicentric tumors occurring simultaneously

Lymph Node (N)

[ ] NX Regional lymph nodes cannot be assessed
[ ] N0 No regional lymph node metastasis
[ ] N1 Regional lymph node metastasis

Distant Metastasis (M)

[ ] MX Presence of disatnt metastasis cannot be assessed
[ ] M0 No distant metastasis
[ ] M1 Distant metastasis

Primary Tumor (pT)

[ ] pTX Primary tumor cannot be assessed
[ ] pT0 No evidence of primary tumor
[ ] pT1 Excision of tumor complete and margins histologically free
[ ] pT2 The category does not apply to neuroblastoma
[ ] pT3 Residual tumor
  [ ] pT3a Microscopic residual tumor
  [ ] pT3b Macroscopic residual tumor or grossly incomplete excision
  [ ] pT3c Surgical exploration only, tumor not resected
[ ] pT4 Multicentric tumors

Lymph Node (pN)

[ ] pNX Regional lymph nodes cannot be assessed
[ ] pN0 No regional lymph node metastasis
[ ] pN1 Regional lymph node metastasis
  [ ] pN1a Regional lymph node metastases completely resected
  [ ] pN1b Regional lymph node metastases incompletely resected

Distant Metastasis (pM)

[ ] pMX Presence of distant metastasis cannot be assessed
[ ] pM0 No distant metastasis
[ ] pM1 Distant metastasis

Clinical Stage Grouping (cTNM)

[ ]	I	T1	N0	M0
[ ]	II	T2	N0	M0
[ ]	III	T1	N1	M0
		T2	N1	M0
		T3	Any N	M0
[ ]	IVA	T1	Any N	M1
		T2	Any N	M1
		T3	Any N	M1
[ ]	IVB	T4	Any N	Any M

Pathologic Stage Grouping (pTNM)

[ ]	I	T1	N0	M0
[ ]	II	T1	N1a	M0
[ ]	IIIA	T3a	N0	M0
		T3a	N1a	M0
[ ]	IIIB	T1	N1b	M0
		T3a	N1b	M0
		T3b	Any N	M0
		T3c	Any N	M0
[ ]	IVA	T1	Any N	M1
		T2	Any N	M1
		T3a	Any N	M1
		T3b	Any N	M1
		T3c	Any N	M1
[ ]	IVB	T4	Any N	Any M

Histopathologic Type

These tumors can be designated by several terms, including sympathicoblastomas, sympathicogoniomas, malignant ganglioneuromas, and gangliosympathicoblastomas, depending on the extent of cellular differentiation. Ganglioneuroma, which apparently is a well differentiated neuroblastoma, is also covered by this staging classification, even though it behaves in a benign fashion.

Staged by _____ M.D.
_____ Registrar
Date _____

Histopathologic Grade (G)

[ ] GX Grade cannot be assessed
[ ] G1 Well differentiated
[ ] G2 Moderately well differentiated
[ ] G3 Poorly differentiated
[ ] G4 Undifferentiated

Sites of Distant Metastasis

Pulmonary   PUL
Osseous   OSS
Hepatic   HEP
Brain   BRA
Lymph nodes LYM
Bone marrow MAR
Pleura   PLE
Peritoneum   PER
Skin   SKI
Other   OTH

49

Soft-Tissue Sarcoma— Pediatric

Soft-tissue tumors can occur in infants and in children. These tumors can be found in many sites, and they include many histologic types. The most important member of this group is the embryonic rhabdomyosarcoma, or sarcoma botryoides, which can involve several organs. A number of the histologic types are found only in children. Very often these tumors have an embryonic appearance histologically. They are usually highly malignant. These tumors can be staged clinically and pathologically.

ANATOMY

Primary Site. Soft-tissue sarcomas can involve nearly all anatomic sites. In children, these tumors may even affect unusual sites, such as the vagina or extrahepatic bile ducts, which are rarely involved in adults.

Connective, subcutaneous and other soft tissues	ICD-O 171
Retroperitoneum	ICD-O 158.0
Mediastinum	ICD-O 164.2, 164.3

The primary tumor site should be indicated according to the following notations:

ORB	Orbit
HEA	Head and neck
LIM	Limbs
PEL	Pelvis (including walls, genital tract, and viscera)
ABD	Abdomen (including walls and viscera)
THO	Thorax (including walls, diaphragm, and viscera)
OTH	Other

Regional Lymph Nodes. The regional lymph nodes are those appropriate to the location of the primary tumor, as in the following:

Head and neck	Cervical and supraclavicular lymph nodes
Abdominal and pelvic	Subdiaphragmatic, intra-abdominal, and ilio-inguinal lymph nodes
Upper limbs	Ipsilateral epitrochlear and axillary lymph nodes
Lower limbs	Ipsilateral popliteal and inguinal lymph nodes

In the case of unilateral tumors, all contralateral involved lymph nodes are considered to be distant metastases and should be coded as M1.

Metastatic Sites. Since these tumors are found in many sites, they can involve a number of organs either by direct extension or by distant spread, usually through the bloodstream.

RULES FOR CLASSIFICATION

Clinical Staging. There is a clinical and pathologic TNM classification for pediatric soft-tissue tumors. Clinical staging is based on clinical examination, including imaging and laboratory studies.

Pathologic Staging. Pathologic classification is based on information obtained from pre-treatment clinical classification and information obtained from surgery and pathologic examination of the resected specimen. In contrast to sarcomas arising in adults, histologic grading is not used in classifying soft-tissue sarcomas in children, although it has a bearing on prognosis.

The classification for soft-tissue sarcomas is designed to apply primarily to rhabdomyosarcomas in childhood, but it may also be used for other soft-tissue sarcomas. In rhabdomyosarcoma, bone marrow examination is recommended.

There should be histologic verification of the disease.

DEFINITION OF TNM

Clinical Classification (cTNM)
Primary Tumor (T)

- TX Primary tumor cannot be assessed
- T0 No evidence of primary tumor
- T1 Tumor limited to the organ or tissue of origin
  - T1a Tumor 5 cm or less in greatest dimension
  - T1b Tumor more than 5 cm in greatest dimension
- T2 Tumor invades contiguous organ(s) or tissue(s) and/or with adjacent malignant effusion
  - T2a Tumor 5 cm or less in greatest dimension
  - T2b Tumor more than 5 cm in greatest dimension

Note: The categories T3 and T4 do not apply. The existence of more than one tumor is generally considered as a primary tumor with distant metastases.

Regional Lymph Nodes (N)

- NX Regional lymph nodes cannot be assessed
- N0 No regional lymph node metastasis
- N1 Regional lymph node metastasis

Distant Metastasis (M)

- MX Presence of distant metastasis cannot be assessed
- M0 No distant metastasis
- M1 Distant metastasis

Pathologic Classification (pTNM)
Primary Tumor (pT)

- pTX Primary tumor cannot be assessed
- pT0 No evidence of primary tumor
- pT1 Tumor limited to organ or tissue of origin; excision complete and margins histologically free
- pT2 Tumor invades beyond the organ or tissue of origin; excision complete and margins histologically free
- pT3 Tumor invades beyond the organ or tissue of origin; excision incomplete
  - pT3a Microscopic residual tumor
  - pT3b Macroscopic residual tumor or adjacent malignant effusion
  - pT3c Surgical exploration only, tumor not resected

Regional Lymph Nodes (pN)

- pNX Regional lymph nodes cannot be assessed
- pN0 No regional lymph node metastasis
- pN1 Regional lymph node metastasis
  - pN1a Regional lymph node metastasis completely resected
  - pN1b Regional lymph node metastasis incompletely resected

Distant Metastasis (pM)

- pMX Presence of distant metastasis cannot be assessed
- pM0 No distant metastasis
- pM1 Distant metastasis

Soft-Tissue Sarcoma—Pediatric

CLINICAL STAGE GROUPING (cTNM)

It is recommended that the full TNM classification always be used.

Stage I	T1a	N0	M0
	T1b	N0	M0
Stage II	T2a	N0	M0
	T2b	N0	M0
Stage III	Any T	N1	M0
Stage IV	Any T	Any N	M1

1. Each of these stage groups may be subdivided by the size of the primary tumor.
2. When the regional lymph nodes cannot be assessed clinically or radiologically, NX should be considered N0 in Stages I and II.
3. Further studies are required to determine the exact significance of N0, N1, and NX in such cases as pelvic tumors.

PATHOLOGIC STAGE GROUPING (pTNM)

Stage I	T1	N0	M0
Stage II	T1	N1a	M0
	T2	N0, N1a	M0
Stage IIIA	T3a	N0, N1a	M0
Stage IIIB	T3b	Any N	M0
	T3c	Any N	M0
	Any T	N1b	M0
Stage IV	Any T	Any N	M1

DIFFERENCES BETWEEN THE 2ND AND 3RD EDITIONS

This classification is the same as that published in the second edition of the *Manual.*

HISTOPATHOLOGIC TYPE

Histology can include the soft-tissue tumors that are found in adults. In general, soft-tissue sarcomas are relatively rare in children. Some sarcomas, for instance, osteogenic sarcomas that are found in children or young teenagers, are classified under the Musculoskeletal System.

HISTOPATHOLOGIC GRADE (G)

GX Grade cannot be assessed
G1 Well differentiated
G2 Moderately well differentiated
G3 Poorly differentiated
G4 Undifferentiated

BIBLIOGRAPHY

1. Bell J, Averette H, Davis J et al: Genital rhabdomyosarcoma: Current management and review of the literature. Obstet Gynecol Surv 41:257–263, 1986
2. Gehan EA, Glover FN, Mauer HM et al: Prognostic factors in children with rhabdomyosarcoma. Natl Cancer Inst Monogr 56:83–92, 1981
3. Hays DM: The management of rhabdomyosarcoma in children and young adults. World J Surg 4:15–28, 1980
4. Horn RC, Enterline HT: Rhabdomyosarcoma: A clinicopathological study and classification of 39 cases. Cancer 11:181–199, 1959
5. Schmidt D, Reimann O, Treuner J et al: Cellular differentiation and prognosis in embryonal rhabdomyosarcoma. Virchows Arch (A):409:183–194, 1986

SOFT-TISSUE SARCOMA—PEDIATRIC

Data Form for Cancer Staging

Patient identification
Name _____
Address _____
Hospital or clinic number _____
Age _____ Sex _____ Race _____

Institution identification
Hospital or clinic _____
Address _____

Oncology Record

Anatomic site of cancer _____
Histologic type _____
Grade (G) _____
Date of classification _____

Chronology of classification
  (use separate form for each time staged)
[ ] Clinical (use all data prior to first treatment)
[ ] Pathologic (if definitively resected specimen available)

Definitions

Primary Tumor (T)

[ ] TX Primary tumor cannot be assessed
[ ] T0 No evidence of primary tumor
[ ] T1 Tumor limited to the organ or tissue of origin
  [ ] T1a Tumor 5 cm or less in greatest dimension
  [ ] T1b Tumor more than 5 cm in greatest dimension
[ ] T2 Tumor invades contiguous organs or tissue(s) and/or with adjacent malignant effusion
  [ ] T2a Tumor 5 cm or less in greatest dimension
  [ ] T2b Tumor more than 5 cm in greatest dimension

Lymph Node (N)

[ ] NX Regional lymph nodes cannot be assessed
[ ] N0 No regional lymph node metastasis
[ ] N1 Regional lymph node metastasis

Distant Metastasis (M)

[ ] MX Presence of distant metastasis cannot be assessed
[ ] M0 No distant metastasis
[ ] M1 Distant metastasis

Primary Tumor (pT)

[ ] pTX Primary tumor cannot be assessed
[ ] pT0 No evidence of primary tumor
[ ] pT1 Tumor limited to organ or tissue of origin; excision complete and margins histologically free
[ ] pT2 Tumor invades beyond the organ or tissue of origin; excision complete and margins histologically free
[ ] pT3 Tumor invades beyond the organ or tissue of origin; excision incomplete
  [ ] pT3a Microscopic residual tumor
  [ ] pT3b Macroscopic residual tumor or adjacent malignant effusion
  [ ] pT3c Surgical exploration only, tumor not resected

Lymph Node (pN)

[ ] pNX Regional lymph nodes cannot be assessed
[ ] pN0 No regional lymph node metastasis
[ ] pN1 Regional lymph node metastasis
  [ ] pN1a Regional lymph node metastasis completely resected
  [ ] pN1b Regional lymph node metastasis incompletely resected

Distant Metastasis (pM)

[ ] pMX Presence of distant metastasis cannot be assessed
[ ] pM0 No distant metastasis
[ ] pM1 Distant metastasis

Clinical Stage Grouping (cTNM)

[ ] I   T1a   N0   M0
          T1b   N0   M0
[ ] II   T2a   N0   M0
          T2b   N0   M0
[ ] III   Any T N1   M0
[ ] IV   Any T Any N M1

Pathologic Stage Grouping (pTNM)

[ ] I   T1   N0   M0
[ ] II   T1   N1a   M0
          T2   N0   M0
          T2   N1a   M0
[ ] IIIA T3a   N0   M0
          T3a   N1a   M0
[ ] IIIB T3b   Any N M0
          T3c   Any N M0
          Any T N1b   M0
[ ] IV   Any T Any N M1

Histopathologic Type

Histology can include the soft-tissue tumors that are found in adults. In general, soft-tissue sarcomas are relatively rare in children. Some sarcomas, for instance, osteogenic sarcomas that are found in children or young teenagers, are classified under the Musculoskeletal System.

Histopathologic Grade (G)

[ ] GX Grade cannot be assessed
[ ] G1 Well differentiated
[ ] G2 Moderately well differentiated
[ ] G3 Poorly differentiated
[ ] G4 Undifferentiated

Staged by _____ M.D.
              _____ Registrar
Date _____

Sites of Distant Metastasis

Pulmonary	PUL
Osseous	OSS
Hepatic	HEP
Brain	BRA
Lymph nodes	LYM
Bone marrow	MAR
Pleura	PLE
Peritoneum	PER
Skin	SKI
Other	OTH

PART III

PERSONNEL OF THE AMERICAN JOINT COMMITTEE ON CANCER

FULL COMMITTEE MEMBERSHIP LISTING FOR THE THIRD EDITION (1959-1986)

W.A.D. Anderson, M.D.
Harvey W. Baker, M.D.
Oliver H. Beahrs, M.D.
David G. Bragg, M.D.
Weldon K. Bullock, M.D.
Paul R. Cannon, M.D.
Paul Carbone, M.D.
David T. Carr, M.D.
William M. Christopherson, M.D.
Murray M. Copeland, M.D.
Michael P. Corder, M.D.
Anthony R. Curreri, M.D.
Sidney J. Cutler, Sc.D.
Herbert Derman, M.D.
Theodore P. Eberhard, M.D.
Jack Edeiken, M.D.
George M. Farrow, M.D.
Eugene P. Frenkel, M.D.
Alfred Gellhorn, M.D.
Donald E. Henson, M.D.
Howard B. Hunt, M.D.
Robert V.P. Hutter, M.D.
B.J. Kennedy, M.D.
Alfred S. Ketcham, M.D.
Howard B. Latourette, M.D.
Edward R. Laws, M.D.
Louis A. Leone, M.D.
Seymour H. Levitt, M.D.
Virgil Loeb, Jr., M.D.
Robert J. McKenna, M.D.
William A. Meissner, M.D.
William C. Moloney, M.D.
William T. Moss, M.D.
Clifton F. Mountain, M.D.
Max H. Myers, Ph.D.
Gregory T. O'Conor, M.D.
John W. Pickren, M.D.
H. Marvin Pollard, M.D.
William E. Powers, M.D.
Antolin Raventos, M.D.
Guy F. Robbins, M.D.
William L. Ross, M.D.
Philip Rubin, M.D.
R. Wayne Rundles, M.D.
William O. Russell, M.D.
Edward F. Scanlon, M.D.
Robert L. Schmitz, M.D.
Milford D. Schultz, M.D.
Wendell G. Scott, M.D.
Paul Sherlock, M.D.
Danely Slaughter, M.D.
Robert R. Smith, M.D.
Edward H. Soule, M.D.
Samuel G. Taylor III, M.D.
Willis J. Taylor, M.D.
Louis B. Thomas, M.D.
Frank Vellios, M.D.
Morris J. Wizenberg, M.D.
David A. Wood, M.D.
John L. Young, Dr.P.H.
Robert C. Young, M.D.
John Ziegler, M.D.

APPENDIX

SITES, SUBSITES, AND ICD-O CODE NUMBERS

| ANATOMIC SITE | ICD-O CODE | PAGE |

Head and Neck Sites

Chapter 3. Lip and Oral Cavity

Alveolar ridge, lower	143.1	28
Alveolar ridge, upper	143.0	28
Buccal mucosa	145.0	28
Floor of the mouth	144	28
Hard palate	145.2	28
Lip	140	28
Retromolar gingiva (retromolar trigone)	145.6	28
Tongue, anterior two thirds (oral tongue)	141.1–141.4	28

Chapter 4. Pharynx (including base of tongue, soft palate and uvula)

Hypopharynx	148	34
Pharyngo-esophageal junction (postcricoid area)	148.0	34
Posterior pharyngeal wall	148.3	34
Pyriform sinus	148.1	34
Nasopharynx	147	33
Inferior (anterior) wall	147.3	33
Lateral wall	147.2	33
Postero-superior wall	147.0, 1	33
Oropharynx	141.0; 145.3, 4; 146.1–146.3; 146.4; 146.6–146.7	33
Anterior wall (glosso-epiglottic area)		
Tongue posterior to the vallate papillae (base of tongue or posterior third)	141.0	33
Vallecula	146.3	33
Lateral wall	146.6	33
Tonsil	146.0	33
Tonsillar fossa	146.1	33
Faucial pillars	146.2	33
Glosso-tonsillar sulci	146.2	33
Posterior wall	146.7	33
Superior wall		
Inferior surface of soft palate	145.3	33
Uvula	145.4	33

Chapter 5. Larynx

Glottis	161.0	40
Subglottis	161.2	40
Supraglottis	161.1	40

Chapter 6. Maxillary Sinus — 160.2 — 45

Chapter 7. Salivary Glands

Parotid	142.0	51
Sublingual glands	142.2	51
Submaxillary	142.1	51

Chapter 8. Thyroid Gland — 193 — 57

Digestive System Sites

Chapter 9. Esophagus

Cervical esophagus	150.0	64
Intrathoracic esophagus	150.1–150.5	64
Abdominal esophagus	150.2	64

ANATOMIC SITE	ICD-O CODE	PAGE
Lower thoracic portion	150.5	64
Mid-thoracic portion	150.4	64
Upper thoracic portion	150.3	64
Chapter 10. Stomach	151	69
Upper third		
Cardiac area	151.0	70
Fundus	151.3	70
Middle third		
Bulk of the corpus	151.4	70
Lower third		
Antral area	151.2	70
Pylorus	151.1	70
Chapter 11. Colon and Rectum		
Appendix	153.5	76
Ascending colon	153.6	76
Cecum	153.4	76
Descending colon	153.2	76
Hepatic flexure	153.0	76
Rectosigmoid	154.0	76
Rectum	154.1	76
Sigmoid colon	153.3	76
Splenic flexure	153.7	76
Transverse colon	153.1	76
Chapter 12. Anal Canal	154.2	81
Chapter 13. Liver	155.0	87
Intrahepatic bile ducts	155.1	87
Chapter 14. Gallbladder	156.0	93
Chapter 15. Extrahepatic Bile Ducts	156.1	99
Chapter 16. Ampulla of Vater	156.2	105
Chapter 17. Exocrine Pancreas	157.0–157.3; 157.9	109

Lung (Chapter 18)

	162.2–162.9	115

Musculoskeletal Sites

Chapter 19. Bone	170	123
Chapter 20. Soft Tissues		
Connective, subcutaneous and other soft tissues	171	127
Mediastinum	164.2, 3	127
Retroperitoneum	158.0	127
Chapter 21. Carcinoma of the Skin (excluding eyelid, vulva and penis)	173.0, 173.2–173.9, 187.7	133
Chapter 22. Melanoma of the Skin (excluding eyelid)		
Penis	187.4	139
Scrotum	187.7	139
Skin	173.0, 173.2–173.9	139
Vulva	184.4	139

Breast (Chapter 23)

	174, 175	145

Sites, Subsites, and ICD-O Code Numbers

ANATOMIC SITE	ICD-O CODE	PAGE
Gynecologic Sites		
Chapter 24. Cervix Uteri	180	151
Chapter 25. Corpus Uteri	182	157
Chapter 26. Ovary	183.0	163
Chapter 27. Vagina	184.0	169
Chapter 28. Vulva	184.4	173
Genitourinary Sites		
Chapter 29. Prostate	185	177
Chapter 30. Testis	186	183
Chapter 31. Penis	187.1, 187.2, 187.4	189
Prepuce	187.1	189
Glans	187.2	189
Skin	187.4	189
Chapter 32. Urinary Bladder	188	193
Chapter 33. Kidney	189.0	199
Chapter 34. Renal Pelvis and Ureter		
Renal pelvis	189.1	205
Ureter	189.2	205
Chapter 35. Urethra		
Female urethra	189.3	209
Male urethra	189.3	209
Ophthalmic Tumors		
Chapter 36. Carcinoma of the Eyelid	173.1	213
Chapter 37. Melanoma of the Eyelid	173.1	217
Chapter 38. Carcinoma of the Conjunctiva	190.3	223
Chapter 39. Melanoma of the Conjunctiva	190.3	227
Chapter 40. Melanoma of the Uvea		
Uvea	190.0	231
Uveal tract	190.6	231
Chapter 41. Retinoblastoma		
Retina	190.5	237
Chapter 42. Sarcoma of the Orbit	190.1	241
Chapter 43. Carcinoma of the Lacrimal Gland	190.2	245
Brain (Chapter 44)	191	249
Meninges	192.1	249
Hodgkin's and Non-Hodgkin's Lymphoma		
Chapter 45. Hodgkin's Disease		
Chapter 46. Non-Hodgkin's Lymphoma		

ANATOMIC SITE	ICD-O CODE	PAGE
Pediatric Cancers		
Chapter 47. Nephroblastoma (Wilms' Tumor)		
Kidneys	189.0	266
Chapter 48. Neuroblastoma		
Adrenal medulla	194.0	271
Chapter 49. Soft-Tissue Sarcoma—Pediatric		
Connective, subcutaneous and other soft tissues	171	277
Mediastinum	164.2, 3	277
Retroperitoneum	158.0	277